Killing with Kindness

Killing with Kindness

Haiti, International Aid, and NGOs

MARK SCHULLER

RUTGERS UNIVERSITY PRESS

NEW BRUNSWICK, NEW JERSEY, AND LONDON

LIBRARY OF CONGRESS CATALOGING-IN-PUBLICATION DATA

Schuller, Mark, 1973–
  Killing with kindness : Haiti, international aid, and NGOs / Mark Schuller.
    p. cm.
  Includes bibliographical references and index.
  ISBN 978–0–8135–5362–7 (hardcover : alk. paper) — ISBN 978–0–8135–5363–4
(pbk. : alk. paper) — ISBN 978–0–8135–5364–1 (e-book)
    1. Social medicine—Haiti.   2. AIDS (Disease)—Haiti—International cooperation.
3. Nonprofit organizations—Haiti. I. Title.
  RA418.3.H35S38   2012
  362.1′0425097294—dc23

                                        2011046938

A British Cataloging-in-Publication record for this book is available
from the British Library.

Visit our website: http://rutgerspress.rutgers.edu

Manufactured in the United States of America

To Mislène

CONTENTS

ILLUSTRATIONS AND TABLES

Figures

Tables

FOREWORD

PAUL FARMER, MD, PHD

In *Killing with Kindness: Haiti, International Aid and NGOs*, Mark Schuller offers nuanced insight into the mechanisms (and failures) of foreign aid in Haiti. Through his extensive field research, recounted here in a clear, practical prose, Dr. Schuller suggests that the most efficient and effective way to engage in this work is to accompany the intended beneficiaries. "Accompaniment" admits many meanings, but it is not infinitely elastic. To accompany someone is to go somewhere with him or her, to break bread together, to be present on a journey with a beginning and an end. It means listening, working alongside communities, walking with them until their goals become their reality.[1]

Foreign assistance is often complicit in the failures of imagination that allow inequities to persist in Haiti and elsewhere. The standard "trickle-down" aid model consistently disappoints those of good will on both sides of the complex donor-recipient equation.[2] But someone must be benefitting; most systems realize the results they were designed to deliver. We need not return to Max Weber to observe that most bureaucracies excel at self-perpetuation (1946b). There are many complexities and gradations to Weber's work, however, and ample reason to extend a hermeneutic of generosity to most nongovernmental organizations operating in post-coup Haiti. But some distinctions can (and must) be made.

Dr. Schuller does this by contrasting two NGOs: one with a top-heavy organizational structure (due in part to its dependence on large bilateral funders), and one that operates with an inclusive, collaborative approach informed by accompaniment. He shows that sharing decisionmaking among NGO directors and staff and, above all, the intended beneficiaries, can improve the likelihood that service delivery will be humane and sustainable. He also highlights the important of integrating efforts into existing programs, building (or rebuilding) local infrastructure, and collaborating with the public sector. Private enterprises are not meant to replace robust public-sector health, water, and sanitation systems. In fact, when foreign aid bypasses the government, evidence suggests that it can weaken the public sector (see, e.g., Collier 2007).

The international humanitarian response—one of the largest in history—to the January 2010 earthquake in Haiti is a case in point: of the more than

$2 billion in acute relief aid, less than 1 percent went to the Haitian government. One could argue that the fragility and lack of so-called "absorptive capacity" of the Haitian government justifies this distribution of resources; after all, twenty-eight out of twenty-nine federal ministries were damaged or destroyed in the afternoon of January 12, 2010. But could less than 1 percent possibly be an acceptable, much less desirable, amount? There is a vicious cycle at work: aid bypasses the government because it is weak, and then further weakens the government. An accompaniment approach starts with partnerships with the government and other Haitian institutions. It prioritizes job creation and local procurement and the transferring of resources to the poor—forms of "capacity building" (jargon that has been divested of any real meaning).

Dr. Schuller regards Rwanda's recovery after the 1994 genocide as a model of how governments and aid organizations can work together. (And I agree [Farmer 2011b:217–235].) The Rwandan government's approach has been clear and firm: NGOs are welcome, but they must work with within the frameworks and strategies the government has developed. It is a sensible plan, and unlike most, it has actually been implemented. Claims of causality are, as ever, rife with problems. But Rwanda's recovery has been nothing short of miraculous: GDP has trebled in the past decade; almost everyone living with AIDS has access to antiretroviral treatment; Kigali is one of the safest places to live in the world. The country has achieved security in two senses: physical security and also human security. Aid organizations and donors and governments would do well to consider how these lessons might be applied elsewhere.

Dr. Schuller's book suggests new rules of the road for foreign assistance. His prescriptions are the result of dedicated fieldwork and years spent in Haiti living with Haitians, learning their language and cultures, listening to their stories. *Killing with Kindness* is fine scholarly work and a compassionate narrative driven by the lived experiences of Mark Schuller, his colleagues, his friends and neighbors. This book is essential reading for all those interested in a peaceful and truly independent Haiti.

ACKNOWLEDGMENTS

A work of this scope is impossible to accomplish without the active support of many. A work of this theme is inconceivable to attempt individually. At the University of California, Santa Barbara, I would like to extend a heartfelt thank-you to my PhD committee—Susan Stonich, Mary Hancock, Christopher McAuley, and M. Catherine Maternowska—for their engagement, challenging questions, encouragement, and feedback. This book would have not been possible without the support of Karl Bryant, Eileen Boris, Claudine Michel, Cedric Robinson, Kum-Kum Bhavnani, Leila Rupp, Barbara Herr-Harthorn, Laury Oaks, Elizabeth Robinson, Sharon Hoshida, Hillary Haldane, Tiffany Willoughby-Herard, Beth Currans, Jeanne Scheper, Molly Talcott, Carlos Alamo, Sylvanna Falcon, and Corina Kellner. I will always be indebted to Jean-Robert Cadely, Leisl Picard, and the staff and invited faculty from Florida International University's Haitian Summer Institute for my introduction to Haiti. The genesis of this research project was in Minnesota, through activism in Morris and the Twin Cities. Members of the now-defunct St. Paul Tenants Union played a central role in my political/activist education.

This education continued and was deepened through the active involvement of and support from many friends and colleagues in Haiti, especially Dawn Pinder, Kathy Wright, Josette Perard, George Werleigh, Ernst Mathurin, Renate Schneider, Joseph Philippe, Anne Hastings, Reed Lindsey, Allande, Anna, Anne and Laurent, Camille, Corasme, Daphne, Denise, Edele, Gerrit, Livingston, Logisse, Maxime, Mirlène, Mislène, Yolette, the staff at Fonkoze-Biwo Alfa, Kay Kapab, Hospice St. Joseph, and especially the generous staff and recipients of the NGOs featured in this book. Finally, thanks go to those who had to remain anonymous but whose courage to tell the truth made this story possible. Colleagues and students at the Faculté d'Ethnologie and Université de Fondwa offered helpful insights. Special thanks to Jimmy Toussaint, Djenane St. Juste, Fabrice Charmant, and Jeremy Dupin for necessary research assistance.

Facilitating this complex research on donors would be impossible without the crucial support of many people: in Haiti, Mme Garçon, Mme Clement, and the USAID librarian Mme Legros and other donor agency staff; in Europe, Greet Schaumans, Alessandra, Charles, Mme Zaugg, Robert, and the European Commission's information specialist Ms. Dias and other donor staff; in Washington,

Stephen DeCanio, Joseph McGee, Melody, Esther, Freda, Alverta, and several anonymous staff at USAID, the World Bank, IMF, IDB, and the State Department.

This research was made possible by financial support from many sources: the National Science Foundation's Graduate Research Fellowship (2002–2007), the African American Studies Program at the University of Florida, Gainesville (2002), the UCSB Department of Anthropology's Pre-dissertation Site Visit Fellowship (2002), the Albert Spaulding Fellowship (2003, 2005, 2006), a dissertation fellowship from the Institute for Global Conflict and Cooperation (2004), the Graduate Division Travel Grant (2007), the Labor and Employment Research Fund (2007), and the CUNY Faculty Fellowship Publishing Program (2009–2010). Reaching Up provided funds for publication.

Offering much-needed critique, probing questions, motivation, and support is the "dissertation liberation front" of Hillary Haldane, Karl Bryant, Francesca Deguili, and Helene Lee, who saw the project from beginning to end. Colleagues in anthropology, Hillary, Valerie Andrushko, and Jackie Eng braved the earliest drafts of my rants. Colleagues at UCSB such as Beth Currans, Sonia Matter, Siobhan Brooks, and Tiffany Willoughby-Herard, and elsewhere, such as Pierre Minn, Salvador Vital-Ortiz, Shaun Cleaver, and Kiran Jayaram, offered very useful feedback on individual chapters. For the support turning this into a book, I am also indebted to my colleagues at the African American Resource Center at York College, especially my sister in struggle, Selena Rodgers. My mentor, Virginia Sanchez-Korrol, and participants at the City University of New York's Faculty Fellowship Publishing Program—Alan Aja, Robin Harper, Miranda Martinez, Hyunhee Park, Michael Sharpe, and Victor Torres-Velez—were the coconspirators in conceptualizing the book proposal and the projects, offering necessary feedback on the work in progress. Faye Harrison, Marilyn Thomas-Houston, and Dave Crawford offered very timely feedback and encouragement. Members of the Columbia Women and Society Colloquium helped work on chapter 1. Special thanks go to my York colleague Michele Gregory, who made this possible, and the discussant María Luisa Ruiz at York's sister college, Medgar Evers. I would also like to give props to my Introduction to Anthropology students during the two semesters I foisted the work in progress on them. Their feedback—and their quizzical looks—were absolutely critical. I am profoundly grateful to three individuals who braved the entire book and helped me back down to earth: Jennie Smith-Pariola, Dawn Pinder, and Mark Snyder.

Three individuals deserve special mention for their constant support, advocacy, patient listening, mentoring, midnight editing phone calls, and swift kicks in the ass whenever I needed to be reminded why I started this in the first place: Karl Bryant, Valerie Kaussen, and Gina Ulysse. Thank you. I love you.

Finally, I would like to thank my editor, Marlie Wasserman, for her support and feedback in the process, the anonymous reviewers, and the Rutgers University Press staff, especially Allyson Fields, for making this book possible.

ABBREVIATIONS

AP	Associated Press
CAC	Community Action Council
CCI	Cadre de Coopération Interimaire (Interim Cooperation Framework)
CCM	Country Coordinating Mechanism
CDC	Centers for Disease Control and Prevention
CIMO	Corps d'Intervention et de Maintien de l'Ordre (Haitian National Police)
FOIA	Freedom of Information Act
FRAPH	Front pour l'Avancement et le Progrès Haïtien (Front for Haitian Advancement and Progress)
GAD	Gender and Development
GDP	Gross domestic product
HOPE	Hemispheric Opportunity Through Partnership Encouragement Act
IDB	Inter-American Development Bank
IDP	Internally displaced person
IFI	International financial institution
IMF	International Monetary Fund
IOM	International Organization for Migration
IRI	International Republican Institute
ISC	Initiative de la Société Civile (Civil Society Initiative)
KOFAVIV	Komisyon Fanm Viktim pou Viktim (Commission of Women Victims for Victims)
KONAP	Kòdinasyon Nasyonal k ap Plede Kòz Fanm (National Coordination of Women's Advocacy Organizations)
MCC	Millennium Challenge Corporation
MINUSTAH	Mission des Nations Unies pour la stabilisation en Haïti (United Nations Stabilization Mission for Haiti)
MPCE	Ministère de la Planification et Coopération Externe (Ministry of Planning and Foreign Cooperation)
NED	National Endowment for Democracy

NGO	Nongovernmental organization
ODA	Official development assistance
OFATMA	Office d'Assurance des Accidents du Travail, Maladies et Maternité (Office of Insurance for Work Accidents, Illness, and Maternity)
ONA	Office National d'Assurance (National Insurance Office)
OTI	Office of Transition Initiatives
PEPFAR	President's Emergency Plan for AIDS Relief
PRSP	Poverty Reduction Strategy Paper
R4	Results Review and Resources Request
S/CRS	State Department coordinator for reconstruction and stabilization
SO	Strategic objective
SONAPI	Société Nationale des Parcs Industriels (National Society of Industrial Parks)
UNDP	United Nations Development Program
USAID	United States Agency for International Development
WID	Women in Development

Killing with Kindness

Introduction

Doing Research during a Coup

They let people die! They take the illness and turn it into a big business.

—Gabrielle, HIV activist

February 27, 2004

The city was on fire. Not the Eternal Flame, a work-in-progress memorial to the Haitian Revolution that had yet to be lit, but thick plumes of charcoal-gray smoke filled the sky, blotting out the sun.

I was rushing. My neighbor Lise[1] had warned me. "Better pick up what you can," she said. "You don't know the next time you'll be able to be out in the street." It was late afternoon, soon to be dark.

The market was unusually crowded, voices elevated an octave higher than usual, the staccato shouting of business transactions louder than usual, devoid of its usual joviality: the taunting, joking, and catching up between friends. People scurried by, clutching black plastic shopping bags full of whatever they could afford, whatever they could still find: candles, mosquito coils, cooking oil, matches, batteries for radios, and bulk food like dried beans, rice, milled corn, potatoes, and carrots.

By the time I made it back down the slippery cobblestone street that led to the market, little was left. Instinct, and Michele, a *timachann* (street merchant) whom I had come to know, told me to seek out the crowds, the long queues, to find what I was looking for. Michele had sold her last candle, and save for the two boxes she stuffed into her halter-top for her own family, she was even out of matches.

Stuck in the long lines, I experienced for myself that indeed it was catch-as-catch-can: get what you could while you still could. After being turned away from three "boutiques,"[2] I was finally able to get matches, mosquito coils, and some cooking oil, but no batteries. The "eau miracle" (French for "miracle water") vendor had already closed up shop by the time I got there. Luckily I had iodine tablets, bleach, and a five-gallon jug of treated water.

The *kriz* (crisis) in Pòtoprens[3] (Port-au-Prince) had finally past the point of no return. For the first time since being teargassed while observing an October protest, I was truly scared. The "insurrection" had finally reached Pòtoprens, just as the "rebel" Guy Philippe had boasted, predicting that he would reach the nation's capital by his birthday (February 29, the same day as Aristide's ouster).

Earlier that day, still in an obstinate effort to abide by Haitian law and get my *permis de sejour*[4]—my "green card," enabling me to legally live and work in Haiti—I saw what I had only heard about from my family in the United States watching CNN: the lines were drawn, the streets empty. Downtown, just across the not-quite-finished monument to the bicentennial to the Haitian Revolution (1791–1804), the Texaco station was smoldering. Three trucks, each with ten to fifteen men all clad in black and some toting semiautomatic weapons, circled the gas station. The driver of our *tap-tap* ("public" transport, in this case an old converted minivan packed with eighteen adults, some with merchandise jammed under their seat or on their lap) went numb for a moment, then slammed on the brakes and made an immediate U-turn, speeding back up the hill.

At the stoplight where the tap-taps were supposed to turn, the Total gas station was not only burning, but the pumps had been ripped from the concrete. Spooked, the chauffeur continued to climb, yelling at the passengers to please remain seated. Ordinarily, such a deviation in the normal route would have triggered loud protests from the passengers, particularly the timachann carrying heavy merchandise. Like me, other passengers were stunned into silence. Eventually, the driver zoomed his way through side roads and deposited us in front of the neighborhood Catholic Church, not even bothering to collect the fare.

On the ten-minute down-then-uphill walk to my house, I heard gunshots coming from several directions. The remains of a young man lying in the street, shot up and surrounded by a pool of deep-purple dried blood, was generating commotion from the neighbors. I didn't get a good glance at him, but I was glad that—unlike with other bodies I had heard of from *radyo trannde* (rumor mill, literally "radio of thirty-two [teeth]") as well as seen in images from the foreign press—neighborhood dogs were not yet feasting on the corpse.

These images flashed through my head as I tried desperately to buy two weeks' worth of rations, having difficulty even imagining what I would need, and having an even harder time getting it. I bought what I could find at the inflated price demanded. "We all have to survive," said a middle-aged merchant matter-of-factly.

Toting a black plastic shopping bag and a wad of small bills and coins in my pants pocket, I shuffled back up the slippery cobblestone street to my house, defeated. My neighbor Lise had told me the obvious: stay home. The sun was quickly making its nosedive into the bay, and soon all would be dark. We hadn't had electricity for the past day and a half. Being relatively new to Haiti, I asked

Lise when it was "safe" to be in the streets. "Look," she pointed to the street I had just climbed. "If you see more than two people walk per minute, it's okay. Safer still if you see ten. Just stay at home if the street is empty."

My middle-income neighborhood of Kriswa (Christ-Roi) was sandwiched between the crowded *bidonvil* (shantytowns) of Pòtoprens, built to accommodate two hundred thousand but home to more than ten times that amount, and the mountain suburb of Petyonvil (Pétion-Ville), home to most of Haiti's banks, credit card companies, restaurants, nightclubs, and world-class resorts.[5] Haiti is the most divided country in the hemisphere, with the most millionaires per capita.[6] In Kriswa, rich and poor lived on top of one another.

The *baryè* ("barriers," metal gates walling off the houses of the middle-class families in the neighborhood)[7] were all closed and locked shut. Inside these houses, the only ones with electricity (some had diesel-powered generators, others, like mine, had an inverter to convert electricity stored on car batteries into AC current), families carried on loud conversations as the blue of the compact fluorescent bulbs cast long, eerie shadows on the street.

In the interstices, between the locked gates and the electric blue lights, the low-income families—the timachann, day laborers, servants, *restavèk* children[8]—also huddled close. Julie, the timachann who sold staple goods and penny candy, had long since hauled off her wooden stand and squirreled away her livelihood. But still she stood in the street, where her store usually was. When I asked what she was doing, she said, "My kid hasn't come back yet." He wasn't in school, I asked. "No, schools have been closed for the past week," and actually, on and off for the better part of three months. "He just went to fetch a pail of water."

Pascal, who always demanded my time whenever he saw me pass (and usually got it), was slumped on the cinder block that held Julie's store in place. He smelled very strongly of *tafya* (hard liquor). When I approached, he stood up on top of the block, greeting me at my eye level. "You don't have to worry, Mark. *Pèp la* [the people][9] are defending our country. We'll all be safe here. You'll see."

"Grann" ("Grandma," the nickname for the matriarch), cigarette in hand, responded as she emerged from her six-by-six home. "Our country! It's not the country, but the president you're defending."

Pascal winked at me and offered his hand. "Yes. That's what I said, my country. My democracy." I gave him my hand, and he shook it vigorously.

Thomas, just emerging from a bath and putting his shirt on, said in his cracked voice, "Democracy! We don't have democracy in this country. We've been waiting for democracy since 1986 [when the popular movement deposed the twenty-nine-year father-and-son Duvalier dictatorship]. We have elections. And we pèp la, what do we get? How have our lives changed? Elections are *koupe dwèt* [literally, 'cutting the finger off,' referring to the practice of stamping election cards with a finger]."

Pascal, looking straight at me, said, "*Kore m.*" Since that was the phrase men use while doing a Haitian version of a "high five" (touching fists briefly), I made a fist. Pascal laughed and said, "I said help me out here" (the other meaning of *kore m*). After he stopped laughing, still looking straight at me, he asked, "Why does the U.S. not like Haiti? Why does Bush want to get rid of Aristide?"

Diverting part of the question, I pointed out that the two were in fact separate questions.

Before I could finish, the ever-conciliatory ("Because I'm a Christian," he once said in explanation, by which he meant an evangelical Protestant) Thomas said, "*Mezanmi!* [An expression like "My God!," from the French "my friends."] Pascal, don't you see that Americans give us a lot of *èd* [foreign aid]?"

Grann coughed a smoker's cough. "Where's that *èd* now, Thomas? Does this *èd* ever end up in the hands of us *pèp la*?"

The spirited conversation continued until Julie's son returned with two old cooking oil containers full of water. Seizing on this break in the conversation, I left. As I did, Pascal shot up and gave me a salute. "*Pa lage nou, tande?*" (Don't let us down, do you hear?) Given his last question, I wasn't sure if he was specifically referring to me individually or as representative of the United States.

"*M pap janm lage nou,*" I replied as I walked down the hill to my house. I will never let you all down.

This book is part of my attempt to keep this promise.

The Aid Apparatus Exposed: The 2010 Earthquake

As I write this introduction, it is now six years later. On January 12, 2010, a 7.0 earthquake struck Haiti, leveling much of Pòtoprens. The National Palace was destroyed. Whole neighborhoods were reduced to rubble, underneath which at least 230,000 people were buried.[10] More than 1.5 million people—one in six—instantly became homeless.

The earthquake destroyed all but five houses on the block, trapping ten people underneath and killing two others, including Lise's father. When I arrived a week after the earthquake, middle-class people like Lise and *pèp la* like Pascal huddled underneath a donated tarp, working together to survive. They set up an emergency clinic in the middle of the street with the doctors who lived on the block. Together, without any outside assistance, and putting aside the differences that ripped the country apart in 2004, people found ways to survive. When I returned three months later, most middle-class neighbors had moved to a cousin's or a friend's house. Some *ti pèp* ("small" people, the poorest) like Julie moved back to their family *lakou* (homestead) in the provinces, joining a reverse exodus of some six hundred thousand people. Many remained, still *chèche lavi* (making a living, literally "searching for life"). The starvation was clear in Grann's and Pascal's emaciated faces. The families slept under a couple of tarps, the same tarps housing the emergency clinic during the first week. The garage where many ti pèp resuscitated cars back to life had reopened, also under the shade of a tarp.

Thomas had switched his tune since 2004. "They said that $2 billion has come to Haiti. Where's all the èd that was supposed to arrive? We pèp haven't seen a cent."

While most of them did not get a tent to sleep under, they at least had a tarp. In the context of the earthquake, they were relatively lucky. A short walk down the hill was a makeshift camp in the neighborhood of Solino. More than 6,800 people slept in the space of a soccer field in tents made of easy-to-rip plastic that traps the Caribbean heat. When we visited, it had just rained the night before, the first time in three nights at the beginning of the rainy season. Pools of slick mud seeped into the tents jammed side by side. Standing water attracted flies and mosquitoes, bearers of infections such as malaria and dengue fever. The stench was overpowering, not only from the mud but because nowhere in the camp was a latrine to be found. When asked how people did their daily business, Magalie, a twenty-six-year-old mother of three young children, held up a small plastic bag that she was about to dump in the nearby ravine. Where are the nongovernmental organizations (NGOs)? I asked. No one knew. Only World Vision came by occasionally to give cards to a handpicked group of three evangelical pastors to distribute to the women in the camp for two weeks' food rations. This was before food aid was stopped in April 2010.

The cards had been distributed between 11:00 P.M. and midnight the night before. Magalie said, "You can't afford to sleep when you hear that there's a card distribution. You never know where and when they will give it out. You just have to follow the noise of the crowd and hope you will get yours." Sylvie, who has fourteen people—including her infant daughter and her sister's family—living in her ripped tent, said that she never got a card because she doesn't know the NGO representatives. "It's all about *moun pa w* [your people] getting the goods," she said. Several people in this camp, and leaders of a group of women victims of violence called KOFAVIV, reported several dozen cases of women being propositioned for sex in exchange for cards.[11]

Despite $2 billion in private aid donated in the first three months after the earthquake, the system was clearly not working, leaving many mainstream commentators puzzled. This earthquake exposed to a general audience the problems with the prevailing system of aid. For the first time, NGOs as a system became a focus of sustained mainstream media coverage in the United States. But mostly the story of Haiti has faded into the background, the latest in a string of bad news laced with tales of heroic foreigners. Rather than encourage understanding, these hit-and-run accounts serve mainly to create and reinforce the image of Haiti being hopelessly beyond the pale, a "basket case" (Potter 2009).

As the noted physician and anthropologist Paul Farmer (2003) and others (e.g., Dash 1997; Lawless 1992; Trouillot 1994b) have noted, Haiti is known by its superlatives as an "exceptional" case. The poet Jean-Claude Martineau calls Haiti the only country with a last name: "the poorest country in the hemisphere" (Bell 2001:9).

"Failures" of Development

Haiti's earthquake thrust the international aid system, particularly NGOs, into the public spotlight. In addition to the increased public scrutiny, the earthquake provided a pedagogical moment for the international aid system. For example, UN Special Envoy Bill Clinton apologized for destroying Haitian rice production through USAID food aid. He and Secretary of State Hillary Clinton also publicly questioned donors' overdependence on NGOs and their circumventing of elected governments. A discourse critical of the humanitarian response has proliferated following this exposure, particularly among aid workers and journalists (e.g., Disaster Accountability Project 2011; Humanitarian Accountability Project 2010; Oxfam International 2011), and even from the representative for the Organization of American States (Robert 2010).

The earthquake also exposed the weakness of the state. In addition to not having authority over the camps and the aid distribution—as only 1 percent of emergency aid passed through the government—the state had no ability to prevent the disaster or coordinate relief efforts. The government had been weakened since the mid-1990s by donors' policies of giving their aid directly to NGOs. Even before the earthquake, more than 80 percent of the health clinics and 90 percent of schools were private, run by individuals, missions, or NGOs. Some NGOs—particularly the large food distribution agencies like World Vision, CARE (Cooperative for American Relief Everywhere), or Catholic Relief Services—became parallel states, even marking off territory to people coming into their area. Many in Haiti scoff at this "cutting the cake" approach, wherein Haiti is sliced up and given to NGOs, ceding near-sovereign control to these NGO "fiefdoms."

These private entities have in many respects eclipsed the Haitian government. Most dramatic was the 2004 coup against Aristide, discussed in chapter 1. The events of February 29, 2004, have been told at length in at least ten English-language books, by my last count. Some analysts focus on the roles the U.S. government and its allies played in destabilizing Haiti, particularly the National Endowment for Democracy (NED) and its politically connected branch funds (Sprague 2007). The stage of the drama usually told is the competition for the National Palace being played out through confrontation on the streets. Escaping attention in this analysis is how Haiti's poor majority survived, and under what conditions. While the political party apparatus of NED received a bright spotlight, the United States Agency for International Development (USAID), the humanitarian and development arm of the State Department, remains in relative shadows. While not making headlines, the ongoing, day-to-day work of USAID in Haiti and elsewhere is just as powerful.

Unlike in Iraq or Afghanistan, where we kill with drones, "smart" bombs, and troop surges, too many people in Haiti are nonetheless dying from the consequences of our aid. Gabrielle exclaims, "They let people die! Maybe when people are in their house, living in luxury, they can understand what we're suffering. And what needs to happen. But they take the illness [AIDS] and turn it into a business." Gabrielle is HIV positive, which still is largely a death sentence in a resource-starved country like Haiti.

Hidden from view in most accounts is a world system that has continually applied pressure on the country, draining its resources and forcing it into the debt bondage that kept it from developing—contributing to the very surplus that allowed "the West" to develop.[12] This world system has adapted and altered throughout the years, responding to crises within colonialism (Chakrabarty 1992; Comaroff 1997; Padmore 1969), then development and imperialism (Harvey 2003; McMichael 1996), then global capitalism (Robinson 2004; Sklair 2001). Despite these challenges, this system is very much present today.

Focusing on the lived experience of those meant to benefit, anthropologists have uncovered the many ways "development" has disempowered them. James Ferguson (1990) noted how development discourse hides the political stakes and inequalities, recasting them as "technical" failures in an "anti-politics machine." Building on this analysis, Arturo Escobar (1995) opened an inquiry into the discourse itself and how it reifies national differences, freezing the "underdeveloped" in a subordinate position, what Michel-Rolph Trouillot (2003) called the "savage slot." A range of critical analyses of development have since appeared, documenting the multitude of abuses, inequalities, failures, and injustices of the development apparatus (e.g., Cooke and Kothari 2001; Crush 1995; Edelman and Haugerud 2005; Ferguson 2005; Gupta and Sharma 2006; Illich 1997; Kamat 2004; Petras 2003).

Haiti's geopolitical position—especially its proximity to the United States—highlights the contradictions and flaws in the system of international aid. As such, the seemingly endless crises, violence, and environmental degradation are not expressions of Haiti's culture or "mentality," but rather a clear example and early warning for other heavily indebted, low-income countries in other parts of the world about what can happen if significant changes are not made to the system. It is a canary in the coal mine: in April 2008, following Haiti, there were food riots in a dozen countries across the global South.[13] This book analyzes a key conduit in these crises, the glue for this globalization: NGOs (Schuller 2009).

The Rise of NGOs

NGOs are playing ever more central roles in Haiti, as elsewhere. The 1990s saw a tenfold increase in their numbers, from six thousand worldwide in 1990 to an estimated sixty thousand by 1998 (Regan 2003:3). Following shifts in aid funding, the numbers of NGOs that worked in more than one country doubled in the decade before 1996 to 38,000 (Scholte and Schnabel 2002:250). Currently, there are so many NGOs that we can't even guess at their number (Riddell 2007:53). This rise in the number of NGOs is matched by an increase in funding flowing through them. Globally, in 2005, it is estimated that NGOs channeled anywhere from $3.7 to $7.8 billion of humanitarian assistance (Development Initiatives 2006:47), and $24 billion in development funding (Riddell 2007:259).

To most people, NGOs are characterized by their "doing good." It has become fashionable to criticize the excesses of government and big bureaucracy, particularly since the 1980s with the advent of what is known in the United States as "Reaganomics" and elsewhere as neoliberalism. This critique of "big government" has taken root in the U.S. Tea Party movement. NGOs, doing humanitarian, charity, or development work, have for the most part escaped this criticism, at least until the earthquake.

NGOs are much more elusive than "development," generating a wide variety of responses from scholars and development practitioners. Many who generally argue that development has failed nonetheless hold hope that NGOs can fix what ails the system (e.g., Dicklitch 1998; Edwards and Hulme 1996a; Macdonald 1997; Ndegwa 1996; Uphoff 1993). NGOs are often characterized as "giving voice" to marginalized sectors of society, such as "the poor" (Bailey 1998; McIlwaine 1998) or women (Alvarez 1999; Lang 2000; Mindry 2001; Thayer 2001). Former UN secretary general Kofi Annan held that the purpose of NGOs was to "hold states' feet to the fire" (Karim 2001:94). Recent ethnographies on NGOs have chipped away at such monolithic understandings, as the many different "stakeholder groups" within them assign different meanings to NGOs' actions (Hilhorst 2003:146). While NGOs' missions primarily motivate some actors, to others these organizations are the means to pursue higher status, travel opportunities, or simply a job (e.g., Fortun and Fortun 2000:214; Hefferan 2007:50; Schade 2005:130).

Building on this anthropological trajectory, this book examines how constituencies like donor groups wield a subtle but nonetheless effective influence on NGOs and their "target populations." While not looking for a "smoking gun," this book analyzes how power operates, and the roles our development aid and agencies administering that aid play in transforming local civic life. This power has real material consequences: the death toll of the earthquake and its aftermath was unfortunately very predictable given the present system of aid (Schuller and Morales 2012).

To be more direct, how are we to evaluate NGOs and their impacts on Haiti and other countries in the global South? (Mosse 2005). Do NGOs democratize development, being closer to the people they serve and offering a better system of governance, as some believe? (Clark 1991; Eyma 1992; Paul and Israel 1991). Or are NGOs a tool of imperialism, a "gentle invasion" of the South by the North, as others assert? (Étienne 1997; Gill 2000; Louis-Juste 2007; Petras 1997). More important, on what bases can we make and evaluate these claims?

Assessing NGOs

Central to understanding these questions are participation and autonomy within NGOs. For example, if a particular NGO empowers local recipient communities to participate in all aspects of their work, from setting priorities to evaluation, and is autonomous from not only the state but also donor agencies, then communities can use this NGO to solve local problems. Conversely, if an NGO lacks local participation and autonomy, international donors can use it to establish foreign priorities and maintain foreign control over the country.

This book is an ethnographically based analysis of the local and global phenomena that promote or inhibit participation and autonomy within NGOs. To identify these phenomena this book offers a comparative frame, discussing two Haitian women's NGOs of similar size, nationality, longevity, and sector prevention, but different donors. The group I call "Sove Lavi" (Kreyòl for "saving lives")[14] received only public development aid, including USAID funds, while the other, "Fanm Tèt Ansanm" ("women united"), received mostly private NGO funding. Whereas Sove Lavi repeatedly brushed aside member concerns in favor of top-down mandates, triggering local conflicts, Fanm Tèt Ansanm enjoyed relatively high levels of autonomy and member participation.

To understand these differences, *Killing with Kindness* traces relationships between various sets of actors, including recipients of services, NGO staff, directors, other NGOs, the Haitian government, and donor agencies, using a framework I call "civic infrastructure" (2006b). Civic infrastructure acknowledges, charts, and analyzes the interrelationship between the various constituencies or "stakeholder groups" involved in NGOs or social movements—even temporary groupings or "assemblages" (Deleuze and Guattari 1987)—as each relationship both affects and is affected by others in the "social field" (Bourdieu 1998). This frame allows for comparisons in relationships, highlighting extreme inequalities, both within Haitian society and across the North–South divide. Civic infrastructure also helps to examine patterns in these relationships and to interrogate observed differences between two or more NGOs.

This study is based primarily on long-term ethnographic fieldwork within these two NGOs, the bulk of which was conducted during twenty months spanning Haiti's protracted political/economic crisis, October 2003 to May 2005.

As mentioned above, I lived in a house in a mixed-income neighborhood with a sizeable middle class. I thus saw daily interactions (or lack thereof) between people of different classes in Haiti, and saw firsthand the tenacious threads of civil society missed by donor representatives and their Haitian proxies, safely concealed in their large houses and driven to work, protected by high walls and armed guards. True, living in Kriswa I was spared most of the horrors that bloggers and CNN alike dutifully highlighted in bidonvil such as Sitesolèy (Cité Soleil) or Bèlè (Bel-Air). But living on my own and walking to public transit, I often found myself in situ not unlike Clifford Geertz happening to be around during a police raid (1973:420). Like many other anthropologists before me (e.g., Behar 1993, 1996), several times a day, the social distance and protection that imperialism provided my white body carrying a U.S. passport would pierce my consciousness as a stranger hailed me as "*blan*."[15] Often, this interpellation as Other came with a request for redistributive justice, albeit on an individual level. Unlike the medical anthropologists Paul Farmer and M. Catherine Maternowska, who cofounded Partners in Health and Lambi Fund, respectively, I had little here-and-now to offer while racing against my depleting computer battery, typing up fieldnotes to try and understand the long-term effects of what was happening.

The pages that follow represent a journey that began long before beginning this particular research. Before becoming a graduate student, I was a full-time community organizer in the Twin Cities, working with low-income tenants to redress injustice in their building, their complex, and their city. The target of our organizing was often the city, which had the power to build more affordable housing and thus ease the burden on tens of thousands of tenants. The city also was a primary funding source for one of our key services—the Tenants Union hotline. My job was thus directly at odds with one of our two funding sources. When the other donor, a corporation, moved south and took their charitable giving portfolio with them mere months after kicking out fifty people from low-income housing to expand their office, the city seized the opportunity to freeze its own funds. We were all laid off. Instead of starting the cycle over again with another grassroots group, I decided to study the dynamics of funding, particularly the power that funders wield. Haiti was to prove a very vivid case of the power of funding agencies.

The information that follows was gathered from a variety of sources using a variety of methods.[16] I recorded more than 120 interviews with people ranging from peasant association leaders; current and former factory workers; NGO janitors, frontline staff, and administrators; Haitian government employees; and donor representatives in Haiti, Brussels, Geneva, and Washington. I constructed an archive of more than 4,200 news stories I read in the period, and collected two boxes of print materials from the two NGOs in their "daily life" and their interactions with other institutions, and another two from donors and other

NGOs. And I attempted, despite my racial and national-identity privilege that spared me from what was to become the worst wave of kidnappings in Haiti in May 2005, to live a "typical" daily life within the NGOs and their communities. As part of my attempt to decolonize anthropology (Harrison 1991, 2008), my conclusions followed a process of dialogue with many of the people and groups I studied, with formal conversations discussing my "findings" in the summer of 2006 and punctuated bursts of dialogue since, within the tradition of "participatory action research."

Outline of the Book

This book unfolds much like a detective story. I begin with the 2004 "crisis" as reported in foreign media, filling in the gaps with long-term ethnographic fieldwork, and outlining the importance of women's empowerment. I then detail how Sove Lavi—with public funding, including USAID—failed to deliver. Explaining this local failure, the following chapter discusses its roots on another level, itself demanding an explanation. Through this discussion, we discover that what seem like "local" failures are quite understandable responses to the political environment in Washington a decade after the fall of the Berlin Wall that heralded the Cold War's end and following the terrorist attacks on September 11, 2001. Two policies in particular reproduce and reward inequality and bureaucratic centralization: "results" or "performance" management, and abstinence-only interventions. The process in which power operates within this system of international aid is neither as rational and visible as Karl Marx or Max Weber declared, nor as individuating and diffuse as Michel Foucault outlined. Grafting these insights together, a process I call "trickle-down imperialism" operates within the system, wherein intermediaries impose defensive interpretations onto subordinates, turning otherwise well-meaning policy into disastrous implementation. Local failures stole the spotlight, shielding policies and agencies such as USAID from criticism in the process.

Chapter 1 offers a lived account of recent political and economic crises in Haiti, a case of "episodic violence" stemming from "structural violence" (Farmer 2004; Harrison 1997). This chapter discusses women's understandings, survival, and resistance strategies within such conditions. It thus highlights the importance of women's organizations such as Sove Lavi and Fanm Tèt Ansanm. While discussing my own position and its effects on the research, this chapter voices the diverse lived perspectives of poor women. As structural violence is gendered, women bear the brunt of the political and economic crisis as heads of households and as *poto mitan*, "center posts" or pillars of Haitian society.

Chapter 2 deconstructs donor discourses of "participation," offering an ethnographically grounded concept that addresses multiple perspectives and processes (see also Cooke and Kothari 2001; Hickey and Mohan 2004a; Paley

2001). The chapter discusses relationships between the two NGOs' aid recipients and their communities, and the communities' relationships with the NGOs. One NGO, Fanm Tèt Ansanm, provided space for relatively high levels of recipient involvement in execution, discussion, planning, and even program design and priority setting, whereas participation at the other, Sove Lavi, when it occurred at all, was primarily limited to minute implementation details.

Chapter 3 theorizes the often-contradictory realities within NGO offices, at once hierarchical and familial. Mirroring and reproducing exaggerated inequalities within Haitian society, NGO offices are organized hierarchically, as reflected in spatial practice and language. Despite this hierarchy, most staff spoke warmly about their collegial relationships, many likening them to a family. The two NGOs had different responses to these pressures of hierarchy and inequality: Fanm Tèt Ansanm staff had more autonomy than did Sove Lavi's, with leadership diffused among frontline staff, whereas Sove Lavi was highly centralized and top-heavy. This chapter argues that these differences are due to the two NGOs' leadership structure and individuality.

Chapter 4 outlines a distinction in the two NGOs' autonomy. Sove Lavi was very dependent on donors who sit on their policymaking board. Donors made decisions about policy, strategy, and implementation details and were listed as coauthors of Sove Lavi publications. By contrast, on paper and somewhat in practice, Fanm Tèt Ansanm enjoyed a certain programmatic autonomy from their Northern (European) NGO funders, who use the language of "partners." But donors played a backstage role in Fanm Tèt Ansanm, only implementing community suggestions that matched donor priorities.

Chapter 5 discusses the historical and political roots of donor policies, explaining the political nature of bilateral aid that shapes interactions with local actors. Following a legitimation crisis in international aid at the end of the Cold War, the U.S. Congress responded by imposing "results-based management" as a practice, while special interest groups—including the religious Right—seized the void to define the national interest according to their vision. This chapter details how rumblings in global capitals are magnified in the South during the process of aid implementation.

The book's conclusion presents three grounded theories that derive from the research. First, *Killing with Kindness* challenges binary framings implicit in many models of "civil society" and "globalization," offering a tripartite analysis that tracks and theorizes multiple sets of actors: transnational agencies, the state, and local communities. Second, it highlights roles played by intermediaries in holding up the system: NGOs as "semi-elites" are inheritors of past world systems and pillars of contemporary globalization. Finally, grafting insights from Foucault's technics of power with a Marxist world systems analysis, the book offers a theory of power, especially in international development, that I call trickle-down imperialism. Following the theoretical conclusion is an afterword, pulling together suggestions for changing this system, beginning at the grass-roots level and following the same levels of analysis discussed in this book.

Like many people, I am confronted with a dual reality about Haiti's earthquake. On the one hand, it is one of the world's most serious humanitarian disasters to date. As a common humanity, we should definitely be supporting Haiti's resurrection. This aid is too important, with too many lives at stake, to deny our support to the victims. Even and especially since the U.S. government bailed out Wall Street to the tune of $1.5 trillion, we should be giving grant aid[17] to the South, and we should increase our total allocation to be 1 percent of our gross domestic product (as proposed by the ONE Campaign in an effort to "make poverty history"; it is currently the lowest of any developed country at 0.16 percent). On the other hand, the failure of the NGO system leading up to and especially following the earthquake is now impossible to ignore. With due respect to the musician–activist Bono and the ONE Campaign, our support should come with a clear set of proposed changes to the way our aid is delivered. If we don't, we just continue our killing with kindness.

1

Violence and Venereal Disease

Structural Violence, Gender, and HIV/AIDS

My friend goes to the industrial park every day on foot. She needs to leave at 5:00 A.M. so she can be at work by 7:00 A.M. And with the insecurity at 5:00 A.M., it's dangerous. Assassins pull their guns, rape them, steal their money, all kinds of things.

—Lisette, women's activist and former factory worker

Monday, May 16, 2005, 9:22 P.M.
The shooting continues. This might be a spillover from this afternoon. There was a ton of shooting in the Nazon/Kafou Ayewopò area. According to Radyo Ginen,[1] several people were injured from gunshots. I saw the effect: a complete *blokis* (traffic jam), so it was faster to walk all the way from Sove Lavi to Kabann Kreyòl (two kilometers), where I got in a taxi that was going to Kafou Ayewopò.[2] I walked in the afternoon sun and rode in a blokis through neighborhoods I am not all that familiar with, all so I could make it in time to a Fanm Tèt Ansanm meeting. I got in the taxi and sat in the fetal position, crammed with six other adults, as the car just sat there. A full forty minutes and only one hundred yards later, we were at the gas station where I take the *tap-tap* (public transport) every day I go to Fanm Tèt Ansanm. Just next to us, there was a round of gunshots and then one really loud boom. CIMO (Haiti's special riot police force, or "stormtroopers") and UN troops shot hundreds of rounds of automatic weapons in the air. Panic quickly ensued, with people running away. Many people got out of their tap-tap or taxi to run. The driver prevented the young woman in the back who wanted to run from getting off. "It's more dangerous!," he screamed. "I will get us out of here." So we drove quickly but not rushed, to the corner where I eat lunch on Sundays. Then we got into another, more severe blokis.

There was no way I was going to get to Fanm Tèt Ansanm by four o'clock, or even close to it. I called, and the secretary Michaëlle answered the phone, scolding me for forgetting my manners when I asked for Jonette, the program supervisor who was hosting the meeting. Another of Jonette's sisters was shot and killed, making Jonette the sole survivor. She wasn't going to be in, and there was a panic at Kafou Ayewopò, so Michaëlle didn't think that the volunteers would be by to meet with Jonette. I thought differently, since the volunteers were supposed to be paid. Regardless, few people were even there.

I walked up the hill to my house, exhausted. On the corner was a trash pile like I'd never seen. I asked "Mami," who sits in her store atop the hill, keeping a watchful eye on all goings-on, if this was normal. She said no.

I was totally out of steam by the time I made it up to the *resto* (enclosed restaurant, a notch up from *chen janbe*, "street food") a half block from my house. I asked the proprietor Charlene if she had any food. She said no. Not a thing. She snapped that I should have called in advance and reserved some. I told her that I didn't call because I didn't expect to be here. I tried to get to work but couldn't. So here I am, home early.

So Maxon, another client who owned a midsize neighborhood business, offered me his plate. He was going to have *mayi moulin* (cornmeal). He was eating his veggies, meat, and boiled plantains. Charlene brought me what would have been his plate, which he had already paid for. Charlene wouldn't let me pay for it. She said, "You are a friend. Every so often you give me gifts. Today it's my turn."

And so I ate it, although I am not a huge fan of cornmeal and despite the fact that it was cold. We talked for a little bit. Like the government staff I interviewed last week, and Fanm Tèt Ansanm staff, both Charlene and Maxon said that Haiti had never been this bad. They couldn't (or didn't want to) pinpoint what was causing the situation, why the country had gone to hell. But Maxon said that in his forty-seven years, things were never like this. When he came to Pòtoprens in 1982, people didn't sleep: they stayed up all night, just hanging out or dancing. If people saw someone that needed help in the street, they offered help. Now they don't, because people are afraid. Someone could be literally yards away—a neighbor—asking for help and people don't do anything. Because they are afraid.[3]

A half hour ago I got a call from Dawn (who runs the Hospice St. Joseph, an NGO guesthouse/clinic in the neighborhood). Apparently, on Saturday, two men were kidnapped in broad daylight where I buy my drinking water. What worries me is that this news hasn't made it to the radio. Two of another NGO's staff have been kidnapped in the past week. In sleepy Tèryewouj (Terrier-Rouge), then a twelve-hour journey from Pòtoprens,[4] thieves broke into the peasants' cooperative compound, disguising themselves as police. They beat up the guard but were still unsuccessful in stealing the cooperative's solar panels.

Tuesday, May 17, 2005, 6:17 P.M.
Helicopters swooped overhead all day long. There was a round-the-clock patrol of CIMO in strategic places. People seemed freaked out.

Someone burned the Tèt Bèf market downtown. I got different takes on the damage, but it seems bad. Poor people, including *timachann* (street merchants), are affected. As someone at Fanm Tèt Ansanm pointed out, the only people who could possibly benefit are the big merchants, who control the market and can raise their prices or ride the short-on-supply increase in prices.

It drizzled this morning and was very muddy. I can only imagine what it was like down by the bay, in the "popular" neighborhoods. Around Fanm Tèt Ansanm's office was absolutely awful, with pools of mud bigger than the hurried SUVs zooming by, soaking the unlucky timachann who are just *chèche lavi*—trying to make a living. I was reminded of the promises to make everything all nice for the 2004 bicentennial, when the government destroyed the houses on the street, rendering fifty families homeless.

Jonette is leaving for the United States for an indeterminate amount of time.[5]

I was aware of being the only visibly white person in all the places I visited today. To say that I stick out is putting the matter mildly (Schuller 2010a).

An Anthropologist's Lens

Because I had a U.S. visa, I was able to leave the country. So I left, three days later, using my privilege and leaving behind the hundreds who were intercepted at sea and sent back and the *ti pèp la* in my neighborhood: the timachann, day laborers, and factory workers as well as people like Lisette and her friend. I began the chapter here to highlight the simple fact that people who can afford to opt out of a bad situation often do. Those left holding things together tend to be people *andeyò*—literally "outside," people marginalized by social inequality, what Patricia Hill Collins (2000:32) called "outsiders within."[6] Not able to leave their responsibilities behind as heads of household and primary caregivers, Haitian women in particular faced the brunt of this violence. I also began with these two episodes from my final fieldnotes to bring into view the often-hidden frame of analysis: the *istwa*. The word "istwa" means both "history" in the academic sense of the word as well as simply "story" (see also Bell 2001). As Michel-Rolph Trouillot reminds us, the act of telling a story/history is always a political event and interpretation, and the storyteller is always a political actor (1995:22). The act of writing history is never "neutral" but rather an act of power (28), "a work of combat" (Nicholls 1974). Bias and a theoretical perspective are implicit in the act of writing history. To deny this fact in the search for "truth" about the past is at best misguided and at worst a deception (or "ideology," in theoretical terms).

As is the case with most other official histories, Haiti's story has been dominated by the political stage, told primarily by ideologically driven political actors and ostensibly disinterested media. Missing from the analysis are the voices of the people most affected yet most silenced: women from Haiti's poor majority. While acknowledging my own position as a white, male anthropologist from the United States who left when things got too hot, this chapter attempts to return women's own voices and their own analyses to the fore, and to at least implicitly critique dominant framings of Haiti's recent "history" by contrasting them to the "stories" told by the women who lived that history every day. As Collins (2000:31) argued, Black feminist knowledge begins with critical analysis and retelling of Black women's own experiences and material reality, a particular application of what feminist scholars call "standpoint theory" (Harding 1991). As the Haitian anthropologist Gina Ulysse (2008:113) reminds us, our racial, gender, and class identities cannot be separated from what the "natives" tell us and what is presented for us to "observe." This same critique of objectivity raised by the double meaning of istwa rings true for anthropologists collecting people's stories. The *griyo* (storytellers) are self-aware, conscious political and historical actors who tell us not only what they think we want to hear, but also what they think we need to hear, using us as a mouthpiece (Ulysse 2002). Our own subject positions—including and especially our activism, what can be called "engaged" or "public" anthropology (Besteman and Gusterson 2005; González 2004; Lamphere 2004; Low and Merry 2010; Sanday 2003)—are therefore inseparable from the istwa that we collaboratively produce, which nonetheless have a shared subjective reality that is useful to counter dominant framings.

The stories written by most journalists who swooped into Haiti as the country careened toward President Aristide's 2004 ouster ended on February 29. Once President Aristide was forced out of the country, news coverage dropped off almost immediately. "History" followed the war correspondents to Darfur, to Lebanon, or back to Iraq.[7] While I was in Haiti from October 2003 to May 2005, the Associated Press employed at least nineteen writers on the ground. This hit-and-run approach—following what my journalist friend called the "if it bleeds, it leads" principle—produces stories wherein Haiti only appears on the news when it's bad (Potter 2009). It's not surprising that only one of 1,200 people I polled while giving guest lectures in the United States had a positive first impression of Haiti, attesting to the power of the dominant istwa.

While the mainstream press was defining February 29 as a conclusion, to the people I came to know it was just a beginning. The "Aristide question" will undoubtedly be debated for years to come, with some arguing that he was a victim of the world system (e.g., Bogdanich and Nordberg 2006; Chomsky et al. 2004; Dupuy 2005; Engler and Fenton 2005; Hallward 2007; Robinson 2007), and others arguing that he was principally to blame for the political crisis (Bohning 2004; Charles 2005; Deibert 2005; Dupuy 2007; Fatton 2007; Girard 2005; Rotberg 2003). The controversy over Aristide—while important as he remains the most potent symbol, particularly to Haiti's excluded poor majority—nonetheless keeps our attention only on the political stage, silencing how this crisis was lived day to day by Haiti's poor majority. To people like Maxon, Charlene, and Grann, and everyone else I talked to of all classes, the two-year transition period that followed was worse. Grann, being the only one of the pèp la—Haiti's poor majority—in the neighborhood who was old enough to remember, recalled only one worse period in Haiti's history: in the late 1950s, when the dictator François Duvalier was consolidating power.

As underscored by my ace-in-the-hole privilege protecting my *blan* body (*blan* is the Haitian term for both "foreign" and "white"), mine is a particular point of view. I will not ever claim to speak "for" Haitian people, in the singular or even plural. As they powerfully demonstrate, these subaltern do speak to those who listen (Spivak 1988). I have had the honor of being asked to help share (and yes, mediate) some of their stories (Bergan and Schuller 2009). But as Nancy Scheper-Hughes (1995) has demonstrated, being a "barefoot anthropologist"— staying as close as possible to the poor majority, talking and spending most of my time with them, while eschewing comforts that would put distance between us— is the next best thing. When AP sent nineteen stringers to Haiti, nearly all of them had to rely on at best a French speaker[8] and a politically connected local journalist "fixer"—and their biases and exclusions—to get the story. Only two were in Haiti long enough to learn Kreyòl, get out of their upscale hotel, and scratch beneath the surface. Anthropological research is much more slow going. I waited thirteen months before my first recorded interview, not just because I wanted to keep my commitments and therefore be someone people could possibly trust with their istwa, but also because I needed to get up with the roosters, grumble about the electricity and water, watch as neighbors moved away, or be awoken in the middle of the night by a low-flying UN helicopter or round of gunshots. I also spoke with people from every class: representatives of international development agencies in Washington, Europe, and Haiti, industrialists, government officials, NGO employees of every rung, peasants, factory workers, and timachann. In all, I conducted 115 recorded interviews in constructing this istwa. Following my twenty months of initial fieldwork, I have returned at least twice a year (with two months in the summers), keeping my promises and learning.

Necessarily, the istwa that I tell here differs from, even as it intersects with, other stories and histories. Nonetheless, to set up the constellation of interpretations and accounts, individual and collective stories, and especially to understand Lisette's story at the beginning of the chapter, we need to begin with a mainstream media istwa, the events leading up to that fateful Sunday morning at the end of February.

A Brief Istwa of the Crisis

The crisis began way before 2004, ironically demonstrated by Colleen, who was working at USAID at the time of an October 2005 interview: "There's some move for truth and reconciliation, but that won't work in Haiti. If you do that in Haiti, then people will be talking about what happened two hundred years ago. How do you reconcile something that happened two hundred years ago? I don't know how you would get at it." Colleen's discourse of "moving on" and "not dwelling in the past" is a familiar refrain among development professionals, including Special UN Envoy Bill Clinton, right up until the earthquake in January 2010. Unfortunately this silencing of the past is a major reason why these agencies fail in places like Haiti. As many scholars familiar with Haiti—not to mention Haitian people—know all too well, Haiti's current situation is in large part structured by its past. As Haitian scholars such as Trouillot (1990), Dupuy (1989, 1997), and Fatton (2004) have argued, Haiti's decline was the result of collusion between local and foreign elite groups. As I argued elsewhere (2007a), Haiti's history is best understood in a tripartite frame, tracking the actions and contradictions of three levels of actors: what is called "the international community," the Haitian government, and the Haitian people. Particularly relevant is the role played by intermediaries, typically Haiti's elite groups.

Once the most productive colony in the world, producing large surpluses for the soon-to-be revolutionary French bourgeoisie, Haiti was the second to gain its independence in the Americas. It was the first, and only, slave revolt to succeed in attaining free nationhood, in 1804. The decline begins shortly following Haiti's 1804 independence. While the black military elite since Jean-Jacques Dessalines (1804–1806) and King Henry Christophe (1807–1820) attempted to compel laborers to work in plantations to accumulate the surplus needed to build a military and the impressive Citadel, still standing today, mulatto leaders since Alexandre Pétion (1807–1818) and Jean Pierre Boyer (1818–1843) attempted accommodation with foreign powers (including negotiating the 150 million francs indemnity to France in 1825, discussed below). Haiti's two main elite groups, a dark-skinned military elite and a light-skinned merchant class, competed with each other for access to the Haitian state (Nicholls 1996; Trouillot 1994a). The merchant class, lightened by migration from Lebanon, Syria, and Jordan, made millions off its monopoly in foreign trade, directly aligning its interests with those of foreign capitalists. Neither group defended the interests of the mass of rural laborers, and both used the state to extract wealth for personal gain from the peasantry (Sheller 2004; Trouillot 1977, 1990).

Both groups derived their power from being intermediaries of the international system. Because the world economy was built off slave labor, Haiti was ostracized by the slave-owning powers surrounding it. In the United States, where several pre–Civil War presidents owned slaves, Congress actually passed a gag order, preventing Haiti from being discussed. "The peace and safety of a large portion forbids us to discuss [Haiti]," bellowed a South Carolina senator in 1824 (Farmer 2003:69). For its part, postrevolutionary France demanded 150 million francs in 1825 as an indemnity in exchange for their recognition of Haitian independence, to repay former planters for their loss of "property." Boyer—who had fought against the revolutionary leader Toussaint Louverture—accepted the terms. This is the only such ransom in world postcolonial history. Since the Haitian state was bankrupt, it accepted a usurious loan from a private French bank and spent as much as 80 percent of its tax base to pay it off for more than 120 years (Gaillard-Pourchet 1990; 2002; Marcelin [1897] 2004). When western Europe and North America were building railroads, cable lines, irrigation systems, sewage systems, schools, and hospitals, Haiti was paying off France because of an economic institution France later self-righteously condemned as a "crime against humanity" in 2001.[9]

With Haiti's racially divided elite groups vying for control of the state apparatus, foreign institutions at times played decisive roles in favoring one group or another, offering them tools to oppress society—especially Haiti's poor majority. In 1915, with its European competitors at war with one another, the United States invaded Haiti. White supremacy in addition to foreign capitalism favored lighter-skinned merchants as trading partners and leaders to represent Haiti. During the nineteen-year occupation, the U.S. Marines installed a series of light-skinned puppet governments, built a modern army to quash dissent and revolt, and imposed a constitution that a young Franklin Roosevelt claims to have written personally, which made French (the language of the elite) Haiti's only official language and opened up land to foreign companies. The occupation triggered understandable rage, nationalism, and racial animosity (Polyné 2010; Renda 2001; Smith 2009). Combine this with the centralized bureaucracy and millions in aid in a Cold War context, and the stage was set for a totalitarian regime (Nicholls 1996; Trouillot 1990). François Duvalier was more than willing to take these reins, and did so in 1957.

The inauguration of the official "development" era with the UN's 1948 Mission to Haiti offered more tools for personal enrichment and oppression of the populace. Duvalier ("Papa Doc") perfected this model, using the Cuban Revolution and his own anticommunism to successfully secure more aid from the United States, especially during a famous 1960 speech referred to as "Cri de Jacmel," when Duvalier threatened to search elsewhere (i.e., the Soviet Union) for aid (Diederich and Burt [1970] 2005; Ferguson 1987). Using international aid money, Duvalier built an infamous secret police called the *tonton makout*,[10] responsible for killing at least thirty thousand Haitian people. Arguably less bloodthirsty than his father, Jean-Claude Duvalier ("Baby Doc") was known as a playboy, more interested in bestowing lavish riches on his wife, a light-skinned member of Haiti's elite. With World Bank and USAID support, Baby Doc built factories for U.S. clothing manufacturers, vowing to turn Haiti into the "Taiwan of the Caribbean." Eric Duhaime (2002) estimated that the Duvaliers stole $900 million, including $5.7 million held in a Swiss account that was frozen. Presumably, getting that money back was the primary motivation for Baby Doc's surprise return to Haiti on January 17, 2011, less than a week after the first anniversary of the earthquake. According to the International Monetary Fund's own accounting, of a $22 million loan in December 1980, $20 million was immediately siphoned off, $4 million for the tonton makout and the remainder in Duvalier's personal accounts (Ferguson 1987:70). By 1987, the first year after Duvalier was uprooted (Haitian people use the Kreyòl *dechoukaj*), Haiti's debt to international financial institutions (IFIs)—who decided to keep this debt on Haiti's people—was $844 million. People in Haiti remember this international support of the Duvalier dictatorship, even as development agencies like those Colleen works for would have people forget in their promotion of Haiti's "clean slate." As the Kreyòl proverb goes, "Bay kou, bliye, pote mak, sonje" (The one who strikes the blow may well forget, but the one who receives the scar remembers).

The Haitian state was called a "kleptocracy" (Lundahl 1989; Rotberg 1997) or "predatory state" (Fatton 2002; Lundahl 1984). Under foreign surveillance and with foreign aid going to support their individual wealth and the tonton makout, the Duvalierist state did not invest in its people. As a result, most of the education and health care were private initiatives: by 1991, following the first democratic election, 90 percent of clinics and 85 percent of schools were run by mission groups and NGOs. Connected to this is the lack of "absorptive capacity," or the ability of public agencies to manage funds, noted by many donor groups (e.g., International Monetary Fund 2002; Morton 1997; World Bank 2002a). This was the state inherited by the democratic regimes, set up in the interests of self-promotion and exclusion, run by technocrats from a small "political class" and underpaid civil service professionals fearful of losing their jobs and pensions.

In the mid-eighties, the foreign-supported dictatorship went too far. Responding to threats of swine fever (recently renamed "H1N1 virus"), the United States demanded that the entire population of Haitian pigs be destroyed.[11] Since Haitian pigs were the de facto bank accounts for the peasantry, this amounted to Haiti's "great stock market crash" (DeWind and Kinley 1988; Diederich 1985; Farmer 1992; Smith 2001). The last straw came when Duvalier shot up a student protest in Gonayiv (Gonaïves) in November 1985. Rather than let the popular struggle gain steam, on February 7, 1986, the United States arranged the safe transport of the Duvaliers out of Haiti, paving the way for a military junta. The new government quickly repaid its debt of gratitude to the United States by imposing a range of neoliberal measures authored by the "Chicago Boy"[12] Leslie Delatour. The currency was floated and immediately lost its value, driving already-low wages through the floor (Deshommes 1995, 2006). Protective tariffs on foreign agricultural goods were slashed. Today, Haiti has the lowest tariffs of anywhere in the hemisphere—for example, 3 percent for rice, compared to a regional average of 20 percent. This destroyed Haiti's peasant economy, and little by little, state-owned businesses began to be privatized (see Bazin's [2008] study for a detailed account and critique).

Transition to Democracy

One cannot understand the 2004 coup[13] without reference to the international stage. On December 16, 1990, despite $12 million in U.S. funds spent on the former World Bank official Marc Bazin's candidacy (Clement 1997:21; Griffin 1992:129), the liberation theology priest Jean-Bertrand Aristide was elected president by an overwhelming majority under the Lavalas movement. "Lavalas" is alternatively translated as landslide or "cleansing flood." The Lavalas campaign was founded on transparency, participation, and an end to what they called the "death plan"—neoliberalism. Aristide was removed from office on September 30, 1991, eight months into his presidency. Bankrolled by the CIA (Weisbrot 1997:27), the International Republican Institute (IRI) (Glick Schiller and Fouron 2001:227), and local elites, the military regime of Raoul Cédras and later the CIA-funded and trained paramilitary organization FRAPH (Front pour l'Avancement et le Progrès Haïtien) targeted popular organizations (Human Rights Watch 1993). The coup regime was arguably more repressive than Duvalier, openly murdering and targeting as many as twenty thousand government members and popular leaders. George H. W. Bush spoke of his disapproval of Aristide, and the Vatican (already critical of Aristide and other activist priests like El Salvador's Oscar Romero) officially recognized Cédras as Haiti's legitimate president. These nods of support encouraged the coup regime and FRAPH to continue killing popular organization leaders and other poor people, presumably Aristide supporters (Clement 1997:31). While still in exile, faced with violence and intense multinational pressure, Aristide signed the Governor's Island Accord and Paris Club Agreement, ceding control to international institutions such as the International Monetary Fund (IMF), World Bank, and Inter-American Development Bank (IDB) through privatization and structural adjustment.

Following a U.S. invasion of thirty thousand troops, Aristide finally returned to power on October 15, 1994, and served the rest of his term but was not allowed to extend the mandate for his three years in exile. Haiti's first democratic transfer of power in 1996 followed the election of René Préval, Haiti's second president (after François Duvalier) to serve his full term. During this period, unprecedented amounts of international aid were poured into Haiti—$1.8 billion from the fiscal years 1995 to 1999 (World Bank 2002b). The majority of this aid flowed through NGOs, which sprung up like never before during this period (Morton 1997:1; Smith 2001:31)—what some Haitian scholars qualified as another form of "invasion" (Étienne 1997; Louis-Juste 2007).

The Lavalas governments of Aristide and Préval continued the neoliberal policies begun after the de facto regimes and military dictatorships. Why did the Lavalas leadership, first elected to end this "death plan," accept this aid and "invasion" of NGOs? In addition to the conditions imposed by the Governor's Island Accord noted above, Haiti was broke. During the mid-1990s, according to the World Bank researcher Alice Morton (1997:vi), 90 percent of Haiti's national budget was financed externally, a figure that fell to 70 percent in the mid-2000s (Mulet 2007). As a peasant in Tissous quoted in Jennie Smith's (2001:38–39) ethnography of NGOs argued, "If you are thirsty, and the only water you've got is putrid, you're obligated to hold your nose and drink"—a point that Paul Farmer (2008) and others repeat to Aristide's critics on the Left, who argued that he had made too many compromises and concessions to the IFIs. A sidelined state offered donors and IFIs a more efficient model for the implantation of programs, with little to no resistance.

Haiti's state was weakened in this period by donor policies. In 1995 the Republican-controlled U.S. Congress forced USAID to stop funding the Haitian government in favor of NGOs. In 1997, citing the lack of an elected parliament, the World Bank (2002a:3) suspended new loans to Haiti. Following a current account balance problem wherein the government was drained of its international reserves of U.S. dollars, triggered by this act as well as Haiti's extreme imbalance of imports to exports,[14] the IMF (2001) imposed austerity measures.[15] When Haiti's government failed to deliver, the IMF triggered a freeze of all multilateral funds to Haiti. Meanwhile, bilateral donor flows directly to NGOs remained high, creating a parallel state (Lwijis 2009), what some call a "nongovernmental government." Donors' policy of circumventing the state fueled a "cold war" between the cash-starved Haitian government and the well-funded NGO sector (Morton 1997:40). USAID-funded NGOs crafted development policies that countered the priorities set by Haiti's elected government, notably in agriculture, food security, and education. U.S.-funded NGOs promoted export-oriented agriculture (USAID 1997), undermined local production by removing import tariffs, encouraged dependency by dumping U.S. agricultural surpluses (Richardson 1997), and funded private schools at the expense of public schools and adult literacy programs (USAID 1999). USAID also sanitized the official human rights record, destroying documents connecting FRAPH to the CIA and diminishing or flatly denying victims' testimonies (James 2010).

Donors also played a direct role in supporting opposition to Aristide since his 2000 reelection. Foreign agencies such as USAID and the European Union funded NGOs that played leadership roles in Aristide's opposition (Dupuy 2005). The Civil Society Initiative (ISC) assembled Haiti's business elites who defined civil society in an explicitly ideological liberal framework, following the model of Adam Smith (Jean 2002:34). ISC was founded in 2000 by Hubert DeRonceray, president of USAID's educational partner (FONHEP), and it included other Rightist bourgeois families like the Boulos[16] and pro-business interest groups like the Center for Free Enterprise and Democracy. This group defined itself as the single, authentic representative of "civil society," even though it lacked legitimacy because it represented only bourgeois interests (Jean 2002:35). As a corrective, the Group of 184[17] was founded at a December 2002 IRI conference, held at a Santo Domingo hotel where the exiled putschist

Guy Philippe was also residing (Bogdanich and Nordberg 2006). A significant difference between the oppositions is that the Group of 184 included women's organizations, labor unions, peasants' organizations, and human rights groups—many of which had received U.S. and other donor agencies' funding—in their list of members.[18] In 2003, USAID allocated $2.9 million for "democracy and governance," up from $2 million in 2002, while the overall USAID portfolio was halved over the previous four years, from $107 to $54 million (USAID 2003). USAID (2003) claimed success: "To date, USAID's support to civil society has empowered and perhaps emboldened groups to engage with government on national interests." USAID further explained: "In FY 2002 USAID launched new programs to help Haitian civil society resist the growing trend toward authoritarian rule by . . . developing new political leadership."

This was still not enough. In February 2004, when the "democratic opposition" failed to bring Aristide down, and after the Group of 184 lost control of the groundswell of student-led protests, an armed "insurrection" took over. Philippe and the convicted former FRAPH leader Louis Jodel Chamblain routed police stations, freeing inmates and forcing police officers to hide. Coming from the Dominican Republic, the "rebels" used U.S.-made M16s (James 2004), possibly the same just given to the Dominican Army to patrol the border (Darion Garcia 2003). Despite the political opposition's insistence on their nonalignment with this armed group, Philippe later revealed that he was in constant contact with both the United States and the political opposition (Jacklin 2007). The "insurrection" succeeded quickly. Before dawn on February 29, 2004, the United States flew Aristide out of Haiti aboard a military plane, following the U.S. government's order that Aristide's private security withdraw (Dumas 2008; Tamayo 2004).

As noted above, this is where most of the foreign media attention—not to mention books, blogs, and activism—stops. Despite the many critical events that have occurred since, all too often the istwa ends in 2004 with Aristide's ouster. To people living in Haiti, however, February 29 was not just the end of one story but also the beginning of another story, a very sad one.

Rise in Violence

By any measure, the interim period was more violent than the "insurrection," including more killings and kidnappings. Monique, an NGO janitor, recalled, "For myself, I see that things are more difficult. Because now you walk on top of cadavers. No one is spared. You go out. If you return, you say, thank you Jesus. You sleep, you wake up in your bed, thank you Jesus. Because . . . other people, they leave their bed and disappear in the streets, in a car. . . . You go out, you are in fear. You enter, you are in fear. You see my hair? I used to have long hair. This stress caused me to lose my hair. Stress!"

This rise in violence occurred under the watch of UN peacekeeping troops. On March 1, 2004, the day after Aristide left, the Security Council adopted UN

Resolution 1529, a proposal France called for authorizing a UN peacekeeping force with troops from the United States, France, Canada, and Chile, called the Multilateral Interim Force. Immediately, foreign troops secured the international airport, the free trade zone, the downtown financial district, and Channmas (Champs-de-Mars),[19] the symbolic center of the nation and seat of government, international organizations, and some NGOs' offices. Troops also patrolled the industrial park surrounding the international airport. The force set up bases in strategic locations. They took over Aristide's private university near his home in Taba (Tabarre) and occupied the Casernes Dessalines—the former headquarters of the demobilized army, adjacent to the National Palace. The United States took command of this temporary force. A second UN Resolution (1542) called for a more permanent peacekeeping presence, called Mission des Nations Unies pour la stabilisation en Haïti (MINUSTAH), to take over in June. As of August 2009, when its mandate was once again renewed, MINUSTAH comprised 9,158 soldiers and police officers from forty-seven countries, rising to 12,651 following the earthquake (United Nations 2011). Echoing statements made public on March 4, 2004, by French President Jacques Chirac and UN Secretary General Kofi Annan, Resolution 1542 specified that Brazil would lead the military unit and Canada the civilian police. MINUSTAH's mandate was to help the interim government in its task of providing security, paving the way for successful elections.

When MINUSTAH took over in June, it continued the U.S.-led forces' occupation of buildings and makeshift camps—including factories and hotels, as it proved more profitable for these parties to rent their space to MINUSTAH than to stay open for business. Initially many welcomed Brazil, a Southern country led by a workers' government and known as stars of the world soccer stage. This goodwill quickly evaporated as it became clear to many that Brazil was a proxy for the United States, serving its interests,[20] as the women's NGO employee Yvette exclaims: "The Americans hide their face. They send Brazilians, Argentines . . . [the Americans] are hidden but they're in command!" This common perception was reinforced symbolically, as the ubiquitous white armored personnel carriers and tanks were emblazoned with the English acronym "UN." (In French, Spanish, or Portuguese, the acronym would be "NU" or "ONU.")

Despite MINUSTAH's presence, the security situation deteriorated over the two-year period following Aristide's departure. According to Reuters in their continuing coverage, some fifty people were killed during the four-month period leading up to the three-week "armed rebellion" that killed about eighty, leading to Aristide's forced resignation. On March 5, Reuters reported that there were eight hundred cadavers in the General Hospital morgue, two hundred of which the Pan American Health Organization estimated to be victims of violence (Bachelet 2004). One hospital, opened in late December 2004 by the French NGO Doctors Without Borders, treated more than 2,500 victims of gun violence during the first sixteen months of operation—one thousand in the first three months alone (MSF 2006). A team of researchers estimated the number of violent deaths from this period to be eight thousand (Kolbe and Hutson 2006).[21]

In addition to violent deaths, the interim period was scarred by kidnapping. After a February 19, 2005, jailbreak in which 481 people escaped the National Penitentiary, the kidnappings increased. Given the ineffective response of the National Police and MINUSTAH, the situation quickly spiraled out of control. Journalists and foreigners—including missionaries, NGO employees, and even French consular officials—were not spared. During the months of April through July 2005, when the outspoken journalist Jacques Roche was kidnapped and murdered, the National Police estimated the number of kidnappings at six hundred, an average of more than five per day (RNDDH 2006). Kidnapping quickly became known as a lucrative business. As noted above, Jonette fled the country because everyone else in her family was kidnapped or killed. During the beginning stages, according to keen observers of the situation, people who drove new automobiles or were being driven by a chauffeur were the likely targets—in other words, individuals who looked like they had money. But especially after the ineffectual response to the prison break, no one was spared. Poor women like Monique, who lived in Sitesolèy, became victims: "Myself, for me . . . they pulled a gun on me. Yes! I had eight [Haitian[22]] dollars [about one U.S. dollar] in my hand. Eight dollars to feed my children. And when they pulled the gun on me, I told them I didn't have anything on me, only eight dollars. So they demanded that I give them five dollars I had on me. I gave the five dollars and kept three!"

Everyone I talked with knew someone who had been the victim of kidnapping or attempted kidnapping. Given kidnappers' willingness to quickly negotiate ransom, and given how low they were willing to go, the motivation behind this wave of kidnapping was clearly economic. Mme Auguste, an NGO veteran, told me a story about a boy of thirteen in her neighborhood. She asked him to bring down some coconuts for her, offering him ten goud[23] (a U.S. quarter). The boy rejected it, saying, "What can I do with the ten goud? Why don't you give me a gun instead?" Recoiling, Mme Auguste asked, "What will you do with the gun?" He said, "You don't have a gun. If I had a gun I wouldn't have to climb the coconut tree for you for ten goud. I would look for money in the streets." An NGO director argued that this class of kidnappers was not "well integrated" into Haitian society, not knowing whom to target, because political and economic elites remained for the most part unscathed.[24] In addition, according to several secondhand accounts, the kidnappers spoke English, suggesting involvement by U.S. deportees—some of whom had never even seen Haiti, having been born in the United States to Haitian parents. More than thirty deportees arrived per month in Port-au-Prince following the passage of the Patriot Act in 2001.[25]

Several commentators connected the economic situation and the violence. According to Carlene, a factory worker, featured in the documentary *Poto Mitan*, "Inequality in the country prevents people from getting a good job, so people fall into a series of things they shouldn't do. That's why either big or small, anyone can become a thief." Carlene's colleague Beatrice, a laid-off factory worker, explains, "You see all the thefts or kidnapping being done out there? You think it's poor people committing these acts? It's not. They put poor people [*ti pèp la*] in visible places. The small people [*ti pèp la*] are hungry. They get some money to commit an act. They're hungry, so they do it. And who dies? Poor people. But they're not the ones responsible. There's a hidden hand." Several other commentators made this link explicit, arguing that inequality and misery[26] are the roots of the violence. The only disagreement concerned emphasis: Yolette Etienne, director of the National Campaign Against Violence, argued, "We won't say that misery and poverty create violence, but misery and poverty facilitate violence. In addition, inequality increases violence."

As the stories highlight, while "hard data" are unavailable, women were the primary targets of this violence, as is true in many other conflict/post-conflict situations. Malya Villard of KOFAVIV, a grassroots women's NGO of victims of violence helping other victims, put it this way: "When one government falls and another takes power, many rapes happen. People decide to target women's bodies." According to the most reliable estimates, as many as one in three women in Pòtoprens were the victims of violence (MCFDF 2004). As I describe below, and like in many cultures, women are more susceptible to violence if they are in a vulnerable economic position. "Rape or violence are directly connected with the country's economy," Malya continued. "Sometimes a woman doesn't have any earning power, which makes her a victim." Lisette offers a friend's story: "[Her husband] looks at her, beats her, slaps her, and bites her. Fed up, she finally goes to the police. The officers arrest the man at 2:00 P.M. Around 6:00 P.M. she comes and says, 'Commander, if you don't let him out, my children are going to die of hunger!' So if she had some means of survival in her own hands, she could have the guy stay in prison. However, the man disfigured her and she asked him to be let out."[27] These and many other poignant analyses I could have selected recall Farmer's (2003:350; 2004) argument that episodic violence is a distal form and expression of structural violence.

Structural Violence

The term "structural violence" arose from the liberation theologian Johan Galtung and was recently revived, refined, and popularized by Paul Farmer. Other scholars, including the peace researcher Gernot Köhler, have used the concept to critique global apartheid and other racialized inequalities (Eckhardt and Köhler 1980; Köhler 1978). The Black feminist anthropologist Faye Harrison

(1997, 2002) engaged this concept in her ethnographic writings about Jamaica at the hands of international development agencies. Farmer (2004:317) defines structural violence as "the natural expression of a political and economic order that seems as old as slavery. This social web of exploitation, in its many different historical forms, has long been global." It "tightens a physical noose around [its victims'] necks, and this garroting determines the way in which resources— food, medicine, even affection—are allocated and experienced" (315). Critically, like most ideological systems and oppression, structural violence depends on its invisibility, the "erasure of historical memory" (307).

Yvette, who works at Sove Lavi, points out the connection between "episodic" and "structural" violence: "If it wasn't in [the UN's] interest, they could have brought about peace already. You come to my country. You take up my space where I used to live. You took it! You raised the prices for the goods I buy that used to be more-or-less affordable. You increased the high cost of living here, in my home."

As the women's istwa[28] highlight so far, the more visible acts of episodic violence were accompanied by a deterioration of the economic situation during Haiti's 2004–2006 interim period. Unlike the episodic violence, this structural violence was barely noticed, even by alternative media sources, until April 2008 when thousands of people took to the streets. Although the media finally paid attention, Haiti was saddled with a new istwa: "food riots" and "dirt cookies" suddenly appeared in headlines. Three major indexes of this economic crisis as lived by lower-income women were the loss of factory jobs, the increase in the already high cost of living, and skyrocketing housing costs. Each in turn had severe social consequences.

Factory jobs, already diminished, plummeted in the interim period. According to the Ministry of Social Affairs and several NGO employees, of the approximately twenty thousand factory jobs in the fall of 2003 before the episodic violence, only an estimated twelve to fourteen thousand remained mid-2005. The most powerful istwa explaining this job loss is that factory owners and merchants were reacting to the violence by protecting their investments from losses, thus decapitalizing the country. But owners and merchants also received substantial gains during the interim period in the form of tax shelter, UN protection of their private property, and money to rent their empty factories to house the UN troops. Meanwhile, the World Trade Organization lifted its quota on Chinese textiles in 2005, opening a huge new competing labor market. This decision negatively affected all garment factories in the Americas, which have higher shipping, labor, and other production costs than their Chinese counterparts that have set up a one-stop-shop. Thus there is evidence that changing economic policies explain the loss of jobs during this period (see Schuller [2008] for further discussion).

In March 2004 the interim government announced that the largest industries and merchants were exempt from paying taxes for a three-year period.

It was among Gérard Latortue's first acts as interim prime minister.[29] While the prices for basic goods and services increased dramatically after 2003, the minimum wage did not increase until a very organized effort in the summer of 2009, which culminated in a unanimous vote in Parliament. A backdoor deal between the manufacturers and the UN, Bill Clinton, and President Préval lowered the agreed-on rate.[30] When I asked workers why they did not speak up during the 2004–2006 interim period, and why the situation deteriorated so much, several people told me the same thing: Owners know they have the upper hand. They can fire everyone or all suspected union members, and replace them with others eagerly awaiting the chance to work for Haiti's low minimum wage. Yvette explained, "They don't want unions in Haiti. When you have a union, they destroy it. They fire everyone because they fear unions." Lisette's coworker refused to join a union because of this fear: "They know if they fire one person, they will find two hundred people standing in line waiting to take her place." Many workers told me that "fifty thousand people are behind you," waiting for the same job. Factory worker and Fanm Tèt Ansanm leader Simone was more pointed in her critique, arguing that the government shared a responsibility with the people: "If there was a government, when workers demand something, we would succeed. [Bosses] would hear us because the government would speak with them. They could raise the minimum wage. They could help us. But I don't see that it will change, because there's no government." This sentiment of not having a government was common during the Latortue period.

These workers not laid off or fired were the "lucky" ones. But even those who worked in the formal sector (about 15–30 percent of the population, depending on estimates) found it difficult to cope with the substantial price hikes in staple goods like rice, corn, beans, and oil during this period.[31] In the mixed, middle-income neighborhood where I lived, a *gwo mamit* (coffee can) of Haitian rice used to sell for seventy-five goud[32] at the beginning of 2004 ($2.00 at the time). At the beginning of 2005, it sold for one hundred twenty-five goud ($3.12). A *ti mamit* (soup can) of Haitian black beans used to sell for forty goud ($1.00), but it soon became sixty goud ($1.50). Prices were lower if bought in large quantities and closer to the port. While there are usually several exchanges from the port to the neighborhood, with each person taking a small profit from which to live, including a few goud to pay for a tap-tap, the Haitian informal market is normally remarkably "efficient" in economic terms, distributing goods quickly and relatively cheaply, as far as possible and to as many people as possible (Fass 1988).

But this market system collapsed during the interim period. Several merchants in the neighborhood closed shop because they could not afford to buy the higher-priced goods, their regular customers could not afford to buy what they sold, or it was too dangerous to risk travel to obtain merchandise. On several occasions—for weeks at a time—the normally busy market in my neighborhood was emptied of half the normal merchants. One in particular, Junia—who always reprimanded me, saying, "I haven't seen you" whenever it had been longer than a day—closed up shop for good in 2005. Operating on the margins of society, many in this class who normally barely eked out a living fell below starvation levels during the coup/Latortue period. Three neighborhood children died from malnutrition. Beatrice, a factory worker, said, "The thing that destroys the country is that you can't buy anything. This *lavi chè a* [high cost of living], Mark, is killing us in Haiti." Lisette was frustrated at government inaction: "Did the high cost of living go up for the government? Because the people, we are suffering and the government doesn't, they act like the cost of living hasn't gone up."

In part, rising fuel costs explained increasing prices for primary subsistence goods. In January 2003 the IMF forced the Aristide government to stop subsidizing the cost of fuel, and this crippled the system, operating as it was with very little profit margin. In addition to triggering protests and strikes from chauffeurs, this action increased prices for transport. Prices for a tap-tap ride within a single route shot up from three to five goud at that time.[33] The fare for one *kous* ("course," equivalent to a route) for shared taxis also doubled, from seven to fifteen goud. During the 2004–2006 crisis, fares increased twice, to as much as ten goud for a tap-tap and twenty-five goud for a taxi. Lisette pointed out that workers earning the stagnant seventy goud ($1.75) minimum wage were not getting anywhere: "If you buy a plate of food for fifty goud, and you pay ten goud for a tap-tap to get to work, ten goud to return . . . that is all your seventy goud." Several people cited a Haitian proverb to explain this situation: "Lave men, siye atè" (Washing your hands, only to wipe them on the ground).

In addition to the rise in prices for staple goods and transport during this period, housing costs skyrocketed almost everywhere (except for the neighborhoods most impacted by violence, such as Bèlè and Sitesolèy). As Yvette suggested, the presence of many foreign troops played a role in this, but more generally, the rise in housing costs resulted from the capitalist logic of supply and demand under extreme duress. Carlene said, "You used to be able to rent a house for 300, 250, now it's 1,600, 3,000, 4,000 for a year."[34] In the twelve months following Aristide's departure, many rents doubled in my mixed-income neighborhood, forcing several people to relocate to neighborhoods such as Bèlè, which were slowly vacated as the violence increased. Several NGO staff and factory workers also reported that their rent in other relatively safe neighborhoods shot up by as much as 150 to 250 percent.[35] Several people have pointed out that rents are artificially inflated in the country because of the constant presence of foreign NGOs and governmental institutions since the 1991 coup, a concrete manifestation of the NGOization of Haitian society (Louis-Juste 2007). Knowing that NGOs have expense accounts and have to spend their money, landlords offer inflated rents to NGO offices and employees. It was not uncommon for foreign NGOs to pay $2,500 for a housing allowance following the earthquake.

Only two people from the lower classes that I talked to owned their homes; they both lived in violence-prone shantytowns within Sitesolèy. Several friends moved into these areas during the interim period because their housing costs became too expensive, another instance of poverty and economic inequality playing a role in the rise in violence. As Carlene explained, "People who could leave [Sitesolèy] already left. We who remain have no choice. It wasn't good, but now things are really bad."

The above stories suggest a direct correlation between the complex sociopolitical crisis and rising housing costs. These increases benefited a small group of landowners. Beatrice explained that her conditions were bad because her landlord "built this house to make money." Some commentators have praised Haiti's informal housing market, unencumbered by legislation, as being one of the most effective, efficient, and fair in the world (deSoto 2000:183). A closer ethnographic look, however, reveals that the vast majority of people of a certain class (e.g., janitor, factory worker, street merchant, day laborer) do not own even their eight-foot-square, dirt-floor, cinderblock, patched-tin-roof houses. Approximately 95 percent of the people I spoke with in these economic brackets rented their house or patch of land, on which they are responsible for building a structure.[36] While it might be true that some landlords originated from a similar class, being lucky enough to squat on empty land before the massive urban migration in the 1980s,[37] most of the land in Pòtoprens is controlled by middle- or upper-income people, some of whom, like my own landlord, live outside Haiti.

Structural violence generally, and particularly lavi chè a, have health consequences as well, which are felt more severely by women. There are only two doctors per ten thousand people, and that number is lower outside Pòtoprens. This means in practice that few people have regular access to health care. Those who do often have to walk hours to see a doctor, who is required to charge for his or her services (since the mid-1990s structural adjustment programs). Most women—three in four—do not have access to trained medical pre- or postnatal care as a result (World Health Organization 2009). As a result, far too many women die in childbirth: 670 out of 100,000 live births. Also, 80 in 1,000, or roughly one in twelve, children die before they reach the age of five. The first experience I had as a houseguest in Haiti taught me the significance of this statistic. Djoni (the Kreyòl spelling of Johnny), my host, chided me for being "too formal" because I used his and others' official first names. A peasant cooperative leader in Tèryewouj, Djoni explained that everyone—at least those with a birth certificate—has an official name.[38] But because survival is far from certain, surviving children are given a nickname. Most people, except schoolteachers and pastors, refer to people by their nickname. Djoni also explained to me that this is why the first big ceremony in a Catholic person's life is traditionally his or her first communion.[39] Djoni himself died of meningitis in 2008. He was thirty-two.

Child mortality rates in Haiti also exacerbate the tradition of valuing boys over girls. Edwidge Danticat (1994:146) beautifully illustrates the simplicity of birth in Haiti, and the tradition of placing a higher value on boys:

> Tante Atie did not come home for supper. My grandmother and I ate in the yard, while Brigitte slept in a blanket in my arms. My grandmother was watching a light move between two distant points on the hill.
>
> "Do you see that light moving yonder?" she asked, pointing to the traveling lantern. "Do you know why it goes to and fro like that?"
>
> She was concentrating on the shift, her pupils traveling with each movement.
>
> "It is a baby," she said, "A baby is being born. The midwife is taking trips from the shack to the yard where the pot is boiling. Soon we will know whether it is a boy or a girl."
>
> "How will we know that?"
>
> "If it's a boy, the lantern will be put outside the shack. If there is a man, he will stay awake all night with the new child."
>
> "What if it is a girl?"
>
> "If it is a girl, the midwife will cut the child's cord and go home. Only the mother will be left in the darkness to hold her child. There will be no lamps, no candles, no more light."
>
> We waited. The light went out in the house about an hour later. By that time, my grandmother had dozed off. Another little girl had come into the world.

As Danticat's narrative illustrates, gender inequality begins at birth.

Gender and Structural Violence

A former factory worker and leader within Fanm Tèt Ansanm, Simone highlights the multiple issues this chapter has discussed thus far: episodic violence, in this case perpetrated by the paramilitary group FRAPH, as well as structural violence:

> I lived in a family for fourteen years without my dad. My father hadn't lived with my mom since I was a baby. So my mother did everything for me. She sent me to school. In 1994 I couldn't go to school anymore because [FRAPH agents] came inside my mother's house, they raped me, they beat me badly, and they killed my grandmother. Then they threw my mother and me out.
>
> You know that my father didn't live with my mother. Sometimes my mother yelled at me when she didn't have money. But she worked dirty jobs, in the factory, to raise me. When I became a young woman,

I couldn't go to school because they beat my skull, but I could still sew. I found a guy who loved me because I wasn't an ugly girl. When I got pregnant, he said it wasn't his, despite the fact that my mother knew about him. I gave him two children like that: when I had the first child, he started helping out, but nine months later, he stopped supporting me. He said that the child wasn't his. I told him that I wouldn't see him anymore. So he told my mother that if I don't see him anymore, this must mean that the child truly isn't his. And after he promised he would help raise his child, I consented to becoming pregnant with his second child.

When I became pregnant with the second child, he beat me even though I didn't do anything. So he just up and left. Remember I had two children. For them to survive I had to work in the factory. I worked hard, but I didn't earn much money. I worked in the factory for 210–220 "Haitian dollars" [1,050–1,100 goud, around $70 at the time] per month, and I had two kids. While working in the factory I found someone who loved me, and he told me he'd help me out and pay for my home. While I was with him I became pregnant with his [my third] child. He said he didn't want a child . . . and I had the child, and this person too said that it wasn't his. . . .

What's more, what destroys me is now I have three children, and I have no one to help me out. I don't have any other job. So I am forced to work in one factory today, tomorrow in another factory, because I know I am never going to make money. All I know is sewing. I work but I can't even open a savings account, because I never have anything left over in my hands. I can't get a better job because I only made it to middle school.

I cite Simone here at length because her story brings the question of gender to the fore. Simone was particularly at risk because gender operates alongside violence, extreme poverty, and inequality to intensify vulnerability to various forms of violence. Dry-eyed and matter-of-fact, Simone held her head up high as she retold her istwa in the volunteer school her women's organization runs. Exceptionally brave and articulate, Simone is like many other very poor women in a resource-starved, foreign-occupied, deliberately underdeveloped, class-divided, male-dominated society like Haiti.

An expression in Haiti declares women to be *poto mitan*, a term literally translated as "center posts," referring to traditional religious spaces (N'Zengou-Tayo 1998). As pillars of society, women bear the brunt of both the episodic and structural violence, in Haiti as in the vast majority of countries. As Faye Harrison (1997) and others have argued, structural violence is gendered. Neoliberal globalization increases burdens on women in several ways. Women are often targeted for low-wage work (Chatterjee 2008; Cravey 1998; Enloe 2000)—in part because of patriarchal norms and the ideology that sees women as more submissive (Benería and Feldman 1992; Churchill 2004; Mills 2003), because women's traditional caregiving role precludes organizing trade unions (Hewamanne 2006; Kim 1997; Mendez 2002), or because of recitations of older gender ideologies of "nimble fingers" that seek to explain why women are particularly well suited to textile factories (Gunewardena 2008; Nash and Fernández-Kelly 1983; Tiano 1994). Transnational feminists argued that while it was problematic, with implicit male biases (Brown 1992; MacKinnon 1989), the social welfare state provided a modicum of legal protection and social services that benefited women and other marginalized populations (Antrobus 2004; Mohanty 2003). The shift toward a neoliberal model erodes these protections, especially through structural adjustment programs (Bergeron 2001; Lind 2000; Moghadam 2005). The privatization of public services, placing greater burden for social reproduction onto individual families, is more greatly felt by women because of their traditional role as family caregivers (Ellis 2003; Gladwin 1991).

In Haiti, gender inequality is grafted onto economic inequality and desperation, an example of what scholars have termed the "feminization of poverty" (Brenner 2000; McLanahan et al. 1989). Marie-Josslyn Lassègue, founder of the feminist NGO Fanm Yo La and minister of women's condition and rights at the time of our 2007 interview, underscored this analysis: "There is also a feminization of unemployment: most unemployed are women. Many people live in poverty, and most of them are women." Edele, a self-described "humanist-feminist activist" who works at Fanm Tèt Ansanm, theorizes women's condition in this vein, saying that women are "double victims." She argues, "There is no justice in the country. The justice apparatus does not work for anyone in the country. A poor woman becomes poorer: women always pay more. I mean, everyone is a victim. Therefore, women are double victims of the situation."

"Women's Life Is Not Pretty": A Life of Inequality

"Women's life is not pretty," began Elizabeth, a leader with Fanm Tèt Ansanm. As the passage from Danticat quoted above reminds us, gender inequality begins at birth. The following section is organized around a life cycle of how gender is made manifest. Edele began her istwa highlighting her own radicalism, her rebellion against gender norms: "There are games for girls and games for boys. The games for boys were active, physical, sports to be done outside. But for girls, the games we were supposed to play kept us inside and taught us to be subservient, to be nurturing." I witnessed a similar phenomenon in my own neighborhood. When I would arrive home from one or the other of the NGO offices, if it wasn't raining and if there wasn't too much violence during the day, I would usually pass a pickup game of soccer on the steep, potholed street. Only one young woman ever played (and even her appearance was rare). Where were the girls? Inside houses that had cement roofs, or (as was the case in my largely middle-class neighborhood) between structures in the bit of space reserved for drying clothes in the heat of the Caribbean sun and the tropical winds. During Lent, children have a tradition of flying kites, mostly handmade with paper scraps or plastic shopping bags. A couple of people explained this to me as a hopeful sign, children raising their hopes and spirits to the sky, to fly free. But this freedom is not universally shared. One time, a neighbor boy's kite string was snagged on the clothesline. Rather than untangle it himself, his younger sister, who was hanging the wash, untangled it for him while continuing to hang up the clothes. This neighbor girl learned at an early age that her place was at home, doing work, so that her brother could play.[40]

A concrete manifestation of this inequality in treatment between boys and girls is unequal access to formal schooling. In turn, this educational discrimination shapes other types of discrimination later in a woman's life. In Haiti, 29 percent of women aged fifteen to forty-nine have not had any formal education, compared to 15 percent of men (Cayemittes et al. 2001:15). The latest reported statistic shows that this inequality is growing, with girls not matriculating at the same rate as boys: girls and women constitute about 40 percent of sixth graders, 33 percent of *philo* (seniors), and 10 percent of science students at the public university (Anglade 1995:62, 68). A report for USAID estimates that only 20 percent of the students finishing high school are young women (Adams et al. 1998:1). Danielle, a peasants' organization leader and recipient of Sove Lavi services, who is also a single mother, explains the difficulties of sending her children to school: "When school begins again, I don't know how, with what means, my children are going to school. I don't sleep at night. I am their mother. I am their father. With what money can I take care of my children? If I don't get my act together, I will become a bad influence on my daughter. It is all up to me, alone, to do all I can to send her to school."

While the Haitian Constitution (in section 32) declares education to be a basic human right, daily practice falls short, with an estimated five hundred thousand children without access to basic education, and only 35 percent of children finishing fifth grade (Interim Government of Haiti 2004:33). Danielle's preoccupation with education derives from the fact that education is not free. In fact, it is her largest expense. In Pòtoprens, to send a child to school costs at the very least a quarter of a factory worker's salary, and these are *lekòl bòlèt*—literally "lottery schools," in other words, take your chances. The high cost of education—combined with poverty and income inequality—exacerbates gender inequality. If parents can afford to send only one child to school because of the expense, this poverty pressures an already-unequal gender ideology, and only the boy is sent to school (Adams et al. 1998:3). As the factory worker and Fanm Tèt Ansanm leader Marquise underscores, "Poverty is linked with discrimination because if the parents have girls and boys, they push the boys farther in school than the girls. My mother and father had eight children. And when I got to third grade my father said that he couldn't pay for me to continue in school. Instead I had to work to help raise the others, so they could go to school" (also quoted in Bergan and Schuller 2009).

This educational discrimination in turn shapes access to jobs, which spells economic discrimination against women. Women contribute 70 percent of the national economy but receive only 38 percent of the goods (MCFDF 2004). Women's participation in the economy, mostly as micro-entrepreneurs, is comparatively high, with 54 percent of women active in the marketplace, as compared to the "less developed country" average (23 percent) and the "developed country" average (27 percent) (United Nations Comité Inter-agences Femmes et Développment and Anglade 1992).[41] However, as in other export-processing zones such as the maquiladoras in Mexico (Churchill 2004; Collins 2003), women are overrepresented in low-paying factory jobs, constituting between 70 and 80 percent of the frontline workers. According to a director at the Ministry of Social Affairs and Labor, interviewed in April 2005, close to the same percentage of supervisory positions are held by men. Minister Lassègue had the following analysis: "Women know that they are in an unemployed country. So she does everything she can to keep her job. If she loses it, many people can replace her. However, when decisions are made they take men as supervisors."

Gender inequality shapes, and is structured by, economic exploitation, as women workers are seen as more docile, and therefore easier to control, than their male counterparts (Sassen 1998). Even within the same strata of workers, Haitian women earn less than their male counterparts, as the NGO educator Jacqueline explains: "You do the same work as the men. The man does not have the right to get paid more than you. You see? And you make people aware that it's a question of sex." This inequality could be a holdover from traditional male "breadwinner" ideologies in Haiti's peasant economy, as Danielle's expression "I am the father, I am the mother" underscores. In the agricultural sector, women are paid 60 to 75 percent of men's salaries (Anglade 1995:82). This is generally true across the economy, as Minister Lassègue reports: "In the banks, you can see that all the frontline service workers are women. And you go to a higher level and the majority of them are men. You look in the hospital, and it's the same thing. You look at the nurses, they're women, and the doctors, they're men."

As prefigured by the gendering of games and social roles in childhood, work is also gender segregated. Women are overrepresented in the lowest-paid informal sector (77 percent of the total workforce) while vastly underrepresented in the professional private sector (11 percent) and public sector (4 percent) (Anglade 1995:80). The bulk of informal sector jobs are as timachann. This association of women with small commerce is so powerful that USAID counts all micro-credit programs as assistance to women, according to a 2004 interview with a USAID program director. The most expensive items on the street, however, such as auto parts or electronics, are sold by men.[42] Domestic labor, centering on reproduction, is traditionally seen as "women's work" (Lamphere 1993; Sacks 1975; Strathern 1985). This traditional equation of women with reproduction reinforces the role of women as the poto mitan of the family.

Given women's traditional role in the household, women formally employed as wage laborers work a "second shift" at home (Hochschild 1989), as the laid-off factory worker Elizabeth argues: "Who does the paid work? Who does the housework, huh? We women, we are everything. It's true, men have their role, but women play the bigger role. Long ago men used to pay for the children's school, but now it's on women's shoulders. Women pay the consequence." This is exacerbated by the feminization of the export-processing sector, where women are disproportionally working in low-paying wage-labor jobs, as Monique tells:

> Whoo. My workday? I get up at 4:00, 4:30 or so. I get water because I don't have a faucet where I live. I use the water to clean house and cook for my children. I finish the work in the house before I come here (to the office), and now I work here all day. Then I go home and buy what food I need, I cook, I clean, and I get the kids to bed, and then it's very, very dark. Women work more than men. It's unjust, but this is how the country functions. It was custom in the country.

This second-shift phenomenon is also exacerbated by the fact that many women are heads of household, "the mother and the father" (Clarke 1957). According to a presentation by the Ministry of Women's Condition and Rights, 59 percent of Pòtoprens households are headed by single women (see also Cayemittes et al. 2001). There are many reasons for this, among them the cultural importance of maternity and the unfortunately widespread cultural practice of *san papa*—unknown or unrecognized paternity (Maternowska 2006). Men are also more likely to migrate out of Haiti for seasonal labor, especially to the Dominican Republic in the *batèy* (sugarcane plantations) (Simmons 2010). This in part explains why women would endure more difficult work on the factory line.

Some women, like Monique's coworker Martha, understand this second-shift situation to be aggravated by the contemporary economic crisis. Martha's husband "does a little work around the house," but "since the crisis in the country, he can't find work. He goes looking for work, but no one has any jobs to give him." Martha's husband became an auto mechanic, a relatively well-paying and high-status job for a man with no formal education. But as a job in the informal sector, it is vulnerable to vast fluctuation. According to Martha, the result is that "I alone provide for our house. Our whole family. And I do most of the work in the house." Martha, like many poor people, was diabetic,[43] and had a limited health care budget. In December 2005 she became blind and unable to travel the slippery, potholed, trash-strewn streets of Pòtoprens to get to work. She died between two of my visits, sometime in late 2008.

Intersectionality

These women's stories challenge simplistic, either/or understandings of race, gender, class, or nationality. None of these systems of inequality is foundational; gender is simultaneously operating with inequalities within both the world system and Haiti itself. This complex situation demands an "intersectional" analysis that understands how these social constructs are interrelated (Chinchilla 1992; Collins 2000; Crenshaw 2001; Davis 1983). These women's own intersectional analyses—without using this terminology—complicate their identification with "feminism," understood by many sectors as middle class, foreign, and—given that "feminists" are all members of the NGO class and therefore recipients of foreign aid—even imperialist (Davis 2003; Nagar 2006). Most women who do not identify as feminist are either critical of foreign imperialism or they prioritize working-class issues. Mme Laurent, an NGO staff person, identifies herself as a feminist, albeit conditionally: "I am a feminist, [but] the principal problem I pose before women's rights (or men's), is what rights do the poor majority [pèp la] have?" Mme Laurent argued that radical economic changes are needed to begin to address women's conditions, particularly given the extreme structural violence discussed earlier in this chapter: "First, you need to start improving the people's economic conditions. Only then can women find a situation to improve her conditions: equal work, equal pay. When there is work, she can demand her rights, things like this. But today, she can't even do that because there's no work." For these and other reasons, Mme Laurent and others are critical of self-described feminist organizations, which tend to attract a middle-class constituency and focus primarily on formal political rights; these skeptical women work instead for "women's organizations," those with a broader agenda that implicitly acknowledges the intersectionality of multiple forms of inequality shaping Haitian women's conditions (Coomaraswamy 2002; Corcoran-Nantes 2000; Hrycak 2002).

    Why do the NGO staff and volunteer leaders recoil at the self-definition of feminist? Unlike suburban college undergraduates who support feminism's major tenets but harbor negative stereotypes resulting from a successful cultural backlash (Faludi 1991), women in Haiti—particularly those from the poor majority—have other, more fundamental critiques. As both women of color in the United States and "third world feminists" have argued, the term "feminist" presupposes and reinforces a single, universal sign of "woman" that is culturally, historically, and sociologically contingent, privileging and universalizing the experiences of white, middle-class, "Western" women. Radical Chicana feminists such as Chela Sandoval, Cherrie Moraga, and Gloria Anzaldúa often found themselves in the place of translating their experiences in a struggle over authenticity (Sandoval 2000; Moraga and Anzaldúa 1983). Universalizing middle-class white women's experiences reverses the locus of oppression for Black women: whereas for a middle-class white woman of the second wave of feminism, work was liberation because home was where she faced oppression, Black women always had to work (in the fields, as nannies, and in the factories), so home was the only place for respite (Collins 2000; Young 1997). Further, Angela Davis (1983) argued that white feminists actively contribute to the negative stereotypes of Black men. Valerie Smith (1990) wrote about the problem of "split affinities" wherein women of color are often forced to choose between allegiance to white feminists and Black men. Mme Laurent voiced this critique for many women of Haiti's pèp la, forced to choose between sisterhood with middle-class women and solidarity with their husbands, fathers, and sons and their class. The mobilization against Aristide included self-named feminist organizations in visible places; they compete with college student activists over which group first called for Aristide's ouster.

This politics of representation is magnified in a transnational, neocolonial context. As Gayatri Spivak (1988) asked, who has the authority to speak for marginalized people, or can they speak for themselves? Other third world feminists, like Chandra Mohanty (1988), have critiqued "Western" feminism as missing the important context of colonialism and imperialism, and therefore not being useful for women in the global South in their multiple struggles. Others have critiqued Western feminism's privileging of liberal, individual civil liberties over collective rights (Coomaraswamy 2002; Jolly 1996). Still others are skeptical about the strategic use of feminism as justification for imperialist intervention (Afary 1997; Jayawardena 1994), exemplified by "Western" outrage over "the veil" as prelude to the U.S. invasion of Afghanistan. This concern of feminism privileging a Western Enlightenment worldview and liberalism being imperialist is underscored by the funding of feminist groups. In Haiti, all the self-described feminist organizations accepted official bilateral aid, mostly from Canada and France but even from the United States. All of them were vocal members of Aristide's opposition, one of them a member of the Group of 184.

Despite the differences in opinion over feminism, women's organizations have a long history of engagement in Haiti. In 1820, Haitian women reversed women's status as minors under their husband's custody, a holdover from French colonial rule (Racine 1995:8). The women's movement advocating for this change predated Seneca Falls by a generation. In 1934, just before U.S. troops pulled out from their nineteen-year occupation, a group of professional women founded Haiti's first formal women's organization, the Ligue Féminine d'Action Sociale, who publicly protested the occupation and played a role in the troops' eventual departure (Charles 1995; N'Zengou-Tayo 1998; Racine 1995). Women played visible leadership roles in the democratic movement in the 1980s, including in the November 1985 protest that sparked Duvalier's eventual downfall. Shortly after his departure, on April 3, 1986, a group of thirty thousand women marched in the streets of Pòtoprens, among the largest demonstrations of the period. As scholars (e.g., Benoit 1995; Charles 1995; Racine 1995) have argued, women's popular organizations—organizing working-class women, peasants, and timachann—have had a dual focus on citizenship, democratization, and economic transformation on the one hand, and on women's participation in civic life, representation, and change in traditional cultural roles and stereotypes on the other. Women played such a central role in the popular movement that Aristide launched his campaign in a gendered space—the Mache Solomon, an open-air market in a low-income Pòtoprens neighborhood (Racine 1995:11)—and many political parties formed women's groups to attract women to their cause (Benoit 1995:27). Also owing to their centrality, women increasingly became the targets for gendered violence, particularly during the 1991–1994 coup d'état, as Simone's istwa highlights (Bell 2001; Racine 1999).

This divergence in feminist understandings of women's NGOs has encouraged several classificatory schema aimed at understanding the vast array of these NGOs and the gender paradigm structuring their practice and funding. Esther Boserup (1970) triggered a sustained critical discourse on gender following a popular critique of mainstream development. A second wave of feminism in the North successfully brought about Women in Development (WID), specifically targeting women for development programs and demanding gender-disaggregated data. Transnational feminists and networks, including Caribbean leaders such as Peggy Antrobus, critiqued WID as representing just an "add women and stir" approach (Antrobus 2004; Moghadam 2005; Mohanty 2003) while gender inequality remains unchallenged. Maxine Molyneux (1985) and others argued that women's "strategic gender interests" needed to be addressed in addition to their "practical" interests. These feminist organizations argued that development interventions should specifically address gender as a category of analysis and system of inequality, leading to a Gender and Development approach.

HIV/AIDS

With all the istwa giving us an intersectional analysis to understand how long-term gender inequalities interact with structural violence, global and local systems of exclusion, as well as income inequality and poverty, we can begin to see how HIV/AIDS has also become feminized (Farmer et al. 1996; Susser 2009). In the early 1990s, men infected with the virus outnumbered women five to two, but in 2004 there were equal numbers of men and women living with HIV (UNAIDS 2007). Why is that? All of these are related: violence, coups d'état, inequality, poverty, underdevelopment, and gender (Farmer 1992; Farmer et al. 1996). The Sove Lavi volunteer Gabrielle explains:

> Okay. My life story. My father died when I was eight years old. He left six children in my mother's hands. My mother couldn't meet the needs of all of us children on her own, because she didn't have enough money. My family members who lived andeyò couldn't make ends meet by working the land. We couldn't feed our children or make a living.
>
> So the children split up. Four went to Pòtoprens to look for a job (chèche lavi). My mother left. I came to Pòtoprens when I was seventeen, eighteen years old. I came looking for work. I found a job to care for my family because my mother was becoming old. My father tried to send his children to school, and he was almost there before he died, but we couldn't.
>
> Now, when I came here, I worked. Because my level of education wasn't really, you understand, very high, I had few options. All the same, I worked with all my kindness, with everything I knew, and gave it to my work.
>
> When I turned twenty-four, I became pregnant. I was still looking for someone who could help me out because I always felt I was by myself. I always felt isolated. My mother's health, how can I say this? I had to find someone who could help me, to help with her medical care. Do you understand? So I became pregnant. So I went to see a doctor. In the center, I went to the doctor, and when I got there, they told me they were going to give me a test.
>
> And I finished taking the test, but I never found out the results. But after I gave birth—I had a Caesarian section because I was having difficulty—and then afterward, when the child was a month old, I went to the doctor with him. But this time, I also asked for the results of the tests they gave me. They told me, you are positive.

Like Simone's istwa, Gabrielle details the multiple axes of inequality and oppression, how gender intersects with poverty, class, and Haiti's lack of resources. The intersectionality of oppression, the gendered structural violence, in turn contribute to vulnerability to violence and contracting HIV/AIDS, underlining the importance of the work of both NGOs profiled in this book. These and other women's NGOs are attempting to address these multiple inequalities that contribute to the spread of HIV/AIDS. How they do so, and how successful they are, is the subject of the rest of this book.

As noted in the introduction, Gabrielle is now dead, even as Haiti made significant progress against HIV/AIDS. Why this is—and how to prevent such deaths from happening to others—will be answered in the chapters that follow. To begin, we need to understand the NGOs themselves and the relationships they build with people "on the ground," the focus of the next chapter.

2

"That's Not Participation!"

Relationships from "Below"

To me, what Sove Lavi does can't be participation. For frank participation, we would need to have common interests.

—Maxime, community leader for Sove Lavi

Sunday, June 27, 2004, 7:39 P.M.
We finally reached our summit, this little town, high enough in the mountains to have a forest of pine among the more tropical mango trees. A church service just let out. About forty or so people were already waiting, milling about. It was chilly by Haitian standards, with several peasant leaders wearing torn hand-me-down sweaters. We were over an hour late from of the official start time for the event.

Across the dirt road from the church, completely dwarfed by it, was the national school, four cinderblock rooms with a tin roof. The team planned for many people, so we had to get the benches from both the school and the church and set them outside. Of course, the first thing that had to happen was hang up two big signs, one of which read "Welcome Sove Lavi," which the NGO had on their Kanaval (Carnival) stand. The other one was quite striking, reading "Sove Lavi is involved in the struggle against AIDS. And you?" It felt accusatory. I was so moved by it that I snapped a photo, much to the delight of Lolo, a journalist contractor for Sove Lavi who publicly harbors ambitions to be president of Haiti.

With many strong hands present and already waiting, getting the wooden school/church benches arranged was not such a big deal, except that there were too many chiefs trying to direct. Notably, all the staff were sitting down, barking orders, one from inside an air-conditioned SUV. I was happy to just lift and put things down where I was told, but the peasant leaders kept deferring to me, calling me *dirèkte* (director).

It took about twenty minutes to set everything up. After that, it took a while for people who had waited for us to actually arrive to show up. The meeting was outdoors, at least until the rain started. The benches were arranged in a semicircle, and there was a hill that made a natural amphitheater. Everyone could see the action.

The seats became full. I would guess that more than two hundred people attended, both men and women. That was actually a very good sign. The *rasanblaman* (meeting) began with a song, "Rasanble," featuring the lyrics, "We're waiting for you. Sit down. Assemble. Assemble." Then another song about the struggle, featuring lyrics like "We're working to save our community." There was a brief scuffle between the guy who led the song and a woman who scolded that he was making this too complicated; according to her, all that extra text should be taken out, as this group is only about AIDS.

Then, of course, a prayer.

After this, all the participating CACs (Community Action Councils) had to be introduced, one by one. That took a long time. I was a little surprised at how old some of the people were, many in their fifties. I thought Sove Lavi worked with "youth." Lolo had to get everything just right—he was videotaping the event—so he would occasionally stop the event to physically move people. Then of course we—minus Lolo—had to get up and present ourselves. After the round of introductions (forty-five minutes into the event), Mme Auguste gave a little speech, thanking the CAC leaders who made this possible. Her speech focused on knowledge: it's important that we pass along the knowledge of AIDS to prevent the disease from spreading.

Then the majority of the forty-five remaining minutes featured a very animated man talking about AIDS, HIV, how it's contracted, and how to prevent it. I was impressed with the detail and depth of his knowledge. The Q-and-A period began with this one guy asking how else the disease is spread. A couple of questions came from the point of view that AIDS is an idea to discourage young men and women from having any sex at all, that it's a politics of control. They made a play on the French acronym of SIDA, calling it Syndrôme Inventée pour Descouragée les Adultes/Adolescentes ("Invented Illness to Discourage Adults/ Adolescents" from having sex or having fun). One question was completely ignored, from a man who wanted to know about the difference between coital and oral sex. The audience erupted in laughter and the CAC people were insulted. They didn't know the answer to that question because Sove Lavi didn't tell them, since it's not from the USAID handbook.

Then it started to rain so we moved into the church, hurriedly hauling the benches inside. The group was incontrollable at this point. Several people got up and left when the rain started. It was getting late, and already the meeting cut into lunchtime.

One more time, the song "Rasanble" was trotted out, though it took a while for it to get going. The song was a wall of sound; it was loud in the church hall with the tin roofs and polished concrete floor both amplifying sound.

The big highlight of the meeting was that one of the CAC women demonstrated how to put on a condom. They presented a brown wooden penis, on the larger end of the spectrum. When it was pulled out, people tittered uncontrollably. Interestingly, people also laughed at the slang phrase *fè bagay* (do it). One of the older women corrected them with the phrase meaning "make love," saying love is love, after all, and sex is sex. Someone asked whether all this about AIDS was just *politik* (politics) that U.S. condom manufacturers are inventing to make money. The CAC people didn't, couldn't, or refused to answer right away, so Mme Auguste had to get up on stage to answer it. In the meantime, this person berated the group: "People can't answer this? Hmph!" But it was an interesting question, saying a lot about how people experience this kind of news. Then this same man asked a specific question to Mme Auguste about her salary and about how much money Sove Lavi has.

Untangling Local Meanings

There are many ways to read this—unedited—entry in my fieldnotes, my first "mission" to the provinces with Sove Lavi. It is reprinted as written, fighting the lack of light and electricity, capturing the jumble, the cacophony, the multiple activities and agendas. It is also before I had the chance to interview people formally to learn their interpretation of events, and before I had the chance to become accustomed to a different pace. It is eminently possible that the questions were akin to Clifford Geertz's (1973) "burlesque" winks, poking fun at the CAC leaders, what James C. Scott (1990) called "hidden transcripts." There is a rich tradition of tricksters in Caribbean folklore, particularly in rural culture, embodied in Haiti as Ti Malice.

All this said, this snapshot of an HIV/AIDS training in a remote province highlights many issues to consider in the fight against the disease. This training was used as a model of successful participation given its high turnout. Lolo's pictures in the report certainly helped, showing full benches in a remote location; some found their way to donors' websites. However, regardless of whether or not the unresponded-to questions were sincere, they expose tensions in the relationship between Sove Lavi and the community that undermine the education effort (see also Robins 2009). This story underscores the critical need for a grounded theory that deconstructs simplistic understandings of participation. How is participation defined? How is it measured? How is it understood by different actors?

Any simplistic notion of participation misses important questions and realities, and also the relationships engendered by NGO projects. The training session described above was officially declared a success because of its high turnout, which was a result of local leaders' participation; however, the training nonetheless reveals tensions and local understandings that will sabotage prevention efforts if unaddressed. Clearly with the prevalence of HIV halved over the previous decade, some of what is being done is working. But much is not, and we don't know which is which. Despite the advances made against the disease, Gabrielle died. What explains this mystery? For clues we need an up-close ethnographic look at the NGOs entrusted with the millions of dollars in HIV/AIDS funding.

This book compares two such women's NGOs, Sove Lavi (Kreyòl for "saving lives") and Fanm Tèt Ansanm (women united, literally "heads together"). Given the powerful structural forces of gender discrimination, extreme poverty and inequality, a coup d'état, and neoliberal globalization, the two NGOs nonetheless have different institutional responses. The differences are most clearly seen in the aid recipients' "participation" within the NGOs. Fanm Tèt Ansanm provided space for relatively high levels of recipients' involvement in execution, discussion, planning, and even program design and priority setting, whereas participation at Sove Lavi, when it occurred at all, was primarily limited to minute implementation details. NGOs—like all other people or social groupings—have idiosyncratic histories and biographies (Fisher 1997; Hilhorst 2003; Mosse and Lewis 2006), demanding what the anthropologists Steven Sampson and Julie Hemment (2001) called "NGO-graphy" to uncover them. This chapter provides these histories—the *istwa*—of the two NGOs, critiquing ideological notions of participation with an approach grounded in relationships, what I call "civic infrastructure."

The Two NGOs' Istwa

Fanm Tèt Ansanm

Fanm Tèt Ansanm began as an initiative of the U.S. government in 1985 as part of the Caribbean Basin Initiative to build offshore apparel factories in the period leading up to Duvalier's ouster. It began as a series of two adult education courses in human development and health aimed at empowering women factory workers. Gradually, different programs were added because of workers' advocacy and suggestions made during their evaluation of training programs. For example, the women asked for courses in rights and literacy, so these were added. Early on, the factory workers asked for a clinic. Leonie, who was among the first workers to attend Fanm Tèt Ansanm training programs and who now works for them as a "motivator," recalls, "The workers asked, since Fanm Tèt Ansanm provided us with health education, and we learned how to take our health in our hands, we need a clinic for us to have consultations. And later, we also needed materials, like family planning." Gradually, in this fashion, Fanm Tèt Ansanm's array of services grew. After the women finished all the trainings, they asked for still more to participate in. Coming out of their discussions of common problems in training sessions, they wanted to have a more structured forum for this kind of *tèt ansanm* (literally "heads together," in this context meaning brainstorming or solution-oriented group meetings). The Women's Vigilance Committee (later Women's Committee) was born.

According to Mme Dominique, Fanm Tèt Ansanm's director, the organization was among the first in Haiti working on HIV/AIDS prevention, "before it became à la mode." This, combined with their long years of service in the same location with the same general population, made Fanm Tèt Ansanm a favorable target for larger streams of HIV/AIDS funding, including the Global Fund to Fight AIDS, Tuberculosis, and Malaria (hereafter the Global Fund). In addition to the program training and mobilizing a network of public health volunteers, Fanm Tèt Ansanm began a program of peer educators to disseminate information and materials about HIV/AIDS prevention to their coworkers, churches, and neighborhoods.

Fanm Tèt Ansanm targeted women factory workers from the industrial park surrounding Haiti's international airport. The industrial park was built in the late 1970s as the centerpiece to Jean-Claude Duvalier's "economic revolution," comprising export-processing zones financed by World Bank and IDB loans, bilateral grants, and some foreign direct investment. Surrounding SONAPI (Société Nationale des Parcs Industriels, or National Society of Industrial Parks)—the Haitian government–owned and –managed industrial park—are privately owned buildings haphazardly built at different times. The export-processing zone stretches several kilometers, from the international airport to Lasalin (La Saline), a very low-income *bidonvil* (shantytown) that is the gateway to Haiti's northern provinces as well as to Sitesolèy, Haiti's largest and most violent bidonvil. During its peak in the 1980s, the export-processing industry in Haiti employed seventy thousand workers (Ferguson 1987:83; Hachette 1981:23). The major industry is offshore export processing for textiles in which local/international subcontractors produce shirts, jeans, underwear, or clothing accessories for U.S.-based corporations such as Levi Strauss, Disney, and Sara Lee (makers of Hanes). Haiti was an early recipient of the aforementioned Caribbean Basin Initiative, providing free-trade incentives to increase the region's "competitiveness" by exploiting its "comparative advantage" (proximity to the United States and low wages). In an October 2003 conversation, a U.S. citizen who owns an electronics factory lamented the fact that other businesses are no longer profitable since the United States lost its manufacturing base to cheaper labor markets such as the Pacific Rim (see also Enloe 2000; Sassen 1998; Wallerstein 2004).

SONAPI, and possibly the privately owned factories, was supposed to be on a power grid that received a full ten hours of electricity during the workday. At least during the period of my research (2003–2005), this rationing did not occur. As a result, factory owners economized electricity usage to the bare essentials on the shop floor, meaning the equipment and only sometimes lighting and almost never fans. Because Fanm Tèt Ansanm rents out a portion of a factory, the Fanm Tèt Ansanm office was also affected by the blackouts. Almost every day I visited the office, middle-and front-office staff were warned to save what they were working on before switching to inverter power. Most factories did not offer treated water for frontline workers to drink. Most workers told me of either nonexistent or inadequate toilet facilities, such as one toilet for several hundred workers on the floor, including both men and women (see figures 2.1 and 2.2). Until Fanm Tèt Ansanm opened one in November 2007, there was no medical clinic in SONAPI and few in the surrounding area. Fanm Tèt Ansanm's clinics were some of the few places where women could receive free medical care in the Pòtoprens area.

This is the general context in which Fanm Tèt Ansanm provided their services. According to criteria established by donors, Fanm Tèt Ansanm performed beyond expectations. For example, they promised to distribute 84,400 condoms in 2003, and they wound up distributing 103,956, according to annual reports to donors. In addition, 485 instead of 420 people completed voluntary AIDS testing. Instead of 5,950 people attending educational seminars on HIV/AIDS as promised, almost double that number attended: 10,129. In the clinic, 1,992 people were counseled on family planning methods between October 1, 2003, and September 30, 2004, one of their donors' fiscal years. Of these people, 239 people accepted condom usage, 59 people accepted Depo-Provera, and 65 people accepted some form of a birth control pill. These acceptance rates are high when compared to other family planning clinics in Haiti, like the Centres pour les Développement et de la Santé (CDS) in Sitesolèy (Maternowska 2006).[1] The generally low rates of acceptance are due in part to the high cultural value attached to motherhood (a pro-natal value system embodied by the phrase *poto mitan*), as well as long-standing Catholic beliefs about birth control. In addition to the organization's family planning services, 3,977 people had a consultation with one of Fanm Tèt Ansanm's doctors during the same period.

Fanm Tèt Ansanm existed in a very specific social milieu that was undergoing rapid change. As described in the previous chapter, the whole export-processing sector was declining. Among other consequences, for Fanm Tèt Ansanm there were fewer factory workers, the "target population" for its programs. Fanm Tèt Ansanm program director Edele explained, "[Our work] is more difficult. I mean, already there weren't enough jobs. Because there aren't enough jobs, workers are mobile. Sometimes they don't even have time to finish and pass trainings, because they already lost their job. This mobility makes reinforcing unions difficult. One moment you hear they were there, then you hear they aren't there anymore. They lost their job." By the time I began my fieldwork in November 2003, attendance had fallen for trainings and for the Women's Committee. Several Fanm Tèt Ansanm staff told me wistfully that in previous years, before the political crisis, all four meeting spaces were full of women

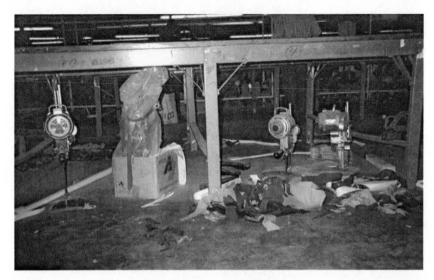

FIGURE 2.1 Garbage on the factory floor. Photo taken by factory worker, used with permission.

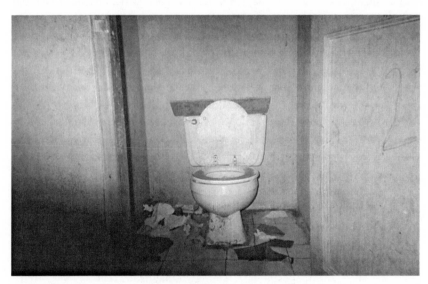

FIGURE 2.2 Toilet for several hundred line workers. Photo taken by worker, used with permission.

taking classes. During the period of my fieldwork (2003–2005), it was rare to see more than one training session concurrently operating; many days there was none.[2] Also owing to the instability in the sector, non- or former-factory workers began to play more visible roles in the organization, especially the clinic and

AIDS-prevention program. For this reason, I use the word that staff people used, *medanm* ("ladies," from the French "mesdames," plural of "madame") when referring to the general population of aid recipients.

Women have historically been, and were at the time of the research, the targets of Fanm Tèt Ansanm's intervention. In addition to this, gender as a category of analysis and intervention has consistently been operant: in the literacy training sessions I attended, women's life histories were used within feminist/Freirian consciousness-raising exercises, in which working-class women's specific problems—both as poor people and as women—were discussed. One in particular, written by a volunteer, discussed the difficulties of confronting sexual harassment on the job and an abusive common-law husband, on top of having to work both at home as an unpaid mother and at work to earn money for the family. Conversations moved from discussing individual "situations" to a shared "condition" as an oppressed group, a process C. Wright Mills (1959) called the "sociological imagination." The gender-equality ideology was typical of the Gender and Development paradigm within international development (discussed in the previous chapter) that addresses the gender roots of social inequality. Further, while not using the language of intersectionality as formulated by Collins (2000) or Crenshaw (1991), Fanm Tèt Ansanm's work targeted multiple inequalities as workers and women.

Around the same time that the factories were closing (and therefore fewer medanm were available to attend training), the newly created Global Fund selected Fanm Tèt Ansanm as a sub-recipient. The signature of AIDS became more pronounced, and Fanm Tèt Ansanm drifted away from other programs. Men became more visible, selected as volunteer trainers. In 2009, at the invitation of a donor agency, Fanm Tèt Ansanm went out of Pòtoprens—far outside the industrial park—to provide HIV/AIDS-prevention training to a small provincial town.

Sove Lavi

Sove Lavi began as a program within a branch of the United Nations in the late 1980s, during Haiti's tumultuous *dechoukaj* period following Duvalier's ouster and before the first democratic elections. Sove Lavi's first and longest-standing program, a network of Community Action Councils (CACs), was also based on one of Paulo Freire's (1985) suggestions. Sove Lavi assembled community leaders, mostly from peasants' organizations but also some rural women's organizations, and trained them to disseminate public health messages, the first concerning hygiene. According to Haitian NGO researchers, the Duvalier regime politicized CACs, using them to collect information and reward people who also served as informants (Gabaud 2000; Mathurin et al. 1989:47). Typical of the WID approach (described in the previous chapter) that specifically targets women in development projects, Sove Lavi practiced a form of *discrimination positive* (a French-language interpretation of "affirmative action") in which the majority of CAC members needed to be women.

Sove Lavi had one, and then two, drop-in centers in the provinces[3] where local youth could receive "counseling."[4] While I did not sit in on these conversations,[5] staff told me that they counseled youth on matters of sexuality, telling them about the dangers of AIDS and other sexually transmitted infections (STIs), early pregnancies, and how to avoid these unwanted outcomes. In one center, local youths also had access to an array of free cultural programming, such as dance, acting, drumming, and English classes. I would often hear youth showing off their English until I came into the room, when they quickly switched to Kreyòl, apparently embarrassed by my native ear. At this center and the main office, youths had access to the Internet so that they could visit the Sove Lavi website and participate in the online forums discussing similar topics.[6]

In addition to the drop-in centers, Sove Lavi managed two major AIDS education projects developed after 2003 with funds from the Global Fund and USAID. The first such project involved "distance learning" in schools. Sove Lavi developed a curriculum for middle schools concerning sexuality with a focus on AIDS, other STIs, and pregnancy prevention. In addition to workbooks, the curriculum had an audio component. Sove Lavi worked with community radio stations for two weekly broadcasts, once during school, when the teacher and students would follow along, and once out of school for parents to follow along with their children. Sove Lavi gave battery-powered radios to participating schools. Especially important for the remotest of areas, Sove Lavi gave tapes of the various lessons to the teachers. Complementing this student education was a parental education component run by Sove Lavi staff. Twice a year, at the beginning and at the end of the program, a team of Sove Lavi staff from Pòtoprens came to visit and evaluate the classrooms. This evaluation consisted of a twenty-one-question multiple-choice and true/false exam. A staff person in Pòtoprens tabulated and analyzed the results to submit to their donors as an evaluation of their outcomes.

When worldwide funds for HIV/AIDS prevention and treatment grew exponentially at the beginning of this century, Sove Lavi was a natural choice for this work because of their CAC model of health education. Almost overnight, beginning in January 2003, Sove Lavi grew from five staff in one office to thirty staff in four offices, a process that development agencies call "scaling up" (Edwards and Hulme 1992; Uvin 1996; Wils 1996).

Growing with their funding portfolio, Sove Lavi set out ambitious goals. Their most grandiose was a Caravan project, where staff would travel to remote communities along with a self-contained sound system to attract crowds to hear the message of HIV/AIDS prevention. Sove Lavi envisioned two to three thousand people attending each Caravan tour, forty-eight tours per year. In short, they had planned to spread the message of HIV/AIDS prevention to

96,000–144,000 people per year. Their desired "milestones" were that half the participants would promise to adopt a "responsible behavior" and practice the responsible behavior within three months. They also promised to donors that all their volunteer CAC members would collaborate with associations of people living with HIV, and half the CACs would include these HIV-positive associations as members. The results of Sove Lavi interventions have been mixed. With some milestones, for example that participants could correctly identify the major means of contraction and prevention of HIV, Sove Lavi met their goals: consistently over 90 percent of people scored 95 percent correct or better. In the case of most other measures, however, including the Caravan just mentioned, Sove Lavi often fell far short. The Caravan began eight quarters late, and only went on a handful of tours that garnered much lower attendance (fewer than a thousand per stop).

Like most NGOs in Haiti[7] Sove Lavi's central office was in Pòtoprens while their aid recipients were scattered throughout several geographic departments. This distance between NGO staff and aid recipients presented logistical challenges, rendering communication more difficult. While a few cyber cafes existed in the provinces, most were to be found in provincial cities. A pronounced digital divide added challenges, contrary to Thomas Freidman's (2005) understanding of the transformative power of technology and globalization. Very few people had access to the Internet long enough to keep an account current, to say nothing about using e-mail as a regular means of communication. For those with a little more means, cell phones became regularly available, especially since 2006 when Digicel opened operations in Haiti. Still, there were wide gaps in rural coverage, as cellular towers were concentrated in cities, especially Pòtoprens. The lack of electricity made it hard for rural leaders to receive calls,[8] since phones need to be charged almost daily. For these reasons, radio and *teledjòl* (literally, "television of the jaw," word of mouth) remained the central means for communication. Occasionally, Sove Lavi staff sent messages via local radio about upcoming CAC meetings and general community meetings. Most often, staff relied on face-to-face communication with CAC members.

Sove Lavi has a wide variety of target populations. It was difficult to glean exactly what Sove Lavi's beneficiary population was: I heard at least eight different answers. Some staff, including the director, defined Sove Lavi as a "women's organization," targeting women. But many staff, including people with several years of experience, disagreed. One attributed the shift to "youth" (which was occurring at the time of my research) to the changing of the guard at the White House: "With Clinton everything was about women: women's equality, and women's concerns. Now it seems, for Bush, AIDS is behind everything." Sove Lavi still preferred working with women, reserving a majority of CAC memberships for this group. Despite this, given traditional gender roles and ideologies, especially during discussions of intimate topics such as sexuality, men and adolescent males dominated Sove Lavi activities. In the two dozen community meetings and trainings I witnessed, only a handful of women spoke. This calls into question the efficacy of the WID, "add women and stir" approach (Antrobus 2004; Moghadam 2005; Mohanty 2003).

Relationships with the Community

As Jennie Marcelle Smith (2001) and others (e.g., Anglade 1974; Barthélémy 1990; Gabaud 2000) have powerfully demonstrated, woven into Haitian social life is a persistent tradition of *youn ede lòt* (people helping one another). Although the period following Aristide's ouster was marked by extreme violence and economic deterioration, many people, especially women, still engaged in this indigenous, grassroots tradition of civil society. I will cite two examples from both NGOs, highlighting the strength of relationships at the grassroots level.

Marie-Ange, a member of one of Sove Lavi's CACs, was in her late fifties, an achievement in a society with a life expectancy of fifty-three years at that time (Interim Government of Haiti 2004). She gave most of her life to serving others. As Marie-Ange explained, first she was a tireless and faithful mother (for the previous ten years a single mother, after she divorced her husband) for her ten children, sending them to school and saving up to buy a house for them in a rural section of Petyonvil, an uphill suburb of Pòtoprens. For the past twenty-two years, Marie-Ange was a community leader with a local NGO and peasants' association.[9] For fifteen years, she walked up and down three eight-thousand-feet mountain peaks to get to work teaching at a small, Catholic Church–run school. Because her efforts were focused on others, she lived modestly, and like many low-income peasants in Haiti, the daily struggle showed on her body. Eating copious amounts sugarcane like many people because it was relatively cheap and widely available, and having no medical care, she spoke her wry wisdom through missing teeth.

Because of her experience, Marie-Ange has been sought out by larger NGOs to act as their facilitator. During our interview, she showed me a piece of paper folded to pocket size that contained her notes about a project, complete with a detailed budget listing the price per pound of seed and the going rate in the locality for human and bovine labor power. Having assumed it was for her peasants' association, I asked her what she was going to plant. She laughed and told me that it was for a neighboring peasants' association. When I asked her why she did that, she did not understand the question. While it was possible that my Kreyòl was too Frenchified by living in the city and associating with NGO professionals, she mainly did not understand because, in her words, "That is what we do." Marie-Ange had the experience writing up projects, and she was literate, so she was obligated to help out and willingly did so. When Sove Lavi came to town looking for leaders, it was neither surprising that Sove Lavi found out about Marie-Ange nor that she volunteered. She recalled, "SL found out that because of my intelligence, they knew I couldn't stay inactive. So they called to invite me to join SL."

In recounting their istwa, some women talked about the need for togetherness. "Helping one another keeps us alive," began Giselle, a factory worker sewing shirts for a company contracting with a U.S. firm who became involved in Fanm Tèt Ansanm. "We are poor. You don't see that? When we help each other, we can survive." Giselle talked about her sòl, an organically organized, no-interest lending system among friends, neighbors, family members, or coworkers, popular all over the Caribbean. Most large expenses in Haiti, most importantly rent,[10] are paid either semiannually or annually. It is extremely difficult for a head of household, even if she has close ties with extended family in Pòtoprens, to come up with enough money to pay her landlord. A sòl was literally the difference between being homeless and having a place to live.

At the end of the two-week pay period, workers are usually paid cash in envelopes, with taxes already taken out, like social security and health insurance. Given Giselle's minimum wage of seventy goud a day (about $1.70 at the time of the interview), she made seven hundred goud per pay period, minus one hundred goud taken out by her employer. With this six hundred goud (about $15.00), Giselle had to buy food and necessary household goods like oil, soap, and laundry detergent. Since she lived in a bidonvil that had been built up during the 1980s with the wave of migration following Haiti's "stock market crash"—USAID's and Duvalier's destruction of the Haitian pig population (Diederich 1985; Farmer 1993; Smith 2001:29)—none of the houses was equipped with running water. She had to buy water, at four goud per gallon,[11] hauling three five-gallon buckets (one in each hand, one on her head) ten minutes up the narrow, slippery, often muddy stairs to her house. After just these necessities, and not even paying for school for her children,[12] Giselle typically had one hundred goud left. She would contribute this amount to her sòl, a pool of people (in Giselle's case, six coworkers). Come payday, everyone paid this same amount, with one person receiving it all to pay for things like rent, school uniforms, school registration fees, health care if someone should fall ill, or a burial if they waited too long. Every three and a half months, Giselle got seven hundred goud. Like many people, Giselle touche ann goud, depanse ann dola ("earned in goud but spent in dollars"; in other words, her expenses vastly outstripped her earnings). Without her sòl, Giselle would not be able to afford to send her children to school, or have her eight-by-eight cinder-block home. Beatrice, Giselle's friend whom she met at Fanm Tèt Ansanm, said, "The sòl saves Haiti!"

A member of Fanm Tèt Ansanm's network of public health volunteers and AIDS peer educators, Giselle was also an active member in her gwoupman katye (neighborhood association). Once a month, she cooked food for the meetings[13] where they sat down and had a tèt ansanm, discussing the problems in their lives and in their community. After everyone was fed, they went out and worked on a concrete solution: installing new PVC that someone managed to obtain so that their community tap would have more water and there would be fewer leaks, or cleaning up trash so that when the next rains come people would not have to walk or live in it. "This is what I am applying from my work at Fanm Tèt Ansanm," Luna, another volunteer member of Fanm Tèt Ansanm, said. "We are *poto mitan* in our neighborhoods. Anyone who has a problem in the area, they ask for us."

Institutional Differences

As Giselle's and Marie Ange's stories show, women in both groups were involved in their communities and invited to take positions of leadership. Despite similarities, a few institutional differences between the NGOs engendered distinctions in these relationships. Sove Lavi chose CAC members as community representatives following an elaborate process, whereas anyone could participate in Fanm Tèt Ansanm. This expresses and reproduces two different orientations to leadership: Fanm Tèt Ansanm "grows" leaders while Sove Lavi "harvests" them. Also owing to institutional differences, the two populations of aid recipients differed in social strata (*kouch sosyal*)—not quite classes in the Marxist sense (Jean 2002:19).[14]

First Contact

Sove Lavi followed an elaborate process for selecting CAC members. First, Sove Lavi staff organized a prescreening mission and met with local health and educational institutions that referred local leaders and groups. During the first meeting, Sove Lavi told local organizations about the process. Local groups selected nine candidates to form a "cellule," whom Sove Lavi staff screened at a public meeting. Candidates were given tests on their knowledge of HIV/AIDS and other community health concerns, their French reading ability, their comfort with public speaking, and their "respectability" in the community. In the screening I attended, this last point was assessed by asking audience members, presumably candidates' friends and family, whether the community holds these people in high esteem. Responses were nothing but positive, either because of this "stacking" or because of politeness in front of strangers (people used the term *etranje*—"foreigner"[15]—to refer to Pòtoprens staff, challenging NGO professionals' status as Haitian). On the way home to Pòtoprens, I asked about this; Sove Lavi took how many friends someone brought to a meeting as a proxy for their leadership abilities. The verb used was *simaye* (disseminate), not *pataje* (share) as in Fanm Tèt Ansanm, suggesting a difference in orientation toward the communities, with Sove Lavi sending information to passive recipients. After a two-and-a-half-hour process of cross-examination, Sove Lavi staff from Pòtoprens selected the five people to invite as CAC members.

By contrast, anyone was welcome to frequent the Fanm Tèt Ansanm center, attend special events, visit the clinic, take classes, or become a member of one of the two committees (the Women's Committee and the HIV/AIDS-Prevention Program peer educators). To join, the only requirement was to complete all necessary training programs. There were two primary modes of contact with Fanm Tèt Ansanm: referral from a current volunteer or "motivation" in the factories described below.[16] Most women I interviewed said that a friend or coworker referred them. Several people in turn told me that they had referred others to the NGO. At public celebrations, such as International Women's Day, Labor Day (May 1 outside the United States), International Day Against Violence Against Women, or World AIDS Day, all in attendance were invited to sign up for training sessions.

Another means of motivation was Leonie and coworkers going inside the industrial park. Workers are usually given a half-hour break from the line, so the pace was frenetic, with thousands of women and men descending on a row of a dozen *timachann* serving up food. Leonie and her coworkers were efficient, usually giving out the entire stack of journals, brochures, or other Fanm Tèt Ansanm materials they brought with them within minutes. Leonie shouted above the crowd noise, repeating phrases about coming to the clinic, or coming to the first day of a new class, until an individual sought her out. At this point, she stopped mid-sentence, called out *"cheri"* (dear), and carried on as personal conversation as possible under the circumstances.

Orientation: Setting Apart or Tying Together

This difference in selection also structures a difference in orientation. People who become committee members at Fanm Tèt Ansanm tend to be peers with their coworkers and neighbors. While they sometimes played specified roles at events, they received no other special treatment. Ritually reinforcing this unity as a community, most public events began and ended with one of four songs, each with a different message. "Rasanble" (Assemble) is the call for women to organize and put their heads together in unity. "Fanm yo, si n pa rele" (Women, if we do not speak up) talks about the importance of women having the courage to defend their rights. "Òganizasyon" (Organization) is about the importance of women being organized, in order to counteract the enormous tasks they face. And the message of "Piti, piti" (Bit by bit), is that we are gaining ground in our struggles for equality and justice, as women and as workers. After large public celebrations, staff handed out little plates of finger food and a cup of Couronne—a popular, syrupy sweet Haitian soft drink—to all present. Staff people viewed this as an important gesture, a ritual of status inversion whereby NGO professionals serve factory workers.[17] Over and over again, the message reinforced was tèt ansanm: unity, dialogue, and working together.

By contrast, Sove Lavi CAC members were treated much differently than ordinary community members. Most of Sove Lavi's activities were only with CAC members, ritually reinforced as "representatives" of the community. They were intermediaries, communicating back and forth between the community and Sove Lavi. Part of the reason for this was the geographical distance. In addition, Sove Lavi daily practice and organizational culture exacerbated this inequality. Instead of the horizontal, community relationship that Fanm Tèt Ansanm rituals reinforced, Sove Lavi ritual practice emphasized the distinction between CAC members and the communities.

An example of this division and vertical relationship occurred on December 1, World AIDS Day. Sove Lavi prepared a skit with youths at their drop-in center, in order to "motivate" surrounding communities, written and choreographed by a university-trained artist. Following a suggestion from the USAID health contractor CDS (Bernard and Desormeaux 1996), Sove Lavi made strategic use of local knowledge, including sexual slang and cultural metaphors such as Bawòn Samdi (in traditional religion, the spirit of death and guardian of the cemetery), to represent AIDS.[18] The skit, which emphasized condom usage (which later was amended by Sove Lavi staff to emphasize abstinence), was quite frank (see figure 2.3). The actors were mostly high school students, which in Haitian terms means that they were among the wealthiest 10 percent.[19] The group traveled by bus to a hamlet, incidentally the location of the first UN project in Haiti and home to their community liaison. After they finished putting on their outfits

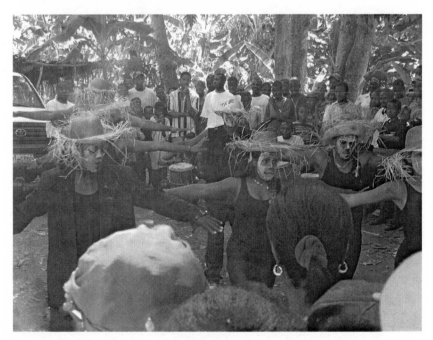

FIGURE 2.3 Sove Lavi educational forum. Photo by author.

and makeup, the group nervously waited for an hour and a half for the market to close. Finally, fed up and hungry, the Pòtoprens staff person in charge decided to go ahead during the market. The youth volunteers performed their skit well, attracting a small crowd. As in most countries, the market is a gendered space, frequented by women buyers and sellers, therefore only men could attend despite Sove Lavi's preference to work with women. After the skit, Sove Lavi had prepared an education forum for the community, complete with two people who were HIV positive to give testimony, a public health nurse they just hired, and a DJ with a very loud sound system.

No one came. The Pòtoprens staff left to return to the provincial center to get the boxed lunches for the youth volunteers, who were growing more irritable and playing with condoms like balloons. The community liaison retreated with the nurse to his house for lunch. I walked around town with Gabrielle, who was one of the two people with HIV Sove Lavi brought in to testify. She was visibly upset, telling me that she felt used, complaining about the lack of motivation done to bring people to the session. Incidentally, we stumbled on a group of local youth practicing a skit they wrote in a public school classroom that was also addressing social messages. They were not invited to participate by the "city kids" or Sove Lavi staff, who hadn't even noticed them. After what seemed like an awkward eternity to everyone, the Pòtoprens staff returned with lunch. I was given one but local youth and the would-be presenters like Gabrielle were not, as they were given a "per diem" that was supposed to include food.[20] I gave my lunch to the presenters to share, but hungry local youth had only chicken bones and whatever else was thrown away as the group dumped their trash in the schoolyard and left in their rented bus.

The message that recipient communities received from these and other practices was that direct beneficiaries of Sove Lavi are set apart from the local community. This puts a strain on local relationships, as Marie Ange explained: "[They say,] 'You're making money off of us! When you talk to us about these things, you will make money.' I explain to them, I don't take the training for money and I don't give it for money. When we ask them to sign, they don't want to. They always say, 'But yes! You will make money and when you make us write [our names], we won't get anything.'" Marie Ange is referring to an attendance sheet that Sove Lavi requires of participants after every event, an expression of what Michel Foucault (1991) called "governmentality," the conduct of conduct, including an obsession with recording official censuses of the population. This census taking may be considered expected and acceptable in "developed" countries whose citizens are accustomed to forms and surveys, but elsewhere this information gathering is often seen as a tool and expression of power. This local fear of the volunteers making money (albeit a volunteer stipend) is deepened by the history of the Duvaliers' collecting people's names in similar fashion to persecute them, using the same CAC model. This ritual act reinforced the differences between the well-paid staff and the beneficiary community. Despite the fact that CAC members were also neighbors, friends, relatives, and members of local churches or other organizations, this act marked CAC members as the chosen elect, along with the Pòtoprens staff. This was especially painful to CAC members because these preexisting relationships were central reasons Sove Lavi chose them in the first place. In chapter 4 I explain some of the roots of this practice.

NGO Class

As even casual observers note, Haiti is an incredibly inegalitarian society. In 2006 it was second to Namibia in income inequality in the world (Jadotte 2006). This inequality presents a barrier in relationships between NGOs and aid recipients. In Haiti there is a popular conception of a *klas ONG*, an NGO class, which is characterized as having certain privileges vis-à-vis the general population. Even chauffeurs are seen as having this privilege, as Fanm Tèt Ansanm's Jean-Baptiste explains, "I am working, and people say, 'Oh! You make money, you work in an NGO.'"

Danielle, a Sove Lavi CAC leader, had this critique: "The leaders [of NGOs] always want to direct an enterprise, a business." Gabrielle was much more critical. According to her, NGOs and foreign aid workers "take the illness [of AIDS] and turn it into a business. They let people die. Thanks to this illness, a lot of people have become bigwigs [*gran nèg*]. A lot of people become rich. Many people drive fancy cars, fancy motorcycles. Many people make a lot of money off the backs of people living with the illness. And many of us living with the illness, we continue to die." Gabrielle is admittedly frustrated, and some of her points may be overstated, but they were echoed by aid recipients from both Sove Lavi and even Fanm Tèt Ansanm. Julie, a volunteer leader at Fanm Tèt Ansanm, complained, "When [foreign donors] release some aid, they come for the bigwigs. They receive the aid. They drive the fancy cars. Yourself, a poor person, when they pass by they only give you a coating of dust. As long as the aid passes through the bigwigs, we poor will never see a cent." In a follow-up meeting in August 2006, CAC members pointed out the hypocrisy of their working for free while Sove Lavi staff are paid well. As I describe below, these differences between professional NGO staff and aid recipients color individuals' perceptions about NGOs, for example differing perceptions about recipients' participation. This is true of both Fanm Tèt Ansanm and Sove Lavi, given the pervasive inequality and social exclusion in the country.

In common usage, *klas* (class) is used in broad strokes, whereas the more fine-grained *kouch* distinguishes "poor" (*pòv*) from "miserable" (*malere*), for example. Given Haitian social organizational criteria, patterns can be seen in the two NGOs' service populations. For example, one of the requirements Sove Lavi imposed for CAC members was mastery of French, the language of the elite.

To speak French requires an education, which in turn requires a considerable portion of a family's income. The average cost of registration and tuition for the cheapest kind of Pòtoprens school, a lekòl bòlèt,[21] was between five and six thousand goud a year—four months' salary working minimum wage. To my knowledge, all but one CAC member—or their family, as most still lived in the traditional, extended family lakou system—owned a house or land.

Comparing the socioeconomic differences in the two populations, as well as the human resources invested in the membership, it can be said that while members of both are community leaders, Fanm Tèt Ansanm "grows" leaders while Sove Lavi "imports" them. Frontline staff person Georges illustrated this point when he said, "Sove Lavi does not create organizations. I mean, we find them in the field, we help them and we work with them." By contrast, Fanm Tèt Ansanm invested as much as two years of educational training in factory workers, many of whom were not literate in Kreyòl before their first visit. After this investment, Fanm Tèt Ansanm invited them to become Women's Committee members or AIDS peer educators. By contrast, Sove Lavi found people with high levels of educational, linguistic, and symbolic capital, including extensive local organizational experience.

Relationships with NGOs

While there are many ways to classify NGOs, one rubric distinguishes between service or membership organizations (e.g., Bebbington and Thiele 1993; Dicklitch 1998; Mathurin et al. 1989; Sen and Grown 1987). The relevant difference involves the relationships between the service population and the NGO: are the aid recipients "clients" or are they "members"? A general distinction concerns the orientation of the relationship: a client only receives services whereas a member is a part of the organization's constitution. Membership and service organizations also differ in the quality of participation, with members having some ownership of the processes by which the work is defined, while clients only participate in the actual delivery of the service (if at all).

Sove Lavi: Clients

Relationships between Sove Lavi and its service population were typical of client–patron arrangements. Sove Lavi practice or habitus (Bourdieu 1980) reproduced clientelism. For one clear example, Sove Lavi organized a three-day national conference bringing together the dual themes of violence against women and the feminization of AIDS, both described in the previous chapter. This was a major undertaking, coordinating more than thirty partner organizations and bringing together people from all over the country. There were more than forty speakers in two concurrent breakout sessions. Speakers included leaders within the interim Haitian government, the NGO sector, and several

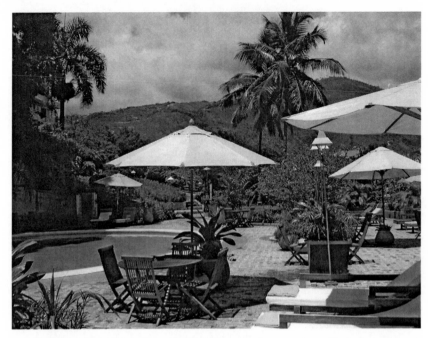

FIGURE 2.4 Hotel Montana, site of the Sove Lavi symposium. Photo by author.

international organizations, including the minister of public health, the minister of women's condition and rights, the UN resident coordinator, a representative from the Canadian development organization (ACDI), and the U.S. ambassador. The conference was well attended; in a press conference Mme Versailles, the director, reported that 350 people participated. In addition, the conference was well discussed; fifteen media outlets—print, radio, and even television—covered the event. Outside the sessions was an exposition where NGOs, community groups, and artists displayed their pictures, pamphlets, T-shirts, and artisanal items for sale.

The conference was held at the Hotel Montana, posh by even U.S. standards. Before it was destroyed by the earthquake in January 2010, the Montana sat atop a mountain, off the road to Petyonvil, featuring large lush terraces and clean swimming pools (see figure 2.4). To most people, especially coming from the provinces, the very space signified exclusion, which is why it was the site of a protest following the 2006 elections, because the poor majority wanted to send a message that their votes should count. Being in the modern, posh, air-conditioned Montana made many uncomfortable, including the Fanm Tèt Ansanm staff and aid recipients with whom I waited in line for the lunch buffet. While factory workers and peasant women patiently waited for their turn to get food, *gran manje* ("big eaters," the Kreyòl equivalent of "fat cats")—most of them men, all of them professional in their titles, their suits, and their use of French—moved to the front of the line and walked past us with their plates overfilled with food that sometimes fell to the floor. By the time our group got to the buffet line, there were only random slices of fruit left—about eight or nine pieces of mango, papaya, and watermelon for more than forty people. The Fanm Tèt Ansanm employee Rose, who also attended the conference, said she had asked the hotel wait staff about the food and was told they would check. Before we could get an answer, we were rushed to the next session, which started an hour late, because all but one of the aforementioned gran manje went over their allotted times to speak.[22] The end of the conference, designed for everyone to participate in the discussion of problems and solutions in workshops, was therefore cut short. The following day, the finale of the symposium, people presenting the summaries of breakout group conversations were set aside to make room for the U.S. ambassador, who had shown up on time and could not wait until his turn in the rotation. Sove Lavi's CAC members and other groups' clients were pushed aside a third time during the conference. At the conclusion of the presentations, during the showing of an educational video by a partner organization, I was pulled aside by Sove Lavi staff. Not wanting to be impolite (this was the first week I had spent with them), I followed the staff into a hotel bar that served as the locale of a reception for "VIPs." The serving tables were extravagantly filled with several non-Haitian dishes, hors d'oeuvres, meats, cheeses, and Haitian beans and rice. I was uncomfortable at the thought that people would be in the same predicament of the previous two days. But two different Sove Lavi staff people assured me that everyone would have enough to eat, that they had learned from the previous days' experience and were on top of things. And in truth, I was really hungry, depleted from the previous two days. So I ate.

After the reception was over, the curtains were opened, revealing a large line of people trying to get food. No additional plates of food were set. The lesson learned was not to have a more equitable distribution of food, but to put up the boundaries and make that privilege invisible, empowering those who are not HIV positive and who generally eat three meals a day to eat even more than they had the previous days. This goes a step beyond the privileging of CAC members discussed above; in this setting, these same CAC members and similar populations for other organizations were left behind. Many of the same people were left on the narrow, winding road down to Pòtoprens to fend for themselves to hail a tap-tap while the gran manje sped by in their white, air-conditioned SUVs emblazoned with their organizations' logos. Down sped some people who had told the audience that we should be working against discrimination because social exclusion increases the prevalence of AIDS. The irony was not lost on the participants who had missed two meals and not been given a chance to speak, as they sang chan pwen—message or "pointing" songs (Averill 1997; Smith

2004)—comparing NGOs to pimps, borrowing language from some of the sessions about the sex trade.[23] As we walked down, laughing, I tried to explain in my still-improving Kreyòl that there is a similar expression in the United States, but I simply couldn't translate "poverty pimp."

Privately, a UN representative—who had spent several thousand dollars of his group's budget—called the conference "a total waste of money." If the point of the conference was to raise awareness, craft an agenda, and organize strategy to combat violence against women and the feminization of HIV/AIDS, it was indeed a failure. But if the point was to get the issue, the organization, and therefore their donors and director in the media, to repost in their reports and websites, it succeeded brilliantly.

"We Don't Depend on Ourselves"

These stories, especially of the symposium, show that the relationships between Sove Lavi and their service population, reinforced through everyday and ritual practices, reproduced and strengthened inequality, hierarchy, and social exclusion. I argue that this is not accidental, but rather characteristic of vertical, client–patron relationships. Said one CAC member, Maxime, "What I see here, I don't want it. Why don't I want it? I don't like their strategy, [and] I don't like their mode of functioning. I don't need for them not to exist, no. But I would like them to change." Said another member, Danielle, "We feel far away from them." Several CAC members put the distance in economic terms, including Julie: "We are already giving of ourselves. We give our bodies, we give our time, we give our talents. It's already a big effort, you understand? We abandon other activities that we had for the benefit of this project, which is a positive project. Today particularly, I had to leave my micro-credit business, which is costing me 150 [Haitian] dollars [nineteen U.S. dollars] to come here because it is a social service. I like supporting social services." Structuring this relationship for many CAC members, reinforcing their perceptions that they were not valued, was that Sove Lavi staff were nearly always late. This frustrated CAC members. Danielle recounted, "They always send for us to let us know when they want a meeting. And they're always late. Sometimes, they give us a time, and when we come to the meeting, when we arrive, we wait, wait, wait, for them. They arrive very late." A focus group evaluation meeting designed for USAID, some eight months after Sove Lavi had last visited CAC members, began with a litany of their complaints about Sove Lavi. Tellingly, the Sove Lavi team I joined showed up two hours later than the meeting was to have begun. Answering the question "What training did you receive at Sove Lavi?," CAC members each responded with a single-phrase answer about the substance of the training and then launched into specific complaints, such as lack of communication, promises broken, lack of follow-up, and the consequences for their relationships with the community.

The lines of communication between Sove Lavi and CAC members were strained. Sove Lavi usually called one CAC member to inform them of an upcoming meeting a couple days in advance. Several CAC members complained about this. Maxime said, "I believe that Sove Lavi should give us two or three days' advance warning to know what we need to do and what we're not doing. Or, will we have time that day? Or also, if Sove Lavi wants to meet with us, they should first ask, because we all might not have time." Danielle was more specific: "Yesterday around four o'clock I got the note" about today's meeting.

CAC members had to pay up front for Sove Lavi training expenses out of their own funds, and the reimbursement process was slow. Djoni complained, "When Sove Lavi suggests that we organize a meeting, they don't reimburse us on time. It's always difficult to get it. We need to beg—how many trips to Pòtoprens?—in order to receive the money." Even given this financial burden, they were more concerned about what they understood as promises Sove Lavi had made to the community. "They proposed a lot of stuff for us: they proposed a community school, a community toilet, things like that," Maxime recalled. "We wrote and gave them a request, but they never responded." Lack of follow-up was a major concern for even otherwise accommodating CAC members, including Marie-Ange: "I would like Sove Lavi to always follow through because when there's no follow-through, it's like you washed your hands very well, only to wipe them on the ground."

This lack of follow-through put a strain on CAC members' relationships with their communities, as outlined by Jimmy: "There are schools that say, 'You never come back anymore.' We say, 'Well, it's not our fault. We don't depend on ourselves. When they send us, we go.'" However dependent they were, CAC members were representatives of Sove Lavi in the eyes of the communities and therefore accountable for Sove Lavi's actions (or lack thereof). Said Junia, "Even now, people always ask us, 'Why was nothing ever done? Is this finished or is it going to continue?'" This creates tension in the community, as Linda explains: "We lose face too, to stand in front of other groups we helped to train."

In both this meeting and the focus group for my own research, the CAC member Djoni[24] assumed leadership, speaking more and more directly to the critiques: "We're not asking for a big thing, but we're asking for mutual respect." As a community leader on the ground—why Sove Lavi chose him in the first place—Djoni felt that his experience, perspective, and time should have been valued. Local leaders know best how to mobilize the community. The failure at World AIDS Day discussed above, especially when compared to the training that began the chapter, is a perfect example of the need for local leadership and ownership. Had local people given their input they would have known when the market and church services would have been in session so as to avoid these times, and known who could generate turnout.

But this social distance and clientelist relationships are not entirely negative from the point of view of the aid recipients. Often, while I was at Sove Lavi's central office, a staff person would introduce me to a CAC member from one or another province. Often, the staff had to translate my Kreyòl to the peasant leader. I would later find out he or she was in town not (or not only) to complain about Sove Lavi, but also to ask for a personal favor from the staff. Often they needed money for a family illness or a burial. Because of the relationships they built with CAC members, Sove Lavi staff felt obliged to help and usually granted these requests. CAC members took other *ti benefis* (fringe benefits) that staff members happily obliged. During missions, CAC members borrowed staff's cell phones, and not just to call other CAC members. After my second or third trip to a particular place, I also received these requests. I too felt obliged to offer my cell phone, for instance. If the CAC member made *kleren* (very strong moonshine from cane juice), charcoal, or other products to sell, Sove Lavi staff people happily bought from them (to "encourage" them). And often, upon our return from being "in the field" to go back into the provincial town, a CAC member would ride along with us. A couple of times the CAC member rode with us all the way to Pòtoprens. Like all acts of patronage, these donations were idiosyncratic, depending on the decision of the donor on a given day.

Fanm Tèt Ansanm: Members?

The situation was different at Fanm Tèt Ansanm. The first contact was either from a friend or coworker's referral, or staff's presence at lunch or on the factory floor. People who become involved in Fanm Tèt Ansanm had either a personal connection or the wherewithal and initiative to seek further contact. Once people visited the space, they chose whether to continue. Many chose to continue. Some staff defined Fanm Tèt Ansanm's continued existence as a matter of factory workers' consent. Many said a variant of the phrase, "If women workers did not come, there would be no need for Fanm Tèt Ansanm." This double negative is worth commenting on further: is this "true, bottom-up" participation, or "participation under control," in Freirian terms (Regan 2003:10), what Gramsci (1971) called "consent"? In the context of Haitian NGOs, Fanm Tèt Ansanm stuck out in its openness to the medanm who wrote individual articles in the journal and sometimes chose the issues to be discussed.

Fanm Tèt Ansanm attempted to provide "backup" (*bak-òp*, not *ankadreman*) to committee leaders, supporting them in their initiatives. While she was working at one of the factories in the industrial park, the Women's Committee leader Lisette fell ill. Knowing her rights to insurance, she visited the OFATMA office and asked to withdraw the funds taken every payday. To her surprise, the government office did not even have a file for her. Lisette called a special meeting of the Women's Committee to discuss this. As a group, they decided they would meet with OFATMA representatives to demand that they fulfill their responsibilities to protect workers, and force Lisette's employer to comply with the law. OFATMA opened an account for Lisette and her coworkers, but they did not charge the company for the taxes taken out of every pay envelope for the previous three years. In response, Lisette and other Women's Committee members wrote an article simply explaining what OFATMA's responsibilities were. This article appeared in an issue of Fanm Tèt Ansanm's Kreyòl-language journal, which has a circulation of five to ten thousand copies and is distributed during the "feeding frenzy" in the industrial park (and also to other NGOs and government agencies). Lisette also contacted local media, volunteering her time even though she was sick. "What could I do?" she asked. "It was unjust." This campaign generated many similar visits to the agency, as workers were empowered to defend their rights. Those individuals[25] who used the information in the journal to plead their case demanded that their accounts be opened as well, and at least some met with success.

Other factory workers found their way to the Women's Committee, like Beatrice, through their frustration with male-dominated unions: "We created a union to improve the factory. Employers don't want to see unions, so our boss fired us all. We hired a lawyer and went to court. The judge declared that the boss owed us a lot of money. But our lawyer took that money and we never saw a dime. I won't say that unions aren't good, but after what they did to me, I won't ever join a union again." In addition to women like Beatrice who left unions in disgust, Fanm Tèt Ansanm provided space for women who are simply afraid to join unions. Yolette said, "In Haiti you can't speak of unions because factory owners don't want you to demand your rights." Beatrice continued, "No matter how we speak with them, if you stand up for your rights, they fire you." Elizabeth argued that simply knowing their rights empowers workers, leveling the relationship a little. "It's not because the boss is unaware of your rights, no. He violates them and you accept it. . . . He has the advantage over you if you don't know your rights." Beatrice explains, "Fanm Tèt Ansanm does a lot for us. They give us knowledge and help us become unafraid, so we can demand our rights." Complementing this was a meeting space away from the boss and from other coworkers who might be in league with them to discuss common issues. During its heyday, the Women's Committee met at least monthly to discuss problems in the factories and would strategize about solutions and offer support to individual committee members in applying them.

Women like Giselle, Lisette, and Beatrice pass the other training programs and apply their knowledge in their neighborhood associations. The training programs' impact is difficult to measure in increasingly popular quantitative calculi, but the women's communities have leaders who read and write Kreyòl, can administer basic first aid, counsel others on HIV/AIDS prevention, can defend their rights, and mobilize community resources. The 2010 earthquake demanded an immediate and effective response from community leaders, so this training meant the difference between life and death in a couple of cases. As Luna said, "The work Fanm Tèt Ansanm does is solid, they trained us, and they help us learn. We have become points of hope where we live." Fanm Tèt Ansanm trains and provides some materials for first aid agents. "For example, a neighbor has a headache or fever," explained Beatrice. "If it's not too serious that they have to go to the doctor you can tell them there's a certain pill you can buy. If it's a mild cut you can bind it for them, and if it is serious you can make a bandage for them and send them to a doctor."

The women appreciate the services they receive, but the situation could be improved, as Marcial explained: "They receive us very well, they speak to us well about women. Everything they tell us is necessary. In Kreyòl class, if they didn't train us we would never understand anything when someone speaks to you. The clinic is totally good, but when they prescribe you a drug, it is expensive to buy elsewhere. So, if you have a problem, it's difficult to resolve it." Especially in the context of other NGOs, being "received well" is important. Factory workers who in Marquise's words "would rather die of thirst because the water makes us sick," were not only given treated water but also cold water, and they were free to take as much as they liked, however the NGO's support was limited. The concern about not having the support to actually solve local problems represents a disconnect between Fanm Tèt Ansanm's priorities and those of the medanm.

Whether this led to a rift is beyond my ability to chart, since interviews were conducted in 2005 and 2006, amid a scale-up at Fanm Tèt Ansanm itself, albeit less dramatic than the one at Sove Lavi. In addition to these common concerns, the medanm discussed others. While the political context and violence kept many services from fully functioning, the clinic's doors remained open most days. When I brought this up as part of my initial findings, staff pointed out that a woman's health is a primary need, unlike training programs. This still did not explain the difference between the Women's Committee and the HIV/AIDS-Prevention Program. At least twice during my twenty months of research, a follow-up meeting of the prevention program preempted the regularly scheduled Women's Committee. In addition, the "promoters" in the prevention program received a monthly transportation stipend while the Women's Committee members did not. Despite the cordial relationship and the medanm's support for Fanm Tèt Ansanm programs, these critiques and distance between staff and medanm grew over time, as outlined below.

Despite these critiques of Fanm Tèt Ansanm, the two NGOs generally have a different orientation toward their aid recipients. Fanm Tèt Ansanm is more cordial, engendering greater participation. Still to be discussed, however, is how to evaluate or measure this participation.

"Carrying Heavy Rocks"

Participation in decision-making processes arose as a social movement strategy to advance marginalized peoples' needs and concerns, particularly for redistribution of power and "democratization" of the state (Castells 1983; Freire 1985). One of the shifts in development discourse, particularly following the failure of large-scale, top-down projects, was a focus on participation. Participation was particularly "mainstreamed" in the 1990s, through the work of the World Bank anthropologist Robert Chambers and his promotion of participatory rural appraisal (Hickey and Mohan 2004b:7). Several scholars, especially anthropologists, have critiqued the on-the-ground realities and practice of this mainstream approach to participation (e.g., Cooke and Kothari 2001; Leve 2001; Paley 2001). One particular argument was that mainstream participatory models failed to transform inequalities because of insufficiently theorized models of power (Parpart 1999), particularly concerning gender (Cornwall 2004; Mansbridge 1999), and because local elites dominate the process (Hickey and Mohan 2004b:13; Mohan 2001). Participation thus becomes a means for legitimizing donor priorities (Brown 2004; Hewamanne 2006; Paley 2001) and can actually strengthen inequalities (Kothari 2001).

In addition to being important to USAID and other donors, participation was one of the three main themes of Aristide's 1990 presidential campaign and the Lavalas social movement. Given the term's wide currency, people have widely divergent understandings of participation, from "a little money" to "giving all of yourself." Donors and NGOs treat it as a simple process that can be measured in a binary, yes/no tick sheet. This represents an unrealistic and unhealthy understanding of NGO projects solely in terms of their "results." Simply put, projects are a process. In an ideal type, NGO projects result from discussions of the problems in the area that generate priorities. In a resource-starved country like Haiti, the weight and diversity of needs can be overwhelming. But community groups often focus on only one or a few problems as priorities at a given time. Once problems are prioritized and made more manageable, solutions can be posed. Turning ideas into action requires planning, organization/coordination, and execution. Ideally once a project is completed local groups evaluate how well they did.

To define and measure participation, I employed a snapshot (table 2.1)—a chart outlining who is involved in the various stages of a development project. For the purposes of this research, I outlined eight such stages: discussion, prioritization, conception, planning, organization, execution, follow-through, and evaluation. I offered a definition originally written in Kreyòl for each stage, so there would be common conceptual understanding. Operationally, I defined the first "discussion" stage as, "What problems exist in our area?" For prioritization, it was "Make decisions—what are the most pressing concerns?" Conception was "What solutions exist for these problems?" For the purposes of the research, planning was described as "Make a plan, assess resources available," and organization, "Tasks and time line finalized—who does what, when?" Execution was outlined as "Put our hands together to work, on the ground working."

TABLE 2.1

Research Tool: Participation Snapshot
Who Does the Following Steps?

	Donor	NGO staff	Beneficiaries
Discussion			
Prioritization			
Conception			
Planning			
Organization			
Execution			
Follow-through			
Evaluation			

Follow-through was defined as "Supervise work, assure that it is being done properly." Finally, evaluation was "Assess how the work was done—what worked well, what needs improvement?" While "conception" or "evaluation" may be differently defined, the terms used were of my own definition. Therefore, I employed a standardized lexicon for research participants, which proved especially useful for people who were not development professionals.

To use this chart, during individual or focus group interviews, I asked people to mark with an X who completed a given step in a development project: NGO staff, donors, or aid recipients. Sometimes in the context of a larger interview, I filled in the chart based on people's answers to questions (all interviews began with life histories but included themes of strengths and weaknesses of the NGOs, participation, autonomy, and Haiti's current situation). In addition to the interviews, I also observed actual practices. Based on a composite of responses from all individual and focus group interviews, corroborated by my observations and informal check-ins with staff and volunteers, the difference in member participation in Sove Lavi and Fanm Tèt Ansanm can be represented graphically. See table 2.2, which shows the difference between the two NGOs in terms of which stakeholder group participates in the eight steps of a development project: donors, NGO staff, or beneficiaries.

As table 2.2 shows, at Sove Lavi, CAC members and other aid recipients participated only in the execution of the project, and sometimes the organization. They were rarely consulted in "planning" the project, as the training that began this chapter highlights. They were just there to set up the tables and present the already-prepared discussion, and were unable to answer the most basic questions. Jennie Smith (2001:34) quoted a peasant as saying, "Participation just

TABLE 2.2

Comparison of Participation between Two NGOs in Several Project Steps

	Sove Lavi			Fanm Tèt Ansanm		
	Donor	NGO staff	Beneficiaries	Donor	NGO staff	Beneficiaries
Discussion					★	★
Prioritization	★	★		★	★	★
Conception	★	★			★	★
Planning	★	★			★	
Organization		★			★	
Execution		★	★		★	★
Follow-through		★			★	
Evaluation	★	★			★	★

means that we have to carry a lot of heavy rocks on our heads." To the best of their knowledge, the project arose from nowhere, as Sove Lavi staff came into their area, described the program, and asked people if they wanted to participate. This ritual was repeated in every new school that Sove Lavi worked with, asking parents for their consent. Especially in remote rural areas, where there is little government or international organization presence, scarce resources, and next to no jobs, few people would oppose a program that offers such resources as tapes, pens, other educational materials, food, money, sometimes even condoms or other birth control methods, and in some cases a youth center complete with satellite Internet and television. "We count on you; you are the only ones who have ever come to see us," a community leader said at a planning meeting. While community members, especially young women, may individually actively support the idea of bringing educational resources, and many like Danielle have personal stories testifying to the importance of HIV education, this consent needs to be understood as "participation under control" (Regan 2003:10), or managed consent (Gramsci 1971).

After the training described at the beginning of this chapter, Sove Lavi held a meeting to plan the following month's activities. Regarding CAC members' participation, they were given a choice of dates for hosting community education forums, and had to sign the attendance roster in order to receive their stipends. There was no space for member questions, and the words members spoke in public were "yes" or "no," or a date and time. As mentioned above, CAC members did not like this approach, seeing it as betraying a lack of respect.

Incidentally, this meeting was rendered moot as USAID had pulled their funding for the project. Front-line staff who went on the mission did not know about this funding shift. Said the team leader Mme Auguste, "I didn't know that it was our last day. I thought we had time to resume again." Meetings that were planned never took place, and promises were broken. Why would Sove Lavi break these promises? I offer some clues in the following chapters.

For an example of the lack of participation, one of Sove Lavi's key programs was education with community groups and schools. This group conducted pre- and post-tests evaluating participants' knowledge of HIV transmission and prevention, focusing on the "ABC" method—abstinence, being faithful, or condom use. At one location in the provinces, all participants had just scored above 95 percent on the test. Sove Lavi staff had returned to Pòtoprens in their SUV, but I stayed on to talk with CAC members. As the dust settled, I asked people—community trainers themselves—what methods of HIV prevention they practiced. Immediately, the group burst into laughter. "My friend, we would very much like to practice HIV prevention," Djoni began. "But they never give us condoms. With all the money they spend on gas and their staff, they could at least give us condoms, no?" Being naive and an anthropologist, I retorted, "But you tell people to practice abstinence," triggering another round of laughter. Speaking over others, Danielle was finally given the chance to finish her thought: "They tell us to not have sex. We tell other people not to have sex. We're okay with not having sex. But for many women here, we don't have the ability to refuse sex when a man wants to. Even if it's just a couple pennies, we need to feed our families. They should focus on reinforcing our economic capacity." Almost everyone chimed in, wanting to add to this analysis, adding their specific suggestions. Maxime argued, "If we are thinking about giving someone knowledge, don't forget that I already said that the knowledge can't advance when the person is hungry. And hunger is the biggest illness there is." Several CAC members pointed this out, citing the Kreyòl proverb, *sak vid pa kanpe* (the empty sack does not stand up). CAC members outlined a plan for a revolving loan fund to create new small businesses as well as a revenue-generating youth activity center that would bring cultural events to the area. They brought these suggestions to Sove Lavi staff, but "nothing happened. All these promises and nothing ever happens." In the following chapters I explain a couple reasons for this. Reflecting on their experience, Maxime said, "For us, there isn't a real collaboration. Our interests are not their interests, they aren't common. Do you see what I am telling you?" Djoni was more direct: "That's not participation! That's 'do [this] for me.'"

By contrast, members of Fanm Tèt Ansanm committees and other medanm participated in agenda setting, the second rung in the "ladder of participation" (e.g., Hart 1997). Most programs existed because of previous advocacy on the part of the medanm: the clinic, the course on legal rights, and the Women's Committee. Members had input on the journal topics, such as during the OFATMA campaign.

The Women's Committee engaged in another campaign, asking the publicly subsidized transport company Service Plus to provide low-cost alternatives for workers to get home from work. Like the more-successful OFATMA campaign, the NGO journal was central to this effort. Lisette discusses another, even more successful campaign in the journal: "We published a journal on March 8 in honor of International Women's Day. We called on all the brave women, all women of conscience, to protest the thirty-six-goud minimum wage. Because of our efforts, [the government] increased it to seventy goud." In other words, members participated in more processes than simply execution, including prioritization and conception. The simple chart presented in table 2.1 was a useful tool to document differences in participation between Sove Lavi and Fanm Tèt Ansanm. Once documented, the differences can be questioned and theorized—which the following chapters offer.

"I Need to Be Able to Help Myself": Similarities

Despite differences between Fanm Tèt Ansanm and Sove Lavi, there are important similarities. One thing that was true across both cases is that volunteer leaders have a different understanding of their own participation than do the NGO staff. Typically, donors—and directors who write reports to donors—state that their beneficiaries participate in several aspects of the development project. Whether this was rhetoric, lack of information, or actual belief, this stands in contrast to how aid recipients themselves see the situation: they do not feel that they had much ownership and say in how the project was conceived or organized, let alone setting priorities or making decisions about interventions.

The snapshot tool was useful to document this difference of perspectives. Because it can be (and was, in my case) used by aid recipients to assess participation, this tool allows a polyvocality missing from most statistically oriented, often donor-funded, NGO research, where one voice (usually the director or designee) speaks for the entire organization. In addition to real-world or perceived pressures to cover up problems or provide positive spin—especially to donors—directors might not know what goes on in the field or after hours. While intuitive, it bears noting that differences in position or social location shape people's understanding. As table 2.3 shows, donors and NGO leadership believe that beneficiaries participate in more steps in the development project than the beneficiaries do themselves. Donors and NGO directors believe that the aid recipients participated far more than they did themselves, the latter only feeling that they participated during execution—in other words, "carrying heavy rocks." It is also interesting that to the aid recipients, projects seemed to appear from out of nowhere, not having arisen from a discussion of problems or priorities. This may not be far from how some NGOs operate. As Marie-Ange said, "They just showed up. They came in their truck and asked to meet with community

TABLE 2.3

Different Perspectives on Participation between NGO Leadership and Beneficiaries

	Donor/director perceptions			Beneficiary perceptions		
	Donor	NGO staff	Beneficiaries	Donor	NGO staff	Beneficiaries
Discussion			★			
Prioritization			★			
Conception		★	★	★	★	
Planning		★	★	★	★	
Organization		★			★	
Execution		★	★		★	★
Follow-through	★	★			★	
Evaluation	★	★	★		★	

leaders. People pointed them in my direction, so they talked with me. I agreed with what they were trying to do, so I became involved." Over time, NGOs' appearing with premade projects adds to citizens' distrust, as NGOs present themselves as parallel states. This distrust is noted in the expression "NGO class" discussed above.

Why did committee members at Fanm Tèt Ansanm, which I characterized as facilitating greater aid-recipient participation, say that they feel like they are only carrying heavy rocks? First of all, it is worth pointing out that several current staff like Leonie began contact with Fanm Tèt Ansanm as a volunteer. Leonie was among the group of people pushing for new directions. Why then did current aid recipients not feel the same? There are two potential explanations. First, socioeconomic differences between staff and aid recipients color people's perceptions. Second, like all models, the chart I used has weaknesses, including that it presents information as if it were ahistorical. That is what is meant by a "snapshot"—it flattens and then fixes an image, freezing it in time. Had I been there earlier, I could have given two such snapshots, comparing Fanm Tèt Ansanm several years apart. A different story emerges because NGOs, like everything else, change over time. In a follow-up meeting I had with Fanm Tèt Ansanm in September 2006, aid recipients critiqued the lack of progress on their ideas and initiatives, such as staff support for obtaining legal documents, support for neighborhood associations, transport, a community cash box based on a sòl model for when the women need medical care, and so forth. They lamented their lack of real participation. In December 2006 the Women's Committee formally presented these and other suggestions to Fanm Tèt Ansanm, including that members receive a stipend similar to that of the HIV/AIDS-Prevention Program. Said one, "The Women's Committee meeting is set for the thirtieth. When the office opens again we will meet with staff to find out if the committee is still happening this year and suggest how things can improve." The lack of communication, and the frustration at not receiving answers from what Women's Committee members felt were simple demands, colored their experiences, causing some to question their relationship with Fanm Tèt Ansanm in similar ways to Sove Lavi's CAC members, as Josette explained: "The salary we get is 250 goud [$6.25]. . . . These things need to change. To get there we need to take a *tap-tap*. When we appear, we need little bread and cola. If I give you my energy [*kouraj*] to help other people, I need to be able to help myself as well. You pay for the transport, but you need to pay for more than that. From the time I leave home, everyone has hope!" that she will come home with money." The Women's Committee has been disbanded since 2007. Actually, as of 2009, Fanm Tèt Ansanm became like other NGOs offering their services about HIV/AIDS in the provinces. Given this, and the increasing intensity of complaints of committee members, it is clear that participation was eroding further. Committee members like Josette identified the AIDS-prevention program as "work" that they do for Fanm Tèt Ansanm (notice her use of the word "salary" in the above quote), and not as a volunteer effort. This is a further clue into volunteers' disaffiliation as "members" and with Fanm Tèt Ansanm's priorities of HIV/AIDS prevention, highlighting how even a generally open NGO can change and how fragile genuine local participation is.

As this chapter clearly shows, simplistic notions of participation do not account for local realities. A more ethnographically grounded, robust understanding of participation based on the relationships NGOs engender with local communities allows us to move ahead. While Sove Lavi's donors deemed the training that began the chapter a success, its ability to change people's understandings and critiques of the HIV/AIDS industry was very limited. If we are to succeed in ending this disease, or rebuild an earthquake-torn Haiti, our efforts need to include real participation. The snapshot model provided in this chapter offers a challenge to NGOs to do so, and a self-assessment to measure their improvement.

Several questions remain, however: What accounts for the different levels of aid-recipient participation seen in Sove Lavi and Fanm Tèt Ansanm? What accounts for the bureaucratic blockages within Sove Lavi, like arriving late or not receiving certificates for their work? What accounts for the gradual erosion of community participation within Fanm Tèt Ansanm? For some answers, in the following chapter I turn to a discussion of the relationships "inside" the NGOs.

3

All in the Family

Relationships "Inside"

We are a family here. That doesn't mean we don't have conflicts from
time to time.

−Mme Auguste, Sove Lavi

Thursday, May 20, 2004 8:36 P.M.
The chairs were all occupied, so people sat on the desks as well. Laughter
drowned out the shouting across the room. Everyone was still waiting for
Mme Dominique, the director, to emerge from her office. Even the doctors were
both there. It was Thursday, the end of the workweek. In the other direction, the
literacy training session was just getting out. Some of the *medanm* visited with
Giselle, who directed the clinic. She peered up from her computer, still trying to
work, but smiled as the medanm streamed in. All of Giselle's coworkers chatted
away, long having turned off their computers.

Leonie stared at the birthday cake, smiling. It was actually her birthday,
unlike Mme Dominique, whose was a couple of weeks ago. Fanm Tèt Ansanm
has a monthly birthday celebration for all staff born that month. Leonie had
begun working with them almost fifteen years ago, a couple years after Fanm Tèt
Ansanm began. She was one of the first women who frequented the center and
one of their first volunteer leaders. As Fanm Tèt Ansanm attracted more funding and increased their programs, Leonie was one of the first new people hired.

Flanking Leonie were the other people who worked in the back office:
all of them had similar stories of being rescued from working in the factories by
displaying some particular talent or leadership abilities to work for Fanm Tèt
Ansanm. The other *ti pèsonnèl* ("small" personnel, manual laborers) stood ready
to carve up the cake and serve the syrupy-sweet Couronne "cola champagne."
They joked with one another, in one corner of the room.

Finally, Mme Dominique came out of her office and gave Leonie a hug.
Vanessa, Mme Dominique's personal secretary, chastised everyone that it was
getting late. She didn't have to remind people about the dangers of arriving

home after dark. It hadn't been three months since Aristide was forced out, and a cloud of fear still hung low over everyone. Immediately after Vanessa spoke, everyone sang a three-language version of "Happy Birthday" that ended with a French phrase for "come on, let's cut the cake," which Monique, a housekeeping worker, did.

The celebration itself lasted all of ten minutes—mostly people talking with their closest colleagues—then people scattered to make it home. The ti pèsonnèl prepared packages of the cake to send home, with everyone receiving the same amount except for the two birthday girls. Leonie took a bigger slice while Mme Dominique, making a comment about her waistline, declined.

Just as four of the ti pèsonnèl, including Leonie, left to pack the company truck to be dropped off en route, the doctors and three middle-office staff people each gave a present to Mme Dominique. She hugged each one of them, and then opened all the boxes one by one. One of them who had recently returned from a conference in Mexico brought back a souvenir. The other gifts—household items like glasses and plates—were purchased at one of the high-end grocery stores, judging by the gift wrap. Everyone there would be driving his or her own car and so didn't have to rush to make it home.

A few of the other staff people had stayed around for the present ceremony. None said anything but all were enthralled with the gifts. Leonie got nothing except for a single card from the whole office.

Jimmy, the driver, honked the horn, signaling for the remaining people getting a wou lib (free ride) to come outside and get in the truck. People said their good-byes, with their paper-towel-wrapped cake tucked under their arm or in their purse.

Within five minutes, everyone but François and Martha, the guard and one of the custodial staff who lived nearby, had left the office. It remained light a little longer, but still night was falling and people needed to get home. François and Martha quickly put everything away and shared the remaining bottles of soda before leaving.

This story highlights the multiple, conflicting realities within the office. Staff clearly shared a sense of being closely knit but people also celebrated within separate spheres, what Jesse Mumm (2008) called "intimate segregation." Discourses and practices of sharing equally sat uncomfortably next to exclusion and privilege just beneath the surface. While everyone got the same slice of cake, sharing the public goods equally, the same is not true of private resources. Tellingly, middle-office staff and the doctors, all solidly middle class in their education and economic status, waited until most of the ti pèsonnèl left before sharing their gifts with Mme Dominique. A couple of times, people in lower-status positions were forced to wait for superiors: the party couldn't start without

Mme Dominique, for example, and the ti pèsonnèl had to wait for their lift home until the "front-office staff" private party was finished.

"Tout moun se moun, men tout moun pa menm"

This chapter explores the connection between discourses of family and realities of hierarchy, manifestations of the difference between "backstage" and "onstage" discourses within NGOs (Doolittle 2006:58; Rossi 2006:47; Sharma 2008). The private gifts were a form of privilege kept hidden (albeit not very well), expressions of the Haitian proverb "*Tout moun se moun, men tout moun pa menm*": everyone is a person (an important corrective to pervasive dehumanization), but not everyone is the same. Forces of centralization and inequality are pervasive in the country. Haiti is an extremely divided society, which is all too apparent in the residential and educational segregation, the use of French as a means to exclude the poor majority, and many other indicators. This inequality can't help but effect the work of NGOs. Despite this, the two NGOs have different responses to this inequality and social exclusion. While far from perfect, Fanm Tèt Ansanm at least had ritual spaces that temporarily suspended hierarchy, at least within the official public sphere. Sove Lavi did not even celebrate birthdays in the office, except for that of its director, Mme Versailles.

This chapter provides an account of how NGOs' daily interactions—what de Certeau (1984, 1998) calls *le quotidien*, the "practice of daily life"—emerge from an inegalitarian *habitus* and augment this inequality (Bourdieu 1980, 1990). As Mary Hancock (1999, 2006), Setha Low (2000, 2006), and others (e.g., Yang 1999) have argued, inequality is structured in spatial design and practice. Therefore, a detailed description of the architecture of the two NGO offices provides the scaffolding for understanding how inequality is structured in day-to-day interactions within them. Using this scaffolding, this chapter presents a "typical" day in the office, from morning to afternoon, highlighting the interactions between the various divisions within the staff that become visible.

Both approaches—a spatial analysis and observation of interactions—highlight many aspects of hierarchy and autonomy, making possible a comparison between Fanm Tèt Ansanm and Sove Lavi. The two NGOs' internal inequality and centralization are different, with Sove Lavi demonstrably more inegalitarian and centralized than Fanm Tèt Ansanm. These differences in hierarchy begin to explain the observable differences in local participation within the NGOs noted in the previous chapter.

Fanm Tèt Ansanm

Fanm Tèt Ansanm's office is situated in a *katye popilè* (low-income or "popular" neighborhood) where the medanm also live and work. Their location thus facilitates much direct contact. At the time of my fieldwork, the office was divided into five distinct zones, with varying degrees of interaction: clinic, administrative office, program office, training rooms, and janitors' closets. These spaces were arranged hierarchically, with the center predictably revolving around the administrative offices, with ti pèsonnèl farthest in distance—in literal and metaphoric senses—from the center. These relatively distinct zones structured a high degree of interaction, cooperation, and interdependence. While these zones were relatively autonomous, the ritual practice discussed in the previous chapter—the annual commemorations—generalized this interdependence and cooperation, with the temporary effect of flattening the hierarchy, at least ideologically, reminiscent of Victor Turner's (1969) *communitas*.

Outside the Office

As mentioned in the previous chapter, Fanm Tèt Ansanm's office is in the export-processing zone by the international airport. President Aristide made renovation of the road to the airport a priority, renaming it (like the airport itself) after Toussaint Louverture, leader of the slave insurrection and progenitor of Haiti's independence.[1] Except for a few potholes, the road stuck out in that it was entirely paved, divided by a median sprouting tropical plants (e.g., coconut trees, banana trees, flowery bushes). Also shooting up were some of Haiti's only traffic lights at the time, optimistically preparing for some future era when electricity would light them. The road is full of several busily painted *tap-tap* of many kinds, for many different routes, filled to the gills with factory workers and supervisors who can afford the five-goud fare, people standing or hanging on (called *sèso*, "coat hanger"). Private vehicles, often large SUVs, transport managers and owners to work. In addition, freight trucks often haul gasoline, tires, produce from the provinces, bolts of fabric to be sent to the factories to be cut and sewed, and boxes of shirts, jeans, underwear, baseballs, baseball caps, and other products to be shipped back to the United States. During the time I conducted fieldwork, a fleet of white "UN" (written in English) tanks and armored personnel carriers often zoomed by. Vehicles drive fast, many of which, especially the tap-tap, suddenly veer to drop off or pick up more passengers.[2] In the mornings and the afternoons, a steady march of skirt-clad factory workers lined both sides of the streets, walking to and from work. Luck, prayer, and a good sprint were required to cross the busy street, as traffic lights did not often work at that time (2003–2005).

To get to Fanm Tèt Ansanm's office, one must leave Boulevard Toussaint Louverture and turn off one of the side streets. During the dry seasons, this trek is a little easier, as the road is made of boulders and mud. During the rainy seasons, in fall and spring, navigating the roads without soiling one's shoes in a four-inch mud pool is often difficult. *Timachann* stands—and often their homes, made of found objects, wooden poles, leftover cinderblock pieces, and tarp—lined both sides of the street, despite the government's action to prepare for Haiti's January 1, 2004, bicentennial by bulldozing the two rows of brick structures. Like most people, I traveled this road by foot. Coming to work is a social affair, as people greet one another, engage in small talk about their relatives, or engage in conversation and debate about the rising gas prices, the price for rice, the general insecurity, or the latest news from *radyo tranndè* (rumor mill). Walking to work, people can see who is preparing which variation of beans, rice, or corn, the charcoal fires already burning and the helpers busy chopping the meat, grating the coconut, or washing the key limes for lemonade. In between, poorer, more recently arrived timachann sold hard candy, crackers, or other snacks for those whose hunger demands attention but who cannot afford a full lunch plate.

Fanm Tèt Ansanm's Lakou

Fanm Tèt Ansanm leased an unused portion of a factory. There were four distinct zones to the office. A cobblestone courtyard about twenty-five feet wide and forty feet deep sat right behind the painted iron double gate that swings open. Like most roads in Haiti and the driveway that it opens into, the courtyard was usually dusty. During the workday, the courtyard housed a small fleet of private and company vehicles, which the guard washed from water dripping from the tank atop the roof. On one side of the courtyard, a chain-link fence separated Fanm Tèt Ansanm's space from the next factory over. Flowers were planted along the other sides, and an assortment of saplings grew in pots made from expired five-gallon water jugs. Fanm Tèt Ansanm's most public rituals, the annual celebrations described in the previous chapter, occurred in the courtyard. Two brightly painted cinder-block buildings flanked both sides of the courtyard. The clinic stood to the right upon entrance, the administrative offices and most of the classrooms to the left.

In the morning, while the hum of the nearby factories' machinery began for the day, the ti pèsonnèl are the only ones in the Fanm Tèt Ansanm office. The guard fills[3] the water tanks, fills the *dèlko* ("Delco," a gas-powered generator) with oil and diesel, primes it for use, and sweeps out the courtyard. Others are sweeping yesterday's dust off the tile floors, wiping it off the desks and computers, and preparing the kitchen for coffee, juice, and lunch. Four of them come in the green company pickup emblazoned with a Japanese flag and the phrase "don du peuple de Japon" (gift of the people of Japan) on both doors. The empty water jugs are taken out and walked over to the local outlet, replaced by full jugs. Beginning around 8:30, the "day" staff begin to stream in, depending on traffic, depending on whether violence made travel difficult or long, and depending on familial duties. The inverter is turned on when the administrator arrives so she can work on her computer. Two other administrative assistants also arrive, turn their computers on, and go to work preparing letters and reports and attempting to return phone calls. In addition to people being away from their office, in Haiti this task is made more difficult by the sorry state of the phone system.[4] The administrator arranges with the chauffeur on call that day what meetings people need to be sent to, what pickups or drop-offs of materials, mail, or office supplies need to be done, and by when. When the electricity is on, medical equipment is washed in boiling water, and the refrigerators are turned on to store necessary items, such as solutions, blood samples, or food, and a block of water to turn into ice for the employees' lunch.

To get into the main office one must walk up a half flight of stairs and come to a small concrete landing. The metal front door often broils because of the sun, sometimes stuck ajar. First-time visitors and slow-to-learn foreign anthropologists often fail to close the door entirely, triggering a *twipe*[5] from Michaëlle, the secretary closest to the door, reminding the offender that the air conditioner is running. A poster, bumper sticker, or sheet of paper adorned nearly all surfaces. Newcomers were given the message that a life without violence is every woman's right, that women are capable of doing any job men are, that justice and peace work together, and that Fanm Tèt Ansanm has been around a long time, participating in conferences about women's rights, workers' rights, population issues, health, AIDS, violence, and development. Michaëlle sat on a cushioned chair with wheels at a large, L-shaped wooden desk that supports a computer, printer, large Rolodex, and a black, ten-line phone. Hovering over the desk is a row of locked, built-in cabinets that traverse the length of the front office. To her left is a large picture window with an A/C unit and usually closed blinds.

Mme Dupuy, the administrator, had a similar setup as Michaëlle, a large, L-shaped Formica desk and computer, a large Rolodex, simple phone, and typewriter. Opposite Mme Dupuy's desk on the way out the door was a very old copier. If double-sided copies are desired, the person has to manually reload the copier, often triggering a jam. The copier was generally only allowed to be on when they "had EDH"—when the state-run electricity (Electricité d'Haïti) was on[6]—but sometimes with the dèlko. At the beginning of my fieldwork, front-office computers were the only ones wired for the Internet, a dial-up modem. By the end of my fieldwork, they had switched to a much faster, satellite-based service that nonetheless did not work properly when the sky was too cloudy, or whenever there was a dip in the average electricity allocation at the network provider's office. Michaëlle and Mme Dupuy are friendly, but they usually worked on their own. Occasionally they engage in conversation with one another or Mme Dominique, the director, especially on Fridays when they and the ti pèsonnèl are the only staff working. In contrast to the business of the walls explicitly proclaiming a women's empowerment orientation, the atmosphere is calm and relaxed, both rare in Haitian NGO offices (I have visited more than thirty before 2007).

To the left of the front office as one walks in the door was a large picture window covered by a curtain. This was Mme Dominique's office, which was darker and cooler than everywhere else. Large windows dominated three walls, one to the outside and two into other offices, the front and middle offices, built to facilitate supervision of the factory floor. Curtains always covered these latter windows. The other wall had a restroom for exclusive use by Mme Dominique and front-office staff when she was away. Mme Dominique has a large swivel chair and a large, L-shaped desk, with pictures of her family and usually piles of file folders. The entrée into Fanm Tèt Ansanm has a generic "professional" office demeanor, reminiscent of "Western" Taylorist bureaucracies (Abramson 1999:241; Sampson 1996:146). This professionalism was reproduced in the frontline staff's daily work rhythm.

Middle Office

Beginning around ten o'clock, Mme Dominique and the middle-office staff begin streaming in, most in their own cars. When they arrive, the mood usually becomes lively, chaotic, or a mixture of both, depending on the big tasks of the day. As people pass others on their way to their desk, they usually exchange greetings. In Haiti, when women, or when a man and a woman, meet up for the first time in a day, they say hello by a *ti bò* (little kiss), as they touch cheeks and kiss in the air.[7] Failure to do so is considered impolite, a sign of a problem or—especially if one is an outsider and a male—choosing favorites, triggering jealousy. During the time I was in Fanm Tèt Ansanm, it often seemed obligatory to recite dangers people saw, ran into, or heard about, to which coworkers would twipe and say "*Mezanmi!*" Some days, in particularly difficult situations or with particularly noteworthy events, salutations would become full-fledged *brase lide* (stirring ideas) where everyone present would contribute her story or analysis, and the volume of the conversation would reach shouting levels, punctuated by laughter or *ò-o* (uh-oh!). These spontaneous brase lide, often lasting for a half hour or more, were the classrooms in which I learned most of what I know about Kreyòl, Haitian culture, history, and especially the contemporary crisis.

The middle office was a crowded, awkward, L-shaped space, home to the four program directors (clinic, health education, human development education, and communication) who make up the Kowòdinasyon Kolejyal (Collegial Coordination), who make programmatic decisions for the agency, and their two support staff. Seven desks, all but one with a phone, are arranged to maximize efficiency, sharing otherwise crowded space and also facilitating conversation by people facing one another other. An aisle led through the middle office to the back office. The communications staff sat to the right of this aisle, with three desks for two people. The configuration of this area changed every so often, especially when one or another of the staff got a new computer. The assistant was the first to get a new computer. Her supervisor worked on a computer so old that it ran Windows 95, which was sent to the back office when she got another one. Edele, the communications director—a *manbo* (traditional religious leader) with long dreadlocks and who usually wears African-inspired dashikis or blue jeans—received a new Macintosh to do graphic design and supposedly develop a website. Ricky Martin looked down at them, his image dominating a French-language poster saying, "AIDS concerns me," until someone covered it up with a Kreyòl poster that discussed women's rights. To the right was a bookshelf with many dusty reports and manuscripts, most of them dating to the 1980s, and a washroom with running water (sometimes), paper towels (sometimes), a roll of toilet paper, and an small mirror on the door.

Immediately to the left of the aisle was Vanessa, Mme Dominique's administrative assistant. Photos of Vanessa's son shared the desk with knickknacks purchased on trips abroad and a couple of small succulents. Unlike the others, Vanessa's desk was relatively free of paperwork. Her computer was one of the first computers in the middle office, which also ran Windows 95, which often gave her problems and was not hooked up to a printer. Vanessa was usually the first person aside from the guard and custodians to arrive, and she worked quietly by herself. She was often not at her desk, however, as she often performed specific tasks to assist Mme Dominique. Vanessa's job was to order office supplies and materials for the celebrations, occasionally meet with funding representatives, and assist with sending off correspondence. A divorcée, she was especially attentive to male visitors. Vanessa locked her desk when she left the office, occasionally dropping the French-language version of the Jehovah's Witness *Watchtower* on Edele's desk as her duty to save a colleague from Satan.

Jonette, the AIDS-prevention program supervisor, was next to Vanessa. Like the other remaining desks, hers was plain and not made of wood. Jonette's desk and even her chair had the largest stack of file folders because she had the most reports to write (she got a computer midway through my fieldwork). To Jonette's right was a window and one of the noisiest and least effective air-conditioning units I have ever encountered. Three oscillating fans, of varying age and quality, changed position depending on who last moved them. The other two supervisors' workspaces had their piles of folders and foreign-purchased trinkets, but no computer. If everyone sat at her desk, these four faced one another, facilitating conversation and a convivial atmosphere. On a rickety desk in the corner sat a communal computer and color ink-jet, the printer of choice for photos of themselves, children, spouses/boyfriends, or wedding/funeral programs. This was a favored spot to conduct Internet research on topics varying from mother-to-child AIDS transmission to Elvis song lyrics, to check e-mail or instant messaging, or to play a backgammon game. But this computer also hosted the institutional memory, with monthly, quarterly, and annual service statistics, reports, guides to the training programs, and programs from past events. During the mornings and early afternoons, whoever sat at this station was presumed to be working on the most pressing institutional business and could command others' attention.

Whenever a monthly, quarterly, or annual report was due, or a representative from one of Fanm Tèt Ansanm's donor groups was scheduled to visit, the mood was chaotic. In addition to the director and the front-office staff, one of the middle-office staff (a program director) was usually glued to her computer and shouted for people to help her find something: a file, a number, a date, or a word. As Giselle, one of the middle-office staff, reported, "Things here aren't done in a one-way street." Most often, other people around stopped what they were doing to lend a hand, or they, in turn, would shout for someone to fetch some document or file from the clinic or the back office, or to get paper for the printer, or to grab the document from the printer. If there were no ti pèsonnèl around to make a delivery, I would try and make myself useful, but usually it took people too long to explain to me what they needed, so they used the intercom phone. People occasionally ran into one another in their comings and goings to help out their coworker. Sometimes there would be a quick, high-pitched argument, followed by laughter as soon as it was resolved. Most of the reports were composed in this *youn-ede-lòt* (one helping the other) way, with many hands touching them. Usually, there were at least a couple of drafts of any given report, and the other middle-office staff people would read the draft and shout out corrections that needed to be made. When the report was finally ready, the staff in charge would celebrate, telling everyone she had finished. The final copy was sent to the printer, saved and saved again, since many times while working, the inverter would discharge and the power would cut out. The *responsab* (person in charge) would with great ceremony walk over herself, pick up the report, and walk into the front office to give it to Mme Dominique. If it was particularly urgent, Mme Dominique didn't wait. She would come into the middle office, offering a quick hello and wave to everyone, and then she would ask where the report was. Despite the air conditioner, Mme Dominique often wore brightly colored, sleeveless dresses, as often kente cloth as out of *Vogue*. Arguably, the middle office is Fanm Tèt Ansanm's communications center, the site for lively interaction. In contrast to the demure and individualist work style of the front office, the middle office is usually spirited and collaborative. While middle-office people were occasionally summoned into the front office, more often front-office staff went to the middle office to make their requests, atypical for hierarchically based organizations.

Back Office

Beginning around 1 o'clock, the "back office" staff members arrive. All except for one had a morning job, so the actual time of arrival depended greatly on traffic. Traffic is especially dense during the school year beginning around noon, when parents pick their children up from school. Aggravating this "normal" situation, the political situation created much more chaotic and unpredictable *blokis* (traffic jams). So back-office staff sometimes do not arrive until much later (three o'clock). The women who work in the back office are the direct contact with the medanm: they are "monitors" who facilitate the four basic training programs. Their job is to prepare lessons—some prepared written handouts—and then to lead discussion. The four have different pedagogical styles. Some monitors have a more hands-on approach than others, which might depend on the subject material. The literacy program is deliberately modeled after Paulo Freire's (1985) *Pedagogy of the Oppressed*. For example, the factory women read life histories actually written by other factory women, or they read sections of the labor code or constitution addressing their civic and political rights. By contrast, much of the women's health seminar information is factual, and the monitor does a bit more lecturing, and draws diagrams and writes out definitions of terms. The monitor does ask questions, however, and tries to put the discussion in a context of the lived experience of the factory workers—for example, by discussing the difficulties associated with a lack of primary health care if a given symptom is not treated right away, followed by a question about why health care is out of their reach.

The back office was the largest, as it was the site for most trainings. A couple of staff reminisced about less insecure times when all four training programs would run concurrently. According to Giselle, "People are afraid to come. To come here for a training is to risk getting home after dark. You never know what is going to happen in these times." The women's health seminar occurs above the clinic when other spaces are used. The room was painted cinderblock, with literally dozens of posters on the walls, many of them made by hand at Fanm Tèt Ansanm, including photos of Fanm Tèt Ansanm events. One poster shows the Maribal sisters, who were all killed by the Dominican dictator Rafael Trujillo on November 25, 1960, and commemorated by the International Day for the Elimination of Violence Against Women.

The four trainers each had a desk with random assortments of items, mostly personal memorabilia, gifts bought in Haiti, or items from someone on a trip overseas. For at least a year and a half, a nonworking computer sat atop a workstation behind the row of desks, dwarfed by the piles of old posters, journals, and other assorted paper stacked on and behind several rusty file cabinets. There was a single phone in this room that couldn't make outside calls.[8] Staff sat on the same metal folding chairs in the classroom, separated by a row of potted plants and detailed ironwork.[9] The usual configuration of metal folding chairs was in a circle, hugging the wood-paneled walls and the room divider, leaving space on the wall shared with the middle office for the monitors, some of whom used an easel for their presentations, especially the dermatologist who lectured once a month. For the entire period of my fieldwork, there was a hole in the lowered, paneled ceiling in the middle of the room, letting the heat in and reminding people who sit or stand nearby that Haiti is indeed in the tropics. The back office, where most of the interactions with the medanm took place, was marginalized, both spatially and in terms of resources allocated, as evidenced by the temperature and the lack of computer equipment.

Lunch and the Ti Pèsonnèl

Lunch was usually a lively communal affair. After the day's meal is cooked, the ti pèsonnèl walk up to the middle- and front-office staff—or call on the intercom—and announce that lunch is ready. The cook also heat lunches for people who brought them from home. Lunch was served in the very back of the office in a room that also doubles as a meeting space for the Women's Committee. A phone could accept incoming calls and make intercom calls. Again, the wood-paneled walls were covered in posters, mostly made by Fanm Tèt Ansanm staff in a pedagogical context, describing the history of international women's rights conventions, the labor code, and the constitution. People ate at a long plywood table that could have come out of a church basement or community center in the United States, surrounded by six fiberglass chairs. Right next to this was a water cooler and a stack of cone cups (when stocked). At the end of the room was the cook Edwidge's closet-sized kitchen, with a sink and cabinets to store her utensils and the dishes. She cooked using two stoves on top of propane tanks. Around eleven o'clock, Edwidge made coffee with a stovetop espresso maker. Her assistant, Martha, took a pewter serving set and four ceramic demitasse cups and walked to Mme Dominique's office to offer her coffee. Then Martha worked her way back to the middle office. The remaining coffee was shared among the ti pèsonnèl. Lunch was usually ready between one and two, depending on many factors that I have only begun to grasp. Cooking Haitian food, almost always done by women, is a very labor-intensive process. Around three, the afternoon coffee was made and distributed.

When one of the front- and middle-office staff sat down to the already-set table to eat (Mme Dominique always worked through lunch, eating in her office), Edwidge or Martha brought out her food, usually starting with the juice of the day or coffee. If the spontaneous morning brase lide sessions were lively, lunchtime conversations were uproarious. Without the constraint of work, the women told full versions of the stories that gripped them. They discussed the latest rumor or news event, such as an incident in someone's neighborhood whereby someone they knew was kidnapped, a story about an illicit organ-donor ring, the capture of a gang leader, or simply a joke. The story was often followed by everyone's analysis. Despite the high energy, and the (what I am told is) traditional conversational style of finishing one another's sentences and then going on, everyone who wanted to participate[10] had a chance to offer her analysis, critique, suggestion, question, or follow-up story. Depending on the day's workload, the lunch brase lide sessions could last as long as an hour or

longer. For the first several weeks, I did not participate in these events, preferring instead to eat outside on the street, thinking I would be able to partake in
the conversation of the day, talking with a different class of people, in an effort
to show allegiance with *pèp la*, the poor majority in the industrial park. It was
a misguided effort, as people inevitably called me *patron* (boss/owner), unable to
understand why I was eating on the street. One day, one of the Fanm Tèt Ansanm
staff chastised me for being aloof, so I started going to the indoor sessions.

When I was there long enough, I noticed that the ti pèsonnèl participated
in these conversations as well, that it was not just the professional middle- or
front-office staff. Edwidge was an excellent storyteller (*griyo*), descriptive and
very witty, and was respected for it. During the analysis portion of the lunchtime
brase lide, staff would often get in heated debates about the political situation
in Haiti and in the United States. It could be argued that the lunch is a kind of
"public sphere" at Fanm Tèt Ansanm, the only space in which people within all
organizational divisions frequent and participate in discussion (Habermas 1989,
1992). Only Mme Dominique and the part-time doctors did not regularly eat their
lunches in the back room. While hierarchies were reproduced and strengthened
by spatial segregation and daily practices within the front offices, it is no acci-
dent that this liminal space—outside the official "work" space—was generally
the most open, deliberative area, where divisions are temporarily suspended
and everyone participates in the brase lide (Turner 1969; Young 1997).

The Clinic

The clinic was a densely packed structure apart from the office. It was next to
the office's dèlko, which often invaded the clinic with engine noise and blue-
black smoke. The courtyard opened into the waiting room, relatively spacious
and well lit, despite there being no lights. Dominating the aural landscape,
often competing with the noisy dèlko, was a television set. The most common
programs were soccer, music videos, news, and foreign movies dubbed into
perfect Parisian French, either Hollywood films—especially starring African
American actors—or Latin American telenovelas. Staff justified this use of electricity as important ambiance: "Here people can relax, not like the hospitals,
which scare people with the smell and feel of death." On the opposite side of the
room was a water cooler and sometimes cone cups. From one o'clock onward,
someone always sits at a front desk, welcoming people and finding the patient's
files for the doctors. The medanm usually began streaming in around three
o'clock. Taped up all over the main waiting room and the anteroom were
glossy—but usually not laminated—posters, discussing the importance of family
planning, HIV/AIDS testing, literacy, and women's rights. Many of the posters
hung askew, and nearly all of the posters were in Kreyòl.

Like doctors' offices in the United States, patients were taken to a nurse's
office, where she took people's temperature, weight, and blood pressure. Unlike

in the United States, the nurse often shouted out the numbers to the reception-ist. Apparently these are not considered private in Haiti, or perhaps poor women do not have privacy in the rest of their lives and so have come to not expect it at the doctor's office. The nurse's office had an operating-room bed for sick patients, including Fanm Tèt Ansanm staff. Across a narrow hallway from the nurse's office is a small bathroom, consisting of a sink basin, a toilet, and a large bucket of water. Users bring their own toilet paper, and often soap. Next was the laboratory, as big as many U.S. closets, stacked with a centrifuge and a sterilizer, where stirrups and other materials for Pap tests were cleaned. Sharing a wall with both the laboratory and the dèlko was a dusty, empty consultation room, doubling as storage for old chairs, hospital beds, stacks of assorted papers, and boxes of stuff I never could identify. Most of the time this room was empty, though this was where the dermatologist, the only woman doctor, met with patients one day a week.

After the patients finished with the nurse, they returned to the waiting room and chatted with one another or the staff, or watched television, sitting in a row of metal folding chairs lining two of the walls. All around this area were boxes of written materials, especially the journals, piled high. Examples of dif-ferent methods of birth control were also piled high: standard condoms, female condoms, Norplant, the pill, the sponge, IUDs, and syringes with Depo-Provera. Plain white boxes of condoms manufactured in India—the only kind approved by the UN because of their effectiveness rates—were here as well, when they were in stock.[11] Often, while a small crowd of eight or so patients waited for the doctor, Leonie gave an impromptu lecture on the various types of STIs or some other women's health issue. She used one of two booklets published by Fanm Tèt Ansanm, with detailed illustrations in full color on glossy paper, passing the booklet around to the patients in the waiting room, who muttered to them-selves or asked questions. When the impromptu lesson finished, Leonie described the courses that Fanm Tèt Ansanm offers: human development, legal rights, women's health, and literacy, as well as a host of other specific programs geared toward practical use, such as first aid and HIV/AIDS prevention. Patients were invited to take literature with them.

To the left of the waiting room were the two consultation rooms for the two lighter-skinned male obstetrician/gynecologists. Since both of them had their own private practice in the mornings, they arrived anywhere between 2:30 and 4:00, depending on their morning case load, traffic, and of course the situation in the streets. Staff met these unexpected occurrences with flexibility, but the medanm, who walked to the clinic, often waited a long time. The consultation rooms were identical, and were the biggest rooms in the clinic. Both have two outside walls and brick "windows" to allow sunlight, in addition to having working light bulbs. The two rooms are both equipped with a wooden desk, old-fashioned hospital bed dividers, and an examining table. One of the rooms had a recently acquired sonogram machine, marked by a sticker identifying it, like the pickup, as a gift from the people of Japan. The other room doubles as an office for Giselle, the clinic director, who preferred to work there on the many days when she had to submit reports. "For one thing," she said, "I don't have to carry the boxes of files very far." In addition, this was the only place in Fanm Tèt Ansanm besides Mme Dominique's office where relative quiet can be found, just the ambient whirring of the sewing machines at a nearby factory, trucks coming and going, and the dèlko. The doors to these rooms are always closed when someone is in them, and often when they are not, in an effort to keep the dust at bay. The clinic and office spheres are usually quite distinct, separated not only by the parking lot but also by daily practice.

The first medanm to arrive were those not currently employed in the export-processing zone because they had a child, the working conditions were too unbearable, or the factory had closed or severely downsized. If unoccupied, the guard and other male ti pèsonnèl greeted the medanm. People seeking the clinic entered it directly, but those attending a training session usually walked around to the back entrance, a grass path between the office building and barbed-wire fence leading onto a platform to the lunchroom. At times, a second gate leading directly to the rear of the office was open. From this entrance, a smaller classroom was to the right, called the "literacy" room because it is where the advanced literacy seminars, smaller than the other sessions, met when space was an issue. Except for one series of seminars I went to at the beginning of my first seven weeks of fieldwork, the training room was largely vacant, a heavy layer of black dust covering the table and the piles of books from the 1980s. Next on the right is a bathroom, with a toilet, a sink, and sometimes a light bulb and paper towels. It is smaller and cleaned less often than the other bathrooms except for the clinic bathroom. But to most medanm, the water cooler and the running water in the toilet and sink are luxuries not available to them at work or at home.

The physical separation kept the zones of activity distinct, as it conserves most resources for the administration. The direct contact with the medanm, the purpose of the NGO, was held within resource-poor areas, without electricity or what it facilitated: Internet, air-conditioning, or cold water. It was truly tout moun pa menm, with people treated unequally.

Commemorations

Exceptions to this state were commemorations of special days, revealing an "anti-structure" or temporary generalization of "communitas" inherent in ritual enactment (Turner 1969). The mood was both lively and chaotic whenever the day included a celebration. In addition to the comings and goings, the shouting for help and the shouting back, everyone had several discrete tasks to accomplish. People's cars were moved from the courtyard and onto the driveway outside the gate. A couple of canvas tents and scores of chairs were set up. The sound system was set up. Decorations made. The food and drinks were picked up, as were the small plastic plates and cups for serving. Programs for the event were designed, typed out, printed, copied, and then folded. Everyone was involved in the process. In the thirteen events that I was in the office the whole day to witness, I never saw a formal planning process. Someone assumed (or was anointed with) the position of leadership and then delegated tasks. A couple of the more computer-savvy people would type up a sheet of tasks. But most of the time, people simply showed up and did whatever preparatory effort was asked of them. Given the frantic pace of activity, and the direct involvement of all the staff, conflicts often arose: the printer jammed or ran out of paper, the chauffeur was late coming back with the balloons, people disagreed over the order of the events, or two people worked on the same task. During times like these, people's latent frustrations or prejudices came out of hiding: remarks laced with sarcasm about Vodou (Haiti's traditional religion), politics, or class antagonism. Once uttered, the parties to the disagreement reacted quickly and in similarly emotional fashion. But the conflicts never lasted more than a few moments, as they usually ended when one of the parties—the one committing the original offence—cracked a joke, laughed, and moved on.

Relationships

The portrait of the Fanm Tèt Ansanm office and the typical daily life inside it suggests several patterns in relationships. Confronted ethnographically, NGOs are fragmented and contradictory (Hilhorst 2003:5,146; Kaag 2008:15). Both this ethnographic sketch and Fanm Tèt Ansanm employees' own analyses testify to two competing sets of characterizations of the intra-office relationships. On the one hand, the work is divided among five distinct spheres: the ti pèsonnèl, the front office, the middle office, the back office, and the clinic. In addition, this division of labor is hierarchical, and relationships are partly shaped by divisions of class. On the other hand, in practice there is also an extraordinary degree of cooperation, especially within each of the five work units but sometimes across them. In addition, most of the staff characterized their relationships with their coworkers and supervisors in familial terms.

First, the five different units within Fanm Tèt Ansanm operated in separate spheres. This separation was particularly evident in the clinic. I spent whole days being absconded in the middle office and did not see a single member of the clinic staff. Occasionally, especially during lunchtime or before the afternoon rush begins, staff from the office, especially back-office staff, visited the clinic and passed time before their shift started (or resumed) by talking with clinic staff. The ti pèsonnèl often congregate in the clinic waiting room when not needed, chatting with the medanm or clinic staff. Only one of the clinic staff, the one with a college degree, frequented the office, especially after the front-office staff left for the day. Sometimes she checked her e-mail (there was no computer in the clinic) while waiting for her coworkers who live in the same city to finish, so they could walk to the tap-tap and ride together. The doctors have been known to visit the front and middle office, especially the female doctor who gave a monthly lecture to the medanm in the back office. But generally the clinic and the other programs operated independently of one another. During the worst periods of the violence, when gunshots were audible and the blokis lasted for hours, the clinic functioned more or less normally, if slightly rushed. But the training programs and meetings of the two committees were often canceled.

To a lesser extent, the three offices—front, middle, and back—were largely autonomous units, with a sharper division between the back office and the rest. Most middle-office staff were supervisors who wrote reports to donors and the government. Front-office staff prepare and submit those reports. Especially on deadline days, there was frequent traffic between the front and middle offices. A large part of NGO life, at least in Haiti, is to attend meetings with government agencies and other NGOs. Because of their long history and successful track record, Fanm Tèt Ansanm was often sought out to partner with other organizations, or at least be represented at meetings. Mme Dominique occasionally went to meetings, however most often middle-office staff represented Fanm Tèt Ansanm. Rarely, one of the back-office staff attended meetings as Fanm Tèt Ansanm's representative. The similarity between front- and middle-office staff is reproduced in the physical environments. Both the front and the middle offices were air-conditioned. Most of the chairs in these two offices had padding. And the computers were all located in the front or middle offices. Mme Dominique or middle-office staff people rarely made contact with the medanm, and the medanm almost never walked through the front or middle offices. The difference in staff and recipients' perceptions about "participation" (discussed in the previous chapter) might be a function of their physical separation and lack of contact, caused by this role specialization.

This distinction in function, collaboration, and physical environment all attest to hierarchy. Much of the physical/infrastructural resources were concentrated in the front and middle offices. The physical temperature is an indicator of status. It was coolest in the director's office, followed by the front office, middle office, back office, and clinic. Working outside, or over a boiling pot, the ti pèsonnèl have the hottest workspace. Everyone in the front office had a computer, and there were five computers for six people in the middle office. Especially considering that Fanm Tèt Ansanm has to pay for diesel to power the electricity, this is a significant distinction in who consumes resources. Interactions between staff of different zones highlight inequality structuring the relationships. The hotter temperature, the less-maintained bathrooms, and the harder chairs for the medanm and the staff who help them, all reinforce "*tout moun se moun, men tout moun pa menm"*: everyone is a person, but not everyone is equal.

In addition to spatial practice, inequality was reinforced by language. Language serves as a marker of class in Haiti. The titles people are given reveal deeply held, persistent practices of inequality. Ti pèsonnèl referred to the front- and middle-office staff people as "Miss" so-and-so, suggesting deference or at least formality. Clinic staff selectively used this title. Many call their supervisor "Miss" (first name), and two of the front office staff people were "Madame" (last name). Back-office staff often hailed their immediate supervisor as "Madame" (last name). This title was most often used in reference to a single middle-office staff person.[12] Interestingly, middle-office staff people often referred to Mme Dominique by her first name. Front- and middle-office staff were all on first-name bases with one another. They only used titles for the doctors.

This hierarchy suggested by language was reproduced through interactions and daily practice. Anytime a ti pèsonnèl happened to walk past a front-, middle-, and even back-office staff person, she can be hailed and given a task. This explains why they would "hide" in the clinic where most of the medanm would hang out. One ti pèsonnèl told me, "Not only one person can reprimand you. Everyone can reprimand you, you understand?" One middle-office staff in particular almost never left her desk. She had the kitchen staff heat up and serve her lunch, which she often brought from home. When she needed something, even from her coworkers in the middle office, they went to her. Another staff person had this critique of Fanm Tèt Ansanm: "People come from different places, they're from different social status [kouch]. You have the impression, there are people, I hear the way they talk that they sound annoyed. It's, I don't feel that at the top perhaps, people who are at the head, take account of this too much." Notice the hesitation in the language; aside from an interview with a particular staff member who later had a conflict with Mme Dominique, and another referenced below, this was the only specific critique voiced in class terms. This might have been a reflection of people's lower level of comfort with me (particularly compared to Sove Lavi, many of whom I had traveled with on several missions), or the fact that I had a formal protocol with Fanm Tèt Ansanm that was communicated via people's supervisors.

Gender is also an organizing principle for staff interaction. All but five employees were women. Tellingly, men performed roles culturally gendered masculine: doctors, guards, and chauffeurs. Fanm Tèt Ansanm hired a female doctor, but she is not a gynecologist, the most important specialty given the organization's focus on women's reproductive health. Previously, they had a female gynecologist who fled the country after being kidnapped. The house-keeping and kitchen staff, traditionally feminine gendered roles, were all women. Interestingly, all the trainers, public health auxiliaries, program managers, and administrators were women, an expression of Fanm Tèt Ansanm's female-empowerment mission. "Gap-filler" NGOs that are replacing feminized social service functions of the state tend also to be feminized. This provides culturally sanctioned leadership roles for women as NGO directors, many of whom, like Mme Dominique, either come from or are married into traditional business elite families.[13]

Despite this inequality reproduced by spatial, linguistic, and interactional practice at Fanm Tèt Ansanm (cf. Bourdieu 1980; de Certeau 1984), there was also a high level of cooperation. One of the ti pèsonnèl told me that "compared to other places in Haiti, there are fewer problems at Fanm Tèt Ansanm." The fact that Haiti's extreme inequalities circumscribed daily life at Fanm Tèt Ansanm is not surprising, given the country's intense social divisions. As one ti pèsonnèl put it, "The main obstacle to development in Haiti is the class struggle." It bears mentioning that most of the medanm think very highly of the group, and that despite the compounded and complex contemporary crisis, Fanm Tèt Ansanm was still highly functional.

Many people told me that Fanm Tèt Ansanm's "team spirit" is its strength and the source of its stability, why people chose to work there for a long time, in direct contrast to Sove Lavi. Written communication from Fanm Tèt Ansanm was a collaborative process. Grant applications, the journal, and the reports are shared, read, discussed, debated, and corrected by all middle-office staff. These exchanges were lively and spirited. In addition, the middle office was mostly egalitarian (beyond the practice of one person holding court, the only one with the "Mme" title). Especially when there were fewer computers, I never knew who was directing the chaotic process of finishing a report. The same cooperation was true of the back office; if someone was sick or if violence in the streets prevented her from being there, others filled in without much of a problem.

And as mentioned above, the celebrations that bring together the medanm and reinforce their solidarity were the products of everyone's labor that day. Additionally, the process appeared organic; people seemed to instinctively know their roles without much formal organization, and the celebration's organizer or emcee changed from event to event. It is true that the ti pèsonnèl did more of the manual labor, and they were the ones serving food and drinks at events. But most everyone was involved in some aspect of the process. The solidarity and unity promoted by the rituals, especially the songs, was prefigured by the collective, seemingly organic labor of putting it together. There was one notable exception to this sharing: except for Mme Dominique's occasional appearance, front-office staff rarely attended the actual events.

All Fanm Tèt Ansanm employees likened it to a family and not just a job. This is related to the cooperation and team spirit just discussed. This familial analogy explains the longevity of employees' tenure at Fanm Tèt Ansanm. Most people worked at Fanm Tèt Ansanm for more than five years, many more than ten, and a few almost twenty. Edele said, "I am a quitter. I usually don't stay along very long at a job. But Fanm Tèt Ansanm is like a family to me. I haven't left. I can't leave because I feel that this is my family, my home." Even during the political crisis, when people "run to return home by five," staff people who lived in neighboring areas waited for others to finish so they could ride the same tap-tap. Middle-office staff with cars gave others rides home or to a place where they could walk home relatively safely, past the dangerous neighborhoods and intersections along the way. A few ti pèsonnèl confided that they had a good relationship with everyone, including the administration. Whenever they were in a financial bind, caused by the crises of poverty and poor health care and educational systems, they felt they could go to front- or middle-office staff for help, similar to Sove Lavi staff helping out CAC members discussed in the previous chapter. Most come from the ranks of the medanm. At least in the eyes of the ti pèsonnèl, the ideology of family implied moral obligations that go beyond the job. As feminists and anthropologists have pointed out, the ideology of family often hides, or provides ideological justification for, systems of inequality (Collier and Yanagisako 1987; Crawford 2008). According to a couple of ti pèsonnèl, however, this is not mere clientelism but a socialist ethos of maternalism, a concern with people's welfare. When I asked people what Fanm Tèt Ansanm's weaknesses were, or what changes they would recommend, some lower-rung employees hoped that Fanm Tèt Ansanm would find more èd (foreign aid), because they believed that it would trickle down to them.[14]

Sove Lavi

While Haiti's extreme inequalities weighed heavily on both NGOs, they undertook different institutional responses. Sove Lavi's office was more divided than Fanm Tèt Ansanm's, with an upstairs and a downstairs staff. Distinctions between trainers — who are the public face of Sove Lavi to the aid recipients — and administration are reinforced by a physical separation. People from the different divisions can and have worked full days without seeing a member of the other. Compounding this, in direct contrast to Mme Dominique's management style that offers staff wide latitude, Mme Versailles has a more centralized approach. Further complicating this is a personnel policy that was written when Sove Lavi was still a small organization housed at their founding agency's office.

Neighborhood

The Sove Lavi office is located off a busy thoroughfare in a more established neighborhood in Pòtoprens, shared with government offices, law offices, schools, a grocery store, churches, and many private houses, many the traditional "gingerbread"—one of Haiti's hidden artistic treasures. Walking through the neighborhood on the way to the Sove Lavi office, one has to contend with fewer potholes and mud puddles, but also less pedestrian space, putting people and cars in direct competition. Several small businesses that cater to professional clients, such as restaurants, copy shops, and cyber cafes where people make Internet-based phone calls to the United States and Canada, dot the landscape. A few timachann sell automobile parts and accessories, and used clothes called "rad Kenedi."[15] Purveyors—usually men—of specialized products such as compact fluorescent light bulbs, flashlights, batteries, garden shears, or jumper cables walk up and down the street with their wares on fading plastic laundry tubs carried on their heads.

The Sove Lavi office is in a lakou protected by an eight-foot-tall rock wall with broken bottles cemented on top, and a ten-foot metal gate. Sitting outside this fence is a group of other timachann selling a variety of articles. A married couple sells cans of salt fish, milk, ketchup, and other sundries, in addition to bottles of soda and Malta (a nonalcoholic malt drink, often considered a meal) that are cooled by a hand-sized block of ice. An elderly woman sells meat, chopped up and ready to be cooked, as well as a large wicker basket full of potatoes, sweet potatoes, carrots, cabbage, eggplant, and breadfruit, depending on what was in season and whether she was able to make it to a downtown market to buy them. Next is a younger woman who sells *fritay* (fried food), such as *pate* (meat and vegetables sandwiched between two dough patties), hot dogs, plantains, bright pink summer sausages, and fish, but not *akra* (root vegetable dough), all fried in a pot of brown grease heated by a handmade charcoal stove. Next to her is a middle-aged woman selling crackers, cookies, and hard candy, and a slight, stooped woman who cooks a pot of beans and rice every day except Sunday.

Inside the lakou, surrounded on all sides by fences of either brick or stone, is a garden centered around a dried-up pool and a worn-down statue. This garden was one of the few places where I saw grass in Pòtoprens. Flowers and fruit-bearing trees also grow. Behind this garden is a cobblestone walkway up to the concrete landing, leading into the building. To the right is a long, wide, semi-paved driveway that leads to the landlord's building, a florist's shop, some seventy yards behind. The lakou is never actually vacant, as one of the timachann families spends the night in the compound, allowed to stay there for free for the measure of security that their presence provides. This is helpful given that the paid armed guard works only twelve hours per day.

The Beginning of the Day

At seven in the morning, the security guard, a tall younger man armed with his own rifle and a single bullet, typically enters the building and takes over the job of watching the place from the family, who mostly have gone outside the gates to begin cooking. The guard sits on a raised porch, on a concrete ledge, and receives visitors. Sitting atop the ledge is a cage of black lattice ironwork, with space left for a metal doorframe and door. Depending on time of day, different people keep the security guard company, most of whom are not Sove Lavi employees but timachann or neighbor day laborer men, who occasionally work for Sove Lavi. The chauffeurs and custodial staff people often hang out in the porch area in between calls for duty.

In addition to the security guard, the only people inside Sove Lavi's office building at this time of the morning are one of two (male) custodial staff, called "logistics," cleaning the office. Like others around it, the building was a traditional gingerbread with fired bricks (not the hand-fashioned cinderblocks common in newer neighborhoods) and wood trim, including beams, archways, doorways, stairways, windows, and shutters. The main entrance led to a spacious foyer, open to the ceiling. On the right was a series of soft-back chairs and double doors that were always closed leading to a conference room. On the left was an unused closet area, the backdrop for a handmade sign about the mission of the organization and a poster of two peasant children looking forlornly upward, asking in Kreyòl, "Do we not have the same right to go to school as everyone?" The children's eyes came up to my midsection. They never quite could fade into the background for me, their eyes seeming to gaze up at everyone and everything. The uneven circular staircase fronted a desk cluttered with individual sheets of paper and a computer. When it was occupied, the head of logistics sat here, dressed in a button-down shirt and often a tie, and gold-looking jewelry, including necklace, bracelet, and fake Rolex. When he was not shouting for one of his two assistants, he spoke an over-enunciated although often grammatically challenged French.

To the right from the front entrance is the conference room, where Sove Lavi held press conferences, meetings with donors or partner organizations, and in the summer of 2006, trainings for local CAC members. Spacious and tile floored, with the windows covered, this room was cool even when the air conditioner was not running. There was a large, rectangular wooden table and some thirty stackable, cushioned aluminum chairs. Until Sove Lavi hired Monsieur Lescot in a new position as director of research and development, the technical team met in the conference room. When the entire Sove Lavi staff convened—twice during my twelve months visiting—they met here. These meetings were all in French, as were the meetings of the technical team before Mme Lejeune's tenure. M. Lescot set up a small office in this room. Working off a laptop that had access to the Internet, and proficient in web searches, he took up very little space. When he began working there at the end of 2004, the room was fitted with a working air conditioner that M. Lescot had running to full capacity while he worked in his office. A self-described "early bird," M. Lescot was usually among the first staff to arrive.

Eight o'clock is the official start of the Sove Lavi workday, but usually only a handful of the thirty staff people arrived by 8:30. Hilhorst (2003:121) argued that rather than merely criticizing NGOs for not following stated rules, anthropologists should be looking for other, symbolic functions that these rules serve.

In periods of new second-tier leadership, or periods of organizational stressors, Sove Lavi administration focused anew on these organizational principles, particularly the normative workday, as concrete manifestations of organizational discipline and solvency. Twice during my period of fieldwork the administration posted an office memo typed in French[16] reminding staff of the official policy regarding work hours. The staff was more punctual for a couple of weeks following this official notice. Not everyone received the same pressure to arrive on time, however. The job of one employee in particular was at stake if he did not arrive on time, so this began his practice of driving on the wrong side of a divided, busy road in order to save some time. After the ti pèsonnèl and chauffeurs, next to arrive were usually the receptionist and the staff in the accounting office, all of whom worked on the second floor.

Upstairs Office

Like many staircases in Haiti, the one at Sove Lavi was uneven and lacked a railing. More than once I tripped as I hurried up the stairs, and I was not the only clumsy victim. The stairway led to a small landing containing an old copier that midway during my participant observation period finally died. Across from the copier sat three metal and cushion chairs, one of which was broken but never removed—so people like me sat on it and fell. This was the formal reception area that faced the office of Anne-Marie, the receptionist, six feet by eight feet, not counting a small supply closet. Anne-Marie sat facing the stairs. She was also the administrative secretary, so she wrote the official correspondence for Mme Versailles, the director (who did not have a computer and never learned to type). Anne-Marie tried to keep her desk neat, but since it was the communications hub for the organization, the spaced acquired papers and files throughout the day. Anne-Marie's desk also housed the only phone that could make calls to cell phones, so often staff came into the office to place phone calls. In addition to the desk that dominated the room, a dorm-room-sized refrigerator kept people's soft drinks cold, next to where the office's water cooler sat, albeit usually empty. Behind Anne-Marie, a usually open, large picture window looked out onto the other private houses in the neighborhood. Every ten minutes or so, Anne-Marie called for one of the logistical staff, beginning with the supervisor. She had a loud voice that could carry to the first floor. When I asked her why she didn't lean over the balcony overlooking the landing, she said with a touch of irony that her job was to staff the phones in case of a call. If the logistical supervisor was unavailable, Anne-Marie yelled for one or another of the logistical staff, beginning with the one who was officially on call (one for the mornings, one for the afternoons).

Coming up from the stairs, the accounting office was to the right. In between the two offices, in a corner of the house, was a large bathroom, with a drum of water and a bucket for flushing the toilet. Sometimes a cut-in-half bar of soap was left on the sink. People brought their own toilet paper, reflective of hyper-individual responsibility or a lack of available funds. The door to the accounting office was always closed to keep in the cold A/C air inside. The office to the left (coming from the outside) was for the administrator[17] and two assistants. The administrator sat in the farthest desk from the door. Closest to the door sat Josue, the "problem solver" or "liaison" between the technical team who went "to the field" and the administration. Josue faced the door, and the other two faced away.

Across the wooden partition sat the two accounting staff, the *chéf comptable* and the *comptable adjoint*. Between the two of them there were three desks. The hand-me-down workspaces were all different from one another. Several pieces of furniture or equipment, including a desk and one of many steel filing cabinets, had a hand-sized USAID sticker attached. A small desk to the side by the front window (this office had ample natural lighting, including a side window, which was good given the state of the city's electricity service) was the official site for the institutional memory. Atop it sat several cardboard boxes stuffed inside of which were numerous file folders.

Walking past the receptionist's alcove there was a dark, narrow hallway flanked by two offices, at the time of fieldwork[18] occupied by the Mme Versailles, the executive director, on the left, and Mme Lejeune, the technical director, on the right. The doors to these offices were nearly always closed, in part because of the newest and most powerful air-conditioning units in the office inside. The walls of Mme Versailles's office were adorned with highbrow Haitian art, original paintings by a renowned Haitian artist. One was a still life; the other two were of idealized natural settings. Mme Versailles set up the desk to face the doorway. Surrounding the recycled USAID aluminum-and-Formica desk were two potted plants. On the left side from when one walked in was a small round table with two folding chairs. This was her meeting area. On the other side of the desk was another desk that housed a computer that never worked. On the wall opposite the two large windows was a long single filing cabinet. In the back corner was another exit, a small door that led to a small restroom that only she used.

By 9:30 most of these offices were already occupied when Mme Lejeune, the technical director, came to her office. Mme Lejeune had arranged an exception to the official work-hours policy because of the distance she had to travel to get to work; she lived in the cool mountains far above Pòtoprens. Unlike at Fanm Tèt Ansanm, there is no ritual of greeting coworkers during the first visit, in part because most of the office doors—individual rooms in an old gingerbread house—were usually closed to keep the A/C inside the offices. The main door to Mme Lejeune's office—leading to the busted copier and the one busted chair (of three) waiting area at the landing of the stairs—had a lock. The office, like most others on the second floor, was well lit. Two large picture windows looked out to a large Catholic church, where many eyes were sometimes glued (including my own) during the long technical team meetings. Despite the small space carved out for the assistant, the technical director's office felt larger than the executive director's office because of its simplicity. Besides the single aluminum-and-Formica work desk, only one wooden bookshelf against an interior wall took up any space. Mme Lejeune changed its orientation, so that while she worked she faced the window, her back to visitors, unlike the previous technical director. A hardly ever used bathroom was carved into the other interior wall. When occupied, this room was cold, even by the Minnesota standards I'm used to. More than a few times, loud protests by several trainers convinced Mme Lejeune to turn down the USAID-donated remote-control air conditioner for the duration of the meeting. The painted wood floors creaked whenever someone walked on them. I often worried that with the full complement of the technical team assembled, we would fall through. But that never happened while I was there, and not since, at least until the earthquake.[19]

At the end of the long hallway was the two-room computer area. One room was for public use, with four older computers (put together with spare parts) lined up on both sides of a hand-fashioned wooden table. This room was often hot: not air-conditioned, poorly ventilated, and collecting four computers' exhaust (not to mention at least four users' sweat). After March 2005 these computers were reserved for local high school students eight hours per week, to be used for an online forum, with two or three people sharing a computer. When the youth were gone, the custodial staff or "friends" of Sove Lavi—all of them men, some of them with regular odd jobs to perform—would use these computers, all of which were wired to the Internet, albeit slow by even Haitian standards. While working at one of these computers, it was easy to tell when the EDH (public electricity) was off. If the office was being powered by a dèlko, one or another staff would kindly request that these computers shut down within the next few minutes. If it was on inverter power, or if Mme Versailles was present, the line feeding this room would be immediately cut without warning.[20]

Behind a glass wall was the mainframe, where the webmaster and a database manager worked.[21] The two windows were shut and covered by curtains when the USAID-stickered air conditioner was on. The three computers in here, two of which also marked by the sticker, were all purchased new, with up-to-date software (e.g., Microsoft Office 2003). Interestingly, we discovered that this software upgrade included automatic translation from languages such as English and French.[22] The chairs, also with stickers, were adjustable, unlike the others. When there was only inverter power on, this room still functioned, because it contained the server and the network connection. Both tech workers were self-taught. When one left to go to school in Canada, he was replaced within the month, the only non–associate director staff to have been replaced within the two prior years. Their job description was primarily to develop Sove Lavi's website, but both were valued for their problem-solving abilities as well.[23] This room was cool enough to keep the computers functional (a sign on the door implored people to close the door behind them), but not uncomfortable to the majority of the staff working there. Reflecting the hierarchy within the organizational chart, the upstairs office staff had more authority and consumed more resources. Also reinforcing their organizational specialization, the individual cellules were physically separated from one another.

Downstairs Office

In the back of the office is a very narrow concrete staircase. If one were not careful, someone of my height[24] would hit his or her head on the ceiling. This staircase led to a back porch where an unused USAID motorcycle sat for a long period. This was also the primary spot for loading and unloading: at different times it held boxes of T-shirts, radios, or office chairs for the next shipment to one of the provincial offices. There was also a giant urn whose function eluded everyone I asked. This was the entrance that timachann would use to visit the trainers, selling bananas, oranges, pineapples, onions, yams, even paintings. At least twice a day, someone would be at the doorstep, *cheche lavi* (literally "looking for life," meaning looking for a buyer), calling out to whoever was inside. As often as not, she was sent away. When she wasn't sent away, the trainers present (all but one were women) would look up from their work writing reports longhand (there were no computers downstairs until late 2005) and negotiate a price for everyone. If mutually agreeable to seller and buyers, the trainers would divide up the produce among all who purchased.

The downstairs office had three open doorways dividing three offices. Only two outlets worked in each office, enough for a single cell phone charger that trainers shared and one fan (usually pointed toward the most senior trainer). There were only two fans for the three rooms, and one did not work well. When the office was on inverter power, which occurred often during the interim period, electricity did not flow downstairs at all. The assorted desks—seven in all, some wood, some more "modern"—faced one another, facilitating conversation. Like at Fanm Tèt Ansanm though to a lesser degree, putting together reports or preparing for the next mission was a task the downstairs staff shared among whoever was present. During subsequent visits I noticed two computers were added downstairs, one relatively new. For lunch, Sove Lavi staff contracted with a timachann's thirteen-year-old child—who came to the office, also his home, after he finished school—to fetch them a Styrofoam box of food and usually a soda. Each staff had his or her favorite drink. Staff usually ate by themselves at their desks, and many continued to work while eating. Squirreled away downstairs were two other storage rooms, containing materials from Sove Lavi projects from the 1990s, but almost never things such as pens. Like toilet paper, people usually bought their own pens, or had this local youth buy one from the street. After a trip to the provinces, if there were leftover pens they would be distributed among the downstairs staff and then quickly stashed away. Often the downstairs was vacant, with staff gone on one or more missions to the provinces. Like Fanm Tèt Ansanm's back office, the structural equivalent of the downstairs office, Sove Lavi trainers functioned more collaboratively than those in the other cellules, and they were similarly marginalized. If they needed to communicate with their supervisor or the administration, downstairs staff had to walk upstairs. They did very often, attesting to a lack of autonomy that they each mentioned during interviews with me. The design of Sove Lavi's office thus engendered individualism, hierarchy, and dependence, reflected in the resources allocated and the physical space itself. This in turn shapes the relationships between coworkers.

Relationships

The first problem that CAC members complained about, Sove Lavi staff showing up late, has its roots in the Sove Lavi office. During my first "mission" to the provinces, I was told that the team would be leaving at 7:30 A.M. Not being a morning person, I took special care to be at the office by 7:30, setting my alarm clock, packing, and preparing the morning coffee the night before. Even so, it was difficult, but I made it. No one else was there besides a shirtless custodial staff person cleaning the desks and moving his makeshift bed into one of the storage areas. The guard had just arrived as I did. Where was everyone else?, I asked. They would be coming, I was assured. So I sat and waited. The majority of the team scheduled to go on the mission arrived at the office by eight o'clock, before the "upstairs" staff. By nine, the newly cleaned, leased SUV was loaded with all the materials, the food, and people's personal effects. We all sat in the trainers' office, chatting about the news of the day, the imminent soccer match between the "gods" of soccer (the Brazilian national team) and the Haitian national team.[25] By ten, most of the rest of the upstairs staff had arrived, and the dèlko was turned on. Seeing nothing else to do, I walked upstairs and turned on one of the four computers in the "lab." At noon, I was called and told that the team was going to be leaving. I ran downstairs and out to the car. No one was there. After another fifteen minutes a driver and the responsab of the mission came to the car. Where were the others?, I asked. They were getting things done; we had to go get a check signed. So we drove up to another NGO's office to get a signature on a check. And then Jeanty (the driver) and I waited while the responsab went to the bank. Jeanty, a former army officer, amused himself by catcalling women as they walked by. This tardiness was not a one-time occurrence. Every single mission that left while I was in the office was similarly late. Mme Pierre, a trainer, explained, "There's a certain slowness in the office, a little blockage. I am not aware of why. There's a whole series of things I know nothing about." Several trainers were adamant. Yvette complained:

> All the time there is a little blockage. Some financial thing. Because of this we spend a lot of time here [in the office]. We lose time. I can't point

my finger, because we all have a role ["finger involved"]. But the biggest reason is an administrative blockage. We *mache twòp* [literally "walk too much," or go from place to place without resolving anything]. We sit in the office for two hours, three hours, even four hours or more. I arrived in a mission in Jakmèl. It isn't too far, but we got there after nine at night. And why? Why? Because we didn't plan it well? We weren't ready? And all these actions have consequences, like I just told you. The institution's image is diminished.

Mme Auguste lamented, "For example, we give the requisition for materials seven days in advance. It's not like the papers appeared the day we leave. Also, they always know we need money for the per diem, for gas, you understand? There's always little expenses. Why are we standing here because someone didn't go to the bank?"

Several staff, especially the "downstairs" staff, pointed to a series of bureaucratic hurdles. Nearing the end of a technical team meeting that was supposed to draft a monthly work plan, Josue came down to talk with Mme Lejeune. He wanted her to tell the group about that week's women's soccer match. Mme Lejeune said that she didn't have enough information about it, and asked if he could talk about it to the group. Dripping with sarcasm, Mme Lejeune said to the trainers that she was sure they were aware of this already, but this week there will be a soccer match. Many people voiced their concern about not being *okouran* (literally "in the current"). This was the first time that staff had heard about it. So Josue, the liaison between the technical team and the administration, began: There is a soccer match. And just like the symposium (discussed in the previous chapter), Mme Versailles is counting on everyone's participation. We need you all involved. When is it?, someone asked. This Thursday (the meeting was on Monday) at 2:30. Josue said that we need to invite all the CAC members from the whole province. It's important. A trainer asked if there were any other details. Josue didn't know them. He had to go back upstairs.

This capped a meeting in which they were discussing the failure to open two of three community centers. In one particular location, schools were dropping out of the program. One reason cited was the lack of respect for meeting times. All three staff in this provincial office commuted from Pòtoprens, and they were all habitually late. This protest by the local community followed others. The center was not yet operational despite the opening ceremony five months prior. This, combined with a new and then energetic technical director, rendered the repeated tardiness a topic of continued discussion. This December 2004 meeting was the first in which trainers attempted to address the structural constraints of their job. The meeting had gone on for two and a half hours at this point, and Mme Lejeune dutifully took notes (with the help of a visiting anthropologist) to take to Mme Versailles.

Josue came back down the stairs, mentioning the name of a consultant Mme Versailles hired to set up the event, and then a list of the activities. Mme Versailles will be giving a word of welcome. We will also give out T-shirts. And trophies. Lunise, the newest trainer hired, brought up the idea that it would be a good opportunity to pass out HIV/AIDS-prevention literature, triggering a discussion about the quality of their materials. One person objected that their materials were only in French, and as such excluded most of the youth they would be targeting. Not appearing to take note, Josue continued by saying they were expecting between three and five thousand people. Georges questioned the logic of the location because Sove Lavi had no ongoing projects in the capital. Ignoring this, Josue said that Sove Lavi needed all the trainers to be able to answer the media calls this week, as we are expecting a rush of media for this event. And then he returned upstairs. Several trainers cited this as a prime example of the brusque communication style in the office, at once highlighting the stakes of the meeting's discussion topic and ending conversation, since they all suddenly had urgent tasks put on their plates.

Three days later this event took place. It garnered some media coverage, especially when Mme Versailles gave the trophy to the winning team (the underdog). She and the captain of the winning team promised to work together to involve "the sports sector" in the fight against HIV/AIDS. The captain of the sports team did not repeat the part of the pledge where Mme Versailles focused on abstinence. To my knowledge (based on the Sove Lavi website and the reports I read), this pledge did not materialize into any ongoing collaboration. Despite this, it was the lead story of the sports broadcast for Radyo Ginen and apparently several others. This success at garnering media attention was facilitated by Sove Lavi's structure, which involved media organizations as members of the alliance. The official report said that four thousand youth attended the event, receiving training on HIV/AIDS education and some other materials (such as a box of three Pantè condoms).[26] The report's declaration flew in the face of the facts, but this ability to rewrite history is a central tool within "bureaucraft" (James 2010).

The soccer match started at 4:30, two hours late and an hour before dusk. Several CAC members—a group of about fifteen women—performed a traditional dance during halftime. Despite the fact that the periods were cut short, there was no time for Sove Lavi staff to conduct the educational portion of the event. December 2004 was one of the scariest months in terms of gun violence, so the crowd did in fact leave before it was too dark. Just before the halftime show, I took a photo (see figure 3.1) that shows no more than three hundred people present. Frustrated, the trainers took it on themselves to do their jobs during the second period while people were watching the game. Judging from the focus of the crowd on the match itself, very few people paid any attention to the trainers, until one of them decided to begin handing out condoms. They had

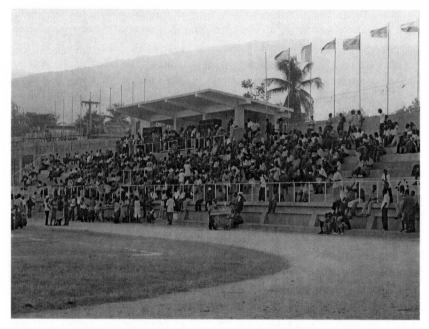

FIGURE 3.1 Crowd reported to be four thousand people at Sove Lavi soccer match/
AIDS training, December 2004. Photo by author.

planned to give them to all "age-appropriate" spectators (i.e., over twenty-three,
since the point was supposedly about abstinence, a fact that Josue told the
group that morning) as they collected the five-goud entrance fee (a little more
than ten cents), an idea they abandoned when staff had arrived almost two
hours after the official start of the match and the crowd was already there.
Suddenly, a noisy group of adolescent males crowded around Lunise, who was by
far the youngest of the staff. In desperation, and to fend off the insults or sexual
come-ons, Lunise threw a box up in the air. All semblance of order shattered at
that point, and the youths took what condoms they could get their hands on.[27]
The French-language materials were trampled on. Mme Versailles declared it
time to return, so the match went into sudden death, with each team attempting penalty shots. It was already dark at this point. One woman managed to
score a goal, edging out the other team, the national women's league champi-
ons, 1–0. Mme Versailles held a brief ceremony and then the Sove Lavi staff
rushed home, leaving the crumpled pamphlets scattered about for the next
crowd to read. Mme Versailles hailed the event a success, and Josue quickly
agreed. The pair left in Sove Lavi's new jeep with Mme Versailles's son. The rest
of the staff took the rented bus back to Pòtoprens, making light of what the rest
of the staff viewed as a clear failure—examples of *chan pwen* (Averill 1997; Smith
2004) or what James C. Scott (1990) called "hidden transcripts."

Staff Analyses: Crisis Management and Lack of Autonomy

This soccer match was to many Sove Lavi staff emblematic of *gestion de crise* (crisis management). According to Lunise, "When things are done in a hierarchical manner, when someone's at the head, you are always waiting. When they need you they will call you, or when you need them you seek them out. Sometimes, the communication isn't sufficient, because there is always some fear or something else stopping you because of the hierarchy." A former Sove Lavi deputy director said that as with many other NGOs in Haiti, Mme Versailles treats it as her own personal business (ARS Progretti 2005:22). This attitude is demonstrated in the way Mme Versailles demands everyone's involvement at the last minute. Mme Lejeune complained, "It's always at the last minute that an urgent question arises. Very often it is a question of money. So, for the moment, I am just managing the day-to-day." This staff concern mirrors the frustration CAC members feel with their lack of participation in the planning, conceptualizing, or defining of the problems and programs on the ground. All these issues have the same source: an autocratic leadership style. During these periods of gestion de crise in which the entire Sove Lavi staff becomes involved in a common task, working overtime for days on end, the organizational chart flattens, making distinctions of rank or seniority less important. These are also times for individual staff to display their loyalty to Mme Versailles. As with Duvalier's dreaded secret police, the *tonton makout* (Diederich and Burt [1970] 2005; Ferguson 1987), this loyalty determined the "latent" or de facto hierarchy, regardless of how the organizational chart outlines the official or "manifest" hierarchy. But unlike at Fanm Tèt Ansanm, individual staff did not have the autonomy to conduct their own planning. Mme Auguste explained, "I am not autonomous because even if you plan out an activity, there's always something that needs to happen: 'Here's what we need to do! Here's how you have to do it!' And we truly lack autonomy." During these periods of crisis management, the only way to command another's time was in the name of Mme Versailles. When two people's directives conflicted, they had to seek her out to resolve the issue, and nothing could be done in the mean time. Autonomy is easier to identify in its absence: people sitting, waiting to talk with Mme Versailles; the downstairs staff's several trips upstairs to resolve a technical issue; or a fully loaded SUV that could not leave the office because the mission responsab had to obtain approval or a signature.

This lack of intra-office autonomy spelled out other problems as well. Internal issues partially explain the conflicts Sove Lavi had with CAC members described in the previous chapter. Lamented Yvette, "My heart is not happy, not only because we let people in the community down, but because there is no reason for it." Mme Auguste said, "We [trainers] are the face of Sove Lavi to the communities." These downstairs staff who go on missions are aware of these conflicts and try to do something. Said Mme Pierre, "They ask you for a badge, a certificate, which is something simple. It's nothing; we could do it ourselves.

In mission reports we write that people were asking for a badge or a certificate that states that they participated in the training. But Sove Lavi never gave them a certificate." I have seen these requests made in several follow-up reports. But in the summer of 2006, two years after the program had ended, this apparent lack of respect still stung for CAC members. Georges continued, "We go to all the small towns. We sit down and speak with people. However, very often, when people present their requests, you are powerless to respond. For example, people complain that the transportation stipend is too small. Sometimes you realize that it really is too small, but that's how the project is written, you understand?" This is related to employees' own frustrations with having to bring their own toilet paper or pens to work because Sove Lavi did not provide them. Regardless of whether it is actually true in practice, staff feel "powerless." When asked to pinpoint the problem or offer solutions, many said that they wished they had more autonomy. Barring this, they wished for better lines of communication between the technical team who represent Sove Lavi to the communities and the unseen administration, working upstairs in the office.

These problems were the subject of the report from a contractor, who had conducted a "SWOT" analysis[28] by interviewing most of the same staff. The French-language report called for open lines of communication, clearly defined roles, and a restructuring of the office. M. Lescot was hired as a result. Some of the contractor's analyses were a bit different, however: "We estimate that even if the institution's structure favors irresponsible behaviors, certain employees profit from this situation to not fulfill their contractual obligations, highlighting a reprehensible indiscipline." "According to certain employees," the report continued in a different section, "the institutional problem-resolution policies create frustrations because most often, in order to resolve a problem, the responsible party is cornered in front of his subordinates." This last quotation suggests that at least some of the responsabs are aware that problems exist. When I was at Sove Lavi from June 2004 to May 2005, six people were let go, and three more left willingly.[29] Given Haitian labor law that grants de jure protections to workers, many NGOs opt to treat new employees as contractors, such as the administrator, technical director, and research and development director. Once the one-year contract expires, the NGO has no legal obligation to the contractor. This had a chilling effect on dissent, as the quote above on hierarchy suggests. This fear of speaking up is by no means unique to Sove Lavi; in a country with a 70 percent employment rate, people lucky enough to have a desk job will very rarely act as whistle-blowers.

Like at Fanm Tèt Ansanm, different zones of the Sove Lavi work space are gendered. But Sove Lavi was much more dependent on men. As with Fanm Tèt Ansanm's director, Mme Versailles was a lighter-skinned member of Haiti's upper classes, but she was surrounded by male managers. In fact, all but one of the administrative staff were men. The only other women "upstairs staff" were

Mme Lejeune[30]—who oversaw the trainers, all but one of whom were women—and the receptionist/secretary, both roles that are traditionally gendered feminine. Like at Fanm Tèt Ansanm, Sove Lavi's chauffeurs and guards were all men, but unlike Fanm Tèt Ansanm, Sove Lavi's janitorial staff were also men. The overall effect, Mme Versailles's post as the executive director notwithstanding, is that most positions of higher authority were staffed by men, whereas women were structurally lower in the hierarchy. Thus Sove Lavi's *discrimination positive* typical of WID has limits.

Like Fanm Tèt Ansanm staff, however, Sove Lavi staff characterize their relationships with their coworkers in familial terms. According to Georges, relationships were "very, very good. We are a family. I can't tell you that we don't have little conflicts from time to time, but we have respect, we can communicate to resolve the problems." His statement was echoed by nearly every other staff member, including the janitors and chauffeurs. Mme Pierre added this following one of her critiques: "You feel like you are living in a family when you are here." Like Fanm Tèt Ansanm staff, Sove Lavi staff celebrate one another's birthdays and weddings, and help out with funerals. Many keep in good contact with one another even when they are done working. Several times when I have been "on mission," a coworker who was not on the clock called to check in on her friends. I have also eaten dinner at a trainer's house with another coworker. And when people left the institution to go to the United States or Canada, or to work at the UN, they still kept in touch.

Comparisons

Both Fanm Tèt Ansanm and Sove Lavi had highly qualified staff who have strong relationships with their coworkers, which many couch in familial terms. And both have some degree of hierarchy within them. This ideology of family and the reality of hierarchy is not a contradiction. At least in "Western" patriarchal families (e.g., Sacks 1975; Strathern 1985), families are hierarchical structures. Some families are more hierarchical than others; some are functional, while others are dysfunctional.

Fanm Tèt Ansanm is more egalitarian, with higher levels of cooperation and a higher degree of autonomy. Labor for celebrations, and even monthly reports, is organized collectively. While this collective team spirit animates the work of Sove Lavi's downstairs staff, there is a persistent divide between upstairs and downstairs staff and different organizational cultures. The upstairs is more formal and businesslike, and they consume the bulk of the organizational resources. The hierarchy within Sove Lavi, the upstairs/downstairs divide, was more noticeable than the front office/back office divide at Fanm Tèt Ansanm. While it is true that some back office or clinic staff at Fanm Tèt Ansanm get to work without passing the front or middle offices, most at least say hello when they arrive. Sove Lavi's upstairs staff can work an entire day without seeing any-one downstairs, unless a trainer comes up to fill out a requisition for an upcom-ing mission. This hierarchy can be heard as well when Mme Versailles opens her door and calls out Anne-Marie's name. Within minutes, Anne-Marie calls for one of the downstairs staff. Often one of the logistical staff is also summoned a few minutes later. Most telling is the differences in autonomy. Work at Sove Lavi is far more centralized than at Fanm Tèt Ansanm. It is possible that these are just idiosyncratic, the differences between two individual working styles. When Fanm Tèt Ansanm's director, Mme Dominique, is away, the only sign is an occasional backlog in reports going out. However, if Mme Versailles is gone for even a couple of days, work all but stops.

These different organizational cultures partially explain differences in the relationships each NGO have with their service populations. Fanm Tèt Ansanm has more space for aid-recipient participation. There seems to be a correlation between this and the internal dynamics of the Fanm Tèt Ansanm staff. On the other hand, at Sove Lavi there are low levels of community participation and similarly low levels of staff autonomy. The same processes—communications and other bureaucratic blockages—diminish community participation and staff autonomy.

What accounts for these differences between Fanm Tèt Ansanm and Sove Lavi? Is it just the question of the personal styles of the directors? Both directors are lighter skinned, both have a master's degree, and both are fluent in both Spanish and French (but not English). Both married into an elite family and even hail from the same part of Haiti. NGO researchers argue that "dysfunc-tional organizational behavior is likely to be a rational response to systematic and predictable institutional pressures" (Cooley and Ron 2002:6). The next chapter explores this question of the differences between the two organizations in greater depth, examining the relationships they have with those "above" them—with the Haitian government and their donor organizations.

4

"We Are Prisoners!"

Relationships from "Above"

We are prisoners!

–Mme Pierre, frontline Sove Lavi staff

Monday, January 17, 2005, 7:12 P.M.

The technical team meeting was postponed to 1:30 to coincide with a 2:30 meeting that was supposed to take place for Kanaval and filling out the weekly work plan. This 2:30 meeting never happened. Josue was supposed to come to the technical team meeting to help the trainers think of what is realistic. But he never did. Instead, he insisted, twice, that people fill out the weekly plan of action, repeating, "It is urgent."

Apparently this meeting cancellation—and the insistence on the weekly action plan—is because the Global Fund called today. Either that or Mme Versailles just told Mme Lejeune about the meeting today. The Global Fund wants a meeting tomorrow. All the staff were shocked that the Global Fund would want to know, week by week, when things are going to be happening. What donor organization wants a weekly work plan as to how a project will be completed? Mme Lejeune, ordinarily a proponent of participation, said, "This isn't a meeting to change the plan. It's a meeting to plan how we're going to execute the project and when. The decisions are already made."

Mme Lejeune asked the downstairs staff to go home and read the already-approved plan for the Global Fund, and read the weekly work plan, so that tomorrow morning at 8:30 people can be ready to have a quick meeting. But there were problems with the printer, so they needed to be sent to a copy shop. But Mme Lejeune didn't have money, so I offered to pay the twenty-five goud. Since it was before four o'clock, it was possible to get it done, but Anne-Marie schooled me, saying that it's too late to make copies and that it can wait until morning. I didn't want to be in the middle of it. "Participation" often means co-optation to do a supervisor's work.

Tuesday, January 18, 2005, 2:42 P.M.

In the Sove Lavi office. Again it's pretty tense. People are complaining.

So the 8:30 meeting actually started around 9:45 and went nonstop until almost 1:00, when people needed to stop to take a break. They were putting together their plan: how many materials they need, when are they doing such and such, week by week.

The plan looked almost unrealistically ambitious. And a lot of work got dumped on Josiane. Josiane and Mme Lejeune had a bit of a run-in every now and again about how things are supposed to work. Again, Mme Lejeune said that it was not the time to revise the plan—since the Global Fund wouldn't allow it—but to specify it. Christian, the database manager, was also at the meeting, to get a sense of what his work was to be. He got a ton of work dumped on him, too, several surveys as well as lots of work collecting statistics about how many people attend the center, the trainings, and so forth. Since it was Christian's first time at a technical team meeting, he interjected over and over again that he was frustrated at the lack of uniformity in the forms, the multiplicity of forms, and mostly their not being filled out. So it appears that they need to have a discussion about these items.

After the meeting broke up, Mme Lejeune was handed a sheet of paper from the Global Fund. Today, they informed Sove Lavi of how they revised the NGO's annual plan—for a meeting later today—even though Sove Lavi had given them a first draft of the annual work plan two months ago, on November 9, and the second, revised plan on November 15. Mme Lejeune said, "Take note of this, Mark. It's very important for your research. Look at the relationship between the NGO and the donor group."

"Decisions Are Already Made"

As we have just seen, Sove Lavi's leadership style tends toward crisis management. We also have seen several bureaucratic blockages. This story directly from my fieldnotes offers a clue as to why: very strict, last-minute, top-down dictates from one of Sove Lavi's donors, the Global Fund to Fight AIDS, Tuberculosis, and Malaria.

What accounts for the vast differences between the hierarchies within Sove Lavi and Fanm Tèt Ansanm? While it is tempting to pin all this on the two directors' personal styles, their behaviors and management approaches are rewarded—or punished—by the institutions "above" them. So for clues to explain the difference in participation and autonomy we need to examine the NGOs' relationships with institutions above them. This chapter completes the analysis of the two NGOs' civic infrastructure, comparing relationships between the two NGOs and the Haitian government, and relationships between the NGOs and their donors.

Relationships with the Government

In a report for the World Bank, Alice Morton (1997:40) characterized the relationship between the NGO sector and the governments of Préval and Aristide as a "cold war." My interviews during preliminary fieldwork in 2002—long before the coup—also attested to this: only one person out of nineteen NGOs reported a constructive relationship with the Haitian government, and two others provided an ambiguous answer. Taking a broader view, this hostility—expressed as noncommunication and a back-and-forth struggle for control—has characterized most of Haiti's history with NGOs (Étienne 1997; Mathurin et al. 1989).

"Cold War"

Morton (1997:40) wrote that since the founding of the office of NGO coordination, the "MPCE [Ministère de la Planification et Coopération Externe, or Ministry of Planning] has been trying ever since to either monitor or control NGO activities in Haiti." On the other hand, a former Haitian minister of social affairs argued that the phenomenon of international funding going directly to NGOs that have no public mandate makes it hard for the government to establish priorities, and ultimately undermines the state's ability to govern: "Haiti's biggest problem is that the tail is wagging the dog" when it comes to foreign aid. When I asked if the MPCE could speed up the process for NGOs—some of whom had been waiting for years for formal recognition, a common complaint—a staff member told me, "Don't forget that the Haitian government does not have much money." MPCE staff had not been paid for seven months. So why not streamline the process, make fewer steps for NGOs to follow? I asked. "Our work is very important," the staff member replied. "The Haitian government alone has the authority to plan for Haitian development. NGOs are good, but they do not have a mandate. Only the government has a mandate."

This conflict over jurisdiction and authority is expressed in many ways. It took months for a container of supplies bound for an organization not officially recognized as an NGO to clear inspections at customs. Recalled the group's executive director, "I was ready to give up, to let them have it," rather than pay the tax on it that only NGOs are exempt from. "We're a charity. Why does the government do this?" The MPCE has the ability to revoke the NGO status of a group if it "does not respect the law." Some NGOs resented the requirements by the Haitian government. Another director said that the government "just wants to know that I was punished with the [annual] report. They just want to feel like they're in control."

The climate of competition is also fostered by practices of large, foreign NGOs. Morton (1997:25) notes a trend in NGOs "raiding" government ministries for employees, "even though the length of [NGO] contracts is short, and there are relatively few good technicians in the government left to 'raid' in the GOH

[Government of Haiti]." NGO staff are better paid than their government counterparts. A twenty-year veteran of the Ministry of Agriculture estimated that
with the same amount of money, the government could do nine times the
amount of work that an NGO could do.[1] Salaries for NGO professionals tend to
be competitive with those for college-educated professionals in the United
States, whereas government salaries are calibrated against Haiti's minimum
wage. Tellingly, this Ministry of Agriculture veteran left his post to work for an
NGO because of a higher salary. Several people have told me that, compared to
government offices, and certainly compared to the majority of Haitians, who
live in poverty, NGO staff are *gran manjè* ("big eaters," the Kreyòl equivalent of
"fat cats"). As one activist passionately explained, "NGOs live in luxury, with
new cars and big air-conditioned offices that just get bigger and bigger, and
what do we get? We're supposed to be grateful for everything." Haiti is not an
outlier case; many world systems theorists see the issue of NGOs taking over
governmental roles as the cornerstone of globalization's erosion of Southern
states' sovereignty (Houtart 1995; Kamat 2003; Leve and Karim 2001; Petras
1997). The situation following the earthquake highlighted donors' near total
exclusion of the Haitian government in favor of NGOs: less than 1 percent of U.S.
funds went to the government (Katz 2010a). Overall, these sets of practices
amount to a "brain drain" of Haiti's public sector. For example, 74.5 percent of
want ads in August 2004 in Haiti's largest and oldest daily newspaper, *Le
Nouvelliste*, were for NGOs or international organizations (Schuller 2009). Of the
remainder, 20 percent were for private-sector jobs and 5.5 percent for positions
within Haiti's government.

This environment of competition is not limited to NGOs and the Haitian
government; on many occasions NGO directors told me that they do not have a
relationship with other NGOs. When I asked why, in some cases the answer was
blunt. One director told me, "There's a fear that they will take our resources and
sources of foreign aid away from us." There may be some interesting sectoral
differences, as staff from all but one women's NGO told me about a vast network
of other women's NGOs, in which they share ideas and strategies. But clearly
there is at least a discourse of competition for limited foreign resources and a
fear of working too closely with other NGOs. As argued in the book's conclusion,
this concern has only magnified since the earthquake.

There was a brief thaw in the cold war in the early 1980s, as Jean-Claude
Duvalier orchestrated a massive restructuring of Haiti's government and economy (Étienne 1997; Mathurin et al. 1989). The ongoing hostility was again
tempered during the Latortue period, at least during the first several months.
One possible reason for this might be the interim government's composition;
some people called it a "nongovernmental government." Several ministers in
the interim government came from high positions in foreign NGOs, including
Bernard Gousse from the International Foundation for Electoral Systems,

Danielle St. Lot from Creative Associates International; and, of course, the government was headed by Gérard Latortue, a UN retiree. It should be emphasized that this period of intentional goodwill did not last, but this was the political context surrounding my research with Fanm Tèt Ansanm and Sove Lavi.

Fanm Tèt Ansanm

Like many NGOs, Fanm Tèt Ansanm had an ambivalent relationship with the government. On the one hand, they worked alongside several agencies, particularly those engaged in HIV/AIDS issues. On the other hand, Fanm Tèt Ansanm denounced what they saw as government's corruption or failure to protect workers, like Lisette's situation with OFATMA discussed in chapter 2.

While Fanm Tèt Ansanm occasionally critiqued particular governmental practices, they refrained from denouncing individuals within the government. Mme Dominique made this distinction perfectly clear: "Extremist feminists [engage in] actions that we can't join. Given their political character, many times we don't participate with them, because there are political actions we can't take because of our NGO status." This noninvolvement stance earned them a degree of respect from both the government and some international donor agencies that I spoke with, and it might help to explain their longevity. But it also drew the ire of other women's organizations, which had sided with Aristide's opposition. KONAP (Kòdinasyon Nasyonal k ap Plede Kòz Fanm, or the National Coordination of Women's Advocacy Organizations) had been an early, vocal critic of Aristide's, hardening its stance throughout his second (often referred to as his third)[2] term (2001–2004). In fact, KONAP had openly called for Aristide to resign, in the name of Haiti's women's movement.[3] Fanm Tèt Ansanm had to pull their support from the coalition as a result. "It wasn't appropriate for us," Mme Dominique explained. "We are here to work." Staff had heated debates on the topic, and while individuals had differing opinions they did not act on them as a group. Eventually, as discussed in chapter 1, the opposition gained momentum, succeeding in their goal of Aristide's removal on February 29, 2004. Throughout the crescendo leading up to Aristide's forced departure, Fanm Tèt Ansanm continued to stay open, providing their educational and health services to *medanm*. They were among the few women's NGOs that continued—or even attempted—to function in this period. Of course there were days when it was not safe to travel in Pòtoprens and Fanm Tèt Ansanm staff could not make it to the office to open the clinic. The factories were also shut down, however, leaving workers at home, so the NGO's closure did not have a big impact.

During the 2004–2006 interim period, Fanm Tèt Ansanm's relationship to the government was distant and professional. According to Mme Dominique, "We do our work, and we let the state do theirs." When I asked if it was hostile or competitive, she quickly said that they do share information, and indeed they are members of a couple of governmental work groups, especially related to public health. Mme Dominique described the relationship as cooperative: "Regarding the government, certainly with Public Health and the Minister of Planning, I can say that, whenever I need, when I call them, they always respond."

Sove Lavi

I first contacted Sove Lavi during the last stage of the 2004 coup. By the time I met with Mme Versailles to discuss my research, the government had already changed, so I only knew about Sove Lavi's relationship with the interim Latortue/Alexandre government. I began my research with Sove Lavi in earnest during May 2004, and maintained close contact for a twelve-month period. During this time, Sove Lavi had an active working relationship with the interim government on many levels. According to Mme Versailles, "I can say that with the state, our relation is very, very good. Very good. And we work, you see, to support what the state is doing. And can't I say in the same way they help us, we help them as well?"

During the symposium discussed in chapter 2, several government ministers and top-level "secretaries" were highlighted, notably the minister of public health, the minister of women's condition and rights, the secretary of state for education, the chief of the inter-sectorial AIDS team, and the secretary of youth and sports. They thanked Sove Lavi, the audience, the donor representatives, and one another for their presence. Their prepared speeches primarily served a ritual function, to give a sense of importance to the event, to show that the interim government was present and accounted for, and to signal the importance to the government of the feminization of AIDS and fighting violence against women. Their presentations, some of which were written by Sove Lavi staff, promised the support and "accompaniment" of the interim government in these matters, in establishing the issues as "national priorities." Sove Lavi's director sat in the center, in between the government officials and the donor representatives, at least one of whom was always present. The president of the republic was unable to attend, and one of the ministers passed along his message of support.[4] The VIP luncheon I was shuttled into during the final day was full of government representatives, a few of whom had attended the entire symposium.

This close collaboration with the interim government existed beyond the scope of the three-day event. Almost once a week Sove Lavi staff met with one of the two ministries with whom they worked most closely, education and health. Usually Mme Versailles did not go, except if it was an event to which the public or the media was invited. Attending these meetings was a task usually delegated to one of the "senior trainers," even though some staff grumbled that it was never a part of their official job description. Three times during my participant observation period, a representative of the government had an official meeting with Mme Versailles. These meetings were usually jovial and lively. Often Mme Versailles would yell across the hall for one of her staff, the technical director, the accountant, or a trainer that happened to be present, to join them, to offer needed information, or to answer a particular question. On several occasions when I went to the office, when I was looking for a *ti benefis* (fringe benefit) of some Internet time, a government employee was on the computer that I was accustomed to using. The first time I saw the person, he (they were always male) would get up and offer me his spot. The Sove Lavi staff on hand pointed out that while I was a *blan*, I was not with the UN or USAID, so he should feel free to continue using the computer. Invariably, the second time I saw this person, he knew that I was not a donor, so there was no need to kowtow. Over the year that I frequented the Sove Lavi office, I encountered eight such government officials.

Sove Lavi also made efforts to incorporate government staff into its work. The "community liaisons" of a couple of its centers were actually local government officials. Like the volunteer CAC members, Sove Lavi staff were chosen to facilitate the NGO's integration into the local community and power structure. Especially during the first contact with schools or other local organizations to discuss the program, the liaison's name recognition and official post indeed helped Sove Lavi accomplish this task. Local people—school directors, pastors, and community leaders—referred to the liaison by a deferential title based on his[5] official government position, "inspector" or "director." Whether the employees were "double dipping" or whether they were doing official government business was unclear, despite my questions. But I was able to observe role conflict, as the person did side business while acting in Sove Lavi's official capacity and on the clock. For example, during a mission to introduce the program in which the community liaison/inspector participated, the other Sove Lavi staff (as well as myself) waited in the SUV for half an hour while he met with the school director regarding his other business. We were therefore late to our next event. The inspector did not even feel it necessary to apologize or even explain to his coworkers what he was doing (but he answered a direct question from a foreign anthropologist). He was just *brase*—maintaining his network ties (literally "stirring").

Structuring the collaboration and the sharing of organizational resources, including human resources, was a juridical/structural relationship between the government and Sove Lavi. In the strictest legal sense, Sove Lavi was not an NGO but a "public utility" granted a license to operate in the government's name. But to the outside world, including donors who did not fund the Aristide government, Sove Lavi functioned like an NGO. M. Lescot had the following analysis: "The way Sove Lavi is now, what I am looking at now, is not Sove Lavi for me. OK? For me, it is like a person at Mardi Gras. In other words, he or she puts on a mask, okay, he or she dances in Carnival. But it is not the person at all. Because the type of organization that Sove Lavi is, is not what it has become today. It does not do what it is supposed to. It is in disaccord, in disharmony, with its mission." M. Lescot, who had over a decade of experience in the NGO and donor sectors, understood this shift of Sove Lavi "masquerading" as an NGO as part of a historical process. Several other coalitions or umbrella organizations in Morton's taxonomy (1997:iii), certainly other donor-funded entities, gradually became NGOs as they began to create their own programs and compete with their member organizations for donor funding. The Haitian Association of Voluntary Agencies (HAVA), a USAID-created coalition group that was founded to coordinate NGO activities, share information, and lobby the Haitian government for regulatory reform, was a highly visible example of this tendency. Yet HAVA too closed its doors after it lost funding. One NGO director was more direct: "Essentially, we follow the money."

As Sove Lavi was founded as a public utility of the Haitian government, three ex officio seats on Sove Lavi's policymaking board were reserved for the same government ministries discussed above, the Ministries of National Education, Youth, and Sports; Social Affairs and Work; and Public Health and Population. According to Sove Lavi's charter and bylaws, this board—the Conseil d'Administration—was required to meet quarterly. Other members of the board were supposed to be elected by the Assemblé Générale (General Assembly) at its annual meeting. During the year that I worked with Sove Lavi, there were no meetings of the board or the General Assembly. According to staff, as of December 2005, there had not been a meeting of the General Assembly since 2003 and probably earlier. While there are several explanations for this, including the political crisis that surrounded Sove Lavi and everything it did, the situation was significant. Sove Lavi's disconnect from its formal decision-making structures occurred during the massive influx of funding from USAID and the Global Fund (Paul and Israel 1991; Thomas-Slayter 1992; Uvin 1996). The last time Sove Lavi's general assembly met to define their policy and strategy, the organization still had only one office, fewer staff, and fewer programs. This meant that all of Sove Lavi's distance learning initiatives, guides, centers, and Caravan took place without formal discussion or approval. As a result, Mme Versailles assumed much greater latitude and control of the organization's operations during this period, which provides a partial explanation for the problems of communication, participation, and autonomy noted in the previous chapter.

Sove Lavi's Relationships with Donors

Similar to the structured collaboration between Sove Lavi and the government, Sove Lavi maintained close ties to donors. As with the three government ministries, three ex officio members of Sove Lavi's board were reserved for donors: USAID, UNICEF, and the World Health Organization. As mentioned in chapter 2, donors were given a prominent place in the symposium, including the U.S.

ambassador, whose schedule had to be accommodated, triggering a reorganization of the program.

In addition to the symposium, donors played a prominent and visible role in many other aspects of Sove Lavi's work. As described in the previous chapter, USAID's presence was literally everywhere. A USAID sticker identified in-kind donations of computers, monitors, printers, chairs, desks, filing cabinets, and a window air-conditioning unit. This use of secondhand office accoutrements is certainly not unique to Haiti. At least when I worked in one, U.S. nonprofit offices are often filled with hand-me-down equipment as well. While Sove Lavi is not the only agency to receive such support from USAID, it was the only NGO office in Haiti that I have visited (of thirty-three) offering such a highly visible symbolic representation of their donor.

This representation was not limited to the Sove Lavi office. For every event, such as the soccer match, World AIDS Day, the Caravan, Kanaval, or other missions to the provinces, Sove Lavi printed T-shirts in its official colors. Every T-shirt included the name and sometimes the organizational logo of the sponsoring agency in large print.[6] When I asked why there were different T-shirts for the same World AIDS Day activities and slogan, I was told that it was to make sure that people knew which donors supported which province. Mme Lejeune sarcastically reported to trainers in a meeting, "We have to make sure we have our donors in big letters," to which one added, "Our masters," a direct reference to slavery. In addition to the T-shirts, donors' names were also printed on the covers of their training manuals. In most of the publications, the donor's name was placed at the same level as Sove Lavi's, identifying them as the guide's coauthor. In at least one guide, the donor's name was given top billing on top of the front cover, identifying them as the primary author. This symbolic action of letting donors mark territory was the subject of conversation in staff meetings. Mme Versailles took a pragmatic approach, telling staff that they had to remember who paid their salaries, and that visible displays of gratitude were effective at generating further support.

This display of gratitude continued on their website. One of the outcomes Sove Lavi promised donors for a given quarter was a certain number of news stories posted on their website (in this case, fifty). The quarter had ended, and there were only three news stories on the website. In addition, fifty youths were supposed to enroll in the online chat forum and write a specified number of postings. By the end of the quarter, only two people had enrolled—both Sove Lavi employees. The following quarter, Sove Lavi solved the problem by having youths come into their office three afternoons per week and use four computers to look at their website and use the online forum. In addition, since there was a dearth of stories, the week after the end of the quarter some donors sent their own stories to be posted, and they all were. One story in particular caught my attention. Fondation Sogebank had taken over all the contracts for the Global

Fund projects concerning AIDS, malaria, and tuberculosis in Haiti. Previously, the United Nations Development Program (UNDP) had administered some of the smaller HIV/AIDS-prevention activities, including Fanm Tèt Ansanm's. This move generated backstage conversation, as no one dared publicly critique either the Global Fund with a $23 million portfolio in Haiti, or Fondation Sogebank, the country's largest foundation and at the time the largest bank. But some HIV/AIDS activists took umbrage, since the foundation was new not only to HIV/AIDS but also to health. And the foundation received criticism for their autocratic management style. Noted at the beginning of the chapter, Mme Lejeune was furious after a meeting with them for sending Sove Lavi changes to their plan—cutting 50 percent of the budget—only hours before their scheduled meeting. One of the stories that Sove Lavi posted late, past the end of the quarter, was a press release by the foundation explaining why they were the best choice to manage all the Global Fund projects.

This display of donor centrality was not accidental but rather quite intentional, emanating from Mme Versailles's formula for success. When I asked her what relationship Sove Lavi had with donors, she replied:

> Well, um. To say, what do I have with donors? Relations I have with them, . . . um . . . they, they are . . . first, you see, in an institution the first person they see is the director. Donors, most often, it is the director they first see. If the director is a person . . . you see, who's . . . valuable . . . a person who is open . . . a person who knows how to lobby, you see, the donors appreciate that. That is to say, they know all the work you do.

Note the hesitation in the conversation. I was not able to get more information or precision during the interview, for reasons I explain below. But this brief exchange outlines Sove Lavi's organizational philosophy and the context in which they work, being open to donor influence and constantly lobbying for further support.

This philosophy was most clearly revealed to several Sove Lavi staff and myself during a series of meetings for the Caravan, mentioned in chapter 2. The Caravan, known to donor groups as "Mobile Health Education/Counselling [*sic*] and Women's Empowerment for HIV/AIDS Prevention" (the original was in English), was supposed to have started in March 2003 with the first disbursement of funds from the Global Fund, as was Sove Lavi's website. Given the sociopolitical situation, many logistical difficulties were outside of Sove Lavi's control. In a memo to Sove Lavi that I translated into Kreyòl for the technical director, the donor had accepted this as an excusable reason for the delay, and pushed back the start date to the fourth quarter of 2004. At a meeting of the technical team in November 2004, the staff who had been given the responsibility for the project was in a panic because nothing had been done, despite the expenses accruing. I helped look for used trucks, and Mme Versailles even asked me to drive one from South Dakota to Miami during one of my trips home because it was cheaper to buy a truck in the United States. I also helped find tent equipment, pricing out various tents, poles, and sound systems. Sove Lavi consistently failed donors' milestones. They were several quarters late in opening the Caravan. Typically they barely get by at the end of a quarter, such as when they planned the grand opening of a provincial center on December 27, 2004, with two days of planning and in between Christmas and New Year's (also Haiti's Independence Day), so it could count as part of the quarter.[7]

Being "Open"

In February 2005, at the end of the day on the Monday before "Fat Tuesday," Mme Versailles called the remaining staff together to view a slide-show presentation about the Caravan for donors that M. Lescot hurriedly cobbled together on his laptop. He was given this assignment only the previous workday. Mme Versailles had asked me to help him with the presentation, especially translating English phrases on images that were borrowed from websites or reports he had found. Later that afternoon, six of us, including a new accounting intern who spoke English, gathered in M. Lescot's ice-cold office that also doubled as Sove Lavi's conference room. The presentation was well organized, and at least in the first half, presented in flawless French. The content was culled from earlier Sove Lavi proposals, discussing the history, purpose, and structure of the Caravan. The practice run and our feedback lasted three hours, well into the evening, consisting of slide-by-slide line editing. Not a single employee brought up the elephant in living room: they had been proposing the Caravan for over two years, and nothing had been done. Instead Mme Versailles made every effort to highlight the technical aspects of the presentation, wanting it to be perfect for the donors who would be assembled in two days. She commented on how well it looked, clearly impressed by the PowerPoint technology, nervously laughing while she did so. Whenever she laughed, Josue and the new intern joined her. Aside from M. Lescot, whose patience was visibly wearing thin as he dutifully made changes, other staff—especially those who had been given responsibility for the Caravan—remained silent. But no one dared leave. While the PowerPoint practice run was occurring, the two janitors led a Tom Sawyer–esque troupe of neighborhood men hurriedly whitewashing the office's exterior and hallways. They had already finished with the chilly office, which now smelled strongly of paint. The amount of preparation, and the careful, almost ritualistic concern about attaining a perfect PowerPoint presentation, resembled religious or magical spaces, and certainly a reverence of donors and their "magic" Western technology (Abramson 1999; Sampson 1996). It most certainly testified to the importance that Mme Versailles, and hence Sove Lavi, attached to appearances, particularly to their donors. While many casual observers of Haiti, such as missionaries, note the profound respect that most people, including (and especially) the poor majority, give to their outward self-presentation (see Ulysse's [2008] nuanced analysis of what she calls "reflexive political economy"), the stakes at Sove Lavi are higher, especially in their relationships with their donors, as appearances can drive reality.

The morning of Ash Wednesday, as I came into the office, final preparations of the space were being made to the whole office, especially M. Lescot's area. The gas-powered generator was turned on. Coffee was brewing on the automatic drip. The floor was being washed. Two white tablecloths were draped over the conference room table. Posters of public health campaigns were hastily put up. Debris and papers were collected in a box and dumped on the floor in the back room. Orders were being barked down the stairs, and people ran upstairs as they were being summoned, sometimes bumping into one another. I offered to help, but no one could tell me what needed to be done, each referring me to another person. One by one, various donor representatives arrived, from the UN, MINUSTAH, the Global Fund, USAID, and the Centers for Disease Control and Prevention (CDC). They were offered coffee and shuffled into the chilly conference room, where the borrowed projector was already shining onto a wooden backdrop. Two of the donor representatives were Haitian, from Fondation Sogebank and the USAID health contractor. One of them wore an ash cross on her forehead, the only one in the room to do so. All the other Haitian people in the room (which included Sove Lavi staff), presumably, were Protestant. Since the majority of Haitian people are Catholic, this could represent a general preponderance of Protestants within the NGO sector, in part because of its missionary history (e.g., Bornstein 2005; Mathurin et. al. 1989).

The room was full, as seven Sove Lavi staff sat in the remaining chairs around the long table. Speaking in French, Mme Versailles introduced everyone around the table, taking special care to introduce Gabrielle, who had happened to stop by the office on Monday to discuss payment for her services rendered in December (discussed in chapter 2).[8] Mme Versailles took the opportunity to invite her to come to the forum (while still not paying her). Following introductions, which lasted a good fifteen minutes, Mme Versailles gave the floor to M. Lescot, who recited his presentation. Occasionally Mme Versailles would add details that M. Lescot as a new hire could not know. After forty-five minutes, the UN representative finally asked the question everyone at Sove Lavi had dreaded: So what exactly is the plan for how to reach the community, who are the partners, and what will be the specific outcome measures? An awkward silence filled the room. Mme Lejeune stepped out.

Mme Versailles finally laughed and explained that they were having this meeting to plan those very elements. She was deploying the strategy that she remain "open" to donor control, which worked for her in the past. The UN representative persisted, explaining that they had two years to work out these details. The USAID contractor intervened, adding that this was a good opportunity to work out such a plan. She cited statistics about how the approach to AIDS prevention was based on faulty assumptions—that 90 percent of Haitians are indeed aware of the disease and the three primary means of prevention,[9] and that more should be done to encourage a change in behavior. Speaking out of turn and in Kreyòl (the rest of the meeting had been in French), Gabrielle said that the major reason people do not practice HIV prevention was the dire economic situation (see chapters 1 and 2 of this volume, and also Farmer 1992; Robins 2009; Susser 2009). The USAID contractor interrupted Gabrielle, saying that they do not want to create dependency, citing a situation with a group called POZ (HIV Positive) that had given bags of rice to members of their support group. Whatever agenda was meticulously planned in advance was abandoned after this point.

Mme Versailles again asked the donor representatives present what they wanted for the Caravan. The UN representative pointed out that such a Caravan had existed in the past, which was news to most Sove Lavi staff. Speaking in poor French, to titters,[10] the American CDC representative said that they were looking for people to do more HIV testing with the President's Emergency Plan for AIDS Relief (PEPFAR), and that the Caravan should focus on that, to which Mme Versailles immediately consented. The USAID representative suggested that it was important that the Caravan encourage people to learn about HIV-prevention measures, particularly abstinence. Again Mme Versailles consented. The MINUSTAH representative, a Sri Lankan who spoke English,[11] suggested that HIV/AIDS was best approached by giving out condoms and having demonstrations on their correct usage. Mme Versailles said they would be open to that if they received materials. And the Global Fund representative said that it was important that the Caravan work with local health organizations, both governmental bureaus and NGOs. Mme Versailles agreed, saying that it was a more effective approach to getting better turnout. As he got up to leave, the UN representative, a former Peace Corps volunteer, pointed out that many of the ideas discussed opposed one another, that the primary point can't be about all these things. Mme Versailles was just agreeing with everyone but they needed to make a decision. And further, if the Caravan was working with local health and youth organizations to assure turnout, the idea of a Caravan would be irrelevant, since they would be preaching to the choir. The whole point of the Caravan, to his mind, was to attract a new audience and funnel them into these local organizations. Again after his intervention, another silence filled the room. It was Mme Versailles who left at this point, saying that lunch was ready.

The awkward silence was broken by a discussion about how to attract large crowds. Gabrielle said that they had to know the terrain, to which everyone agreed, each adding his or her own analysis about why local involvement was best. Returning to the table, Mme Versailles said that Haitians love to dance and listen to music. Styrofoam lunch boxes of beans and rice, chicken, and macaroni were passed around to everyone, beginning with the foreigners and then the Haitian donor representatives.[12] Josue suggested touring with the band that he managed. One of the donors disagreed, saying that it should be a group that was better known and could attract a crowd. Mme Versailles suggested touring with a *konpa* (a popular Haitian style of music) group like Tropicana, who hailed from her part of Haiti and had just celebrated their fiftieth anniversary. Georges politely intervened by saying that Tropicana appealed to a "different slice of society" than their target population—meaning it appealed to older people. Several agencies mentioned the pro bono work they had done with one or another group for public service announcements. Everyone agreed that a big name celebrity—like the Haitian American hip-hop artist Wyclef Jean, who had just started the NGO Yéle Haiti to do public service work—would bring a crowd. (Wyclef built this Yéle Haiti into a platform for a run for president that was derailed on a technicality. Yéle Haiti was also under fire for financial misman-agement of the millions collected after the earthquake.) One of the U.S. agency reps mentioned that they had actually worked with Yéle Haiti and promised to pass along the contact information to Mme Versailles. As everyone ate, Mme Versailles made jokes, triggering loud, forced laughter on the part of some of the Sove Lavi staff, especially Josue. Mme Versailles suggested that they reconvene in a couple of weeks. The remaining donor representatives agreed that it would be a good idea.[13] They returned to their offices with full bellies, some with extra lunch boxes. When the last donor representative left, Mme Versailles expressed satisfaction with the forum's outcome. She explained how important it was to make the donor groups feel like they are involved. Josue and the new intern quickly and vocally agreed. Everyone else stared at his or her plate in silence.

Mme Versailles managed to involve the donors in the planning, in effect selling the vision of the group in exchange for donor funding. As evidenced by the fact that the Caravan eventually did get off the ground, Sove Lavi was able to secure financing. But this came at a price. First, it undermined the time and energy that the technical team had spent working on the project for the previ-ous two years. It also cost the Sove Lavi staff—possibly the most well-educated of any NGO in Haiti (nineteen out of thirty-seven staff members had college degrees, and seven had at least a master's degree)[14]—its dignity. According to M. Lescot:

> Considering the type of activity like that [the forum], we should have been better prepared. You don't give a reference document to someone like we did, and then right away, we re-propose this project. The two con-tradict each other, but [Mme Versailles] did not see that. These things bother me very much, because I feel that we give an impression of a lack of professionalism. However, there are some very good professionals here. Many people have their master's degree! Therefore, for me, what

I see, these questions shouldn't have been asked here. In meetings with people like this, we should come up with solutions for these things. We should have already asked these questions.

Three other staff people specifically mentioned this meeting as an eye-opener for them. This strategy of pulling donors into the planning process, exposing that Sove Lavi had not decided on its own policies, had the effect of giving donors even further control of the program: its goals, objectives, and specific activities. This parallels Sove Lavi using their website as PR for Fondation Sogebank following their failure to complete a specified objective on time. In a sense, Sove Lavi's failures were useful because they offered donors openings for greater control. It also on some level might work for Sove Lavi, in that they do not have to assume responsibility. Several trainers in a technical team meeting said, "We're always running behind them." Exasperated, Mme Pierre exclaimed, "We are prisoners!"

Problems with Donors

However strategic or genuine this strategy of being "open" or allowing donors to "brand" themselves on their T-shirts, computers, and educational materials may have been, it was not always successful. Mme Versailles's relationship strategy deliberately focused on cultivating personal friendships with individual donor representatives.[15] This strategy had previously worked for her; she inherited an organization with three staff members and successfully turned it into a large institution employing more than thirty people, comprising four offices in three departments. A danger with this strategy is that personalities can change within all institutions, and particularly often in development institutions. For example, of all the staff in charge of USAID programs in January 2004 when I conducted a round of interviews, only one person was still there that October. This has a ripple effect on NGOs, as Mme Versailles explains: "But, well, our disadvantage is that most often, people who work for donor groups, often they change their leadership. Every time they do that, you need to begin again. But our relationship is very good. I am not saying it is not hard, [that] we do not have any real problems with them. [Long pause. Then, very quietly] Well, we had problems with them." Every time a donor organization changes their staff, recipient NGOs need to begin cultivating relationships with the new staff people. Unfortunately for this research, Mme Versailles did not elaborate on what problems she saw that Sove Lavi had with donor groups, as she ended the interview following this question, saying, "Ah! We need to say, can't we finish this another day? . . . Because it is, it has become five o'clock." We never completed the interview. While I did not have access to her perspective, the problems that Sove Lavi encountered with donor groups were readily apparent, and other staff spoke quite freely about them.

Given the frequency with which Mme Versailles met with outside agencies in her office, it was at first difficult to guess which types of institutions were meeting with Sove Lavi. But the smell of coffee before the meeting and cigarette smoke after signaled a meeting with a donor group, testifying to Mme Versailles' emotional investment and stress level.

The problem Danielle and others noted about Sove Lavi staff arriving late, discussed in chapter 2, explained in chapter 3 as a problem about waiting on a check to clear, had roots in Sove Lavi's structure. The procedure for releasing organizational funds required that a member of the board sign all checks. This is common in small nonprofit organizations. As the board treasurer for a neighborhood association in Minneapolis, I was required to sign off on checks. But in 2003, when overnight the organization grew exponentially, these procedures proved outdated. Mme Versailles acknowledged this as Sove Lavi's weakness: "We have weaknesses like all other institutions. It functioned in the past, you see, in a certain manner. Now, you see, we are changing it. And all changes are made with a certain difficulty. So, this is why that now, we have . . . you see, I'm working on institutional reinforcement." This was behind the management consultant's SWOT analysis noted in the previous chapter. This consultant also made recommendations for restructuring the organization. Among the recommendations was that Sove Lavi change their charter and bylaws to be in line with their current practice, in effect identifying M. Lescot's "mask" as the real person. Policies and procedures about releasing funds were also specifically mentioned but not implemented, at least not by 2007 when I last inquired. Two recommendations that bore fruit were the creation of the post of research and development director and the adoption of a personnel manual. In addition to hiring M. Lescot in his new post, Mme Versailles replaced the two deputy directors. USAID had given them a template personnel manual authored by a USAID contractor. The remaining suggestions appeared to be boilerplate, such as the making and following of a "checklist" before going on missions, which trainers showed me they habitually did even before this suggestion. Many of the suggestions did not follow from the discussion of the problems, and many problems did not appear to be resolved in the contractor report's conclusion.[16] These discrepancies, and the fact that the report had not been disseminated to employees in the form of a workshop after at least six months of promising to do so (by the time I left Haiti), suggest that the conclusions were preconceived, either on the part of Mme Versailles or the donors. It could also be further evidence of the focus on appearances, to show that they had taken action to solve a problem.

Results-Based Management

When Sove Lavi was a project of a UN agency, housed within its offices, there was never a problem finding signatures. And expenses for this organization were minimal. When Sove Lavi became independent because it no longer worked on family hygiene education, Mme Versailles slowly obtained funding for other projects, gradually growing to a staff of ten over the course of ten years. According to Mme Auguste, these problems of waiting for checks to clear and always starting out late did not exist to the same degree when it was a small organization. This is also not a unique problem to Sove Lavi; several studies address these very problems in scaling up.[17] While it is impossible to isolate whether it was the increase in funds, increase in employees, or the political crisis surrounding Sove Lavi's work, the "scale" of the scaling up in 2003 was quite different than before. There might also have been jealousy and competition on the part of a board member who was also the director of another organization with Global Fund and USAID HIV/AIDS-prevention funding. As a result of applying for the windfall of such funding, Sove Lavi as a "partnership" was becoming an NGO, thrust into direct competition with several of its constituent organizations, as M. Lescot's critique outlined. In addition, the new funds from USAID and the Global Fund came with a policy of "results-based management." Central to this new management style is the donor practice of reimbursing NGOs after they have spent the funds, based on achieving "milestones" or service targets (Pollock 2003).

According to a preliminary study by the USAID contractor Management Sciences for Health (incidentally in Haiti), results-based management was successful, encouraging more cost-effective service delivery. According to the study (Pollock 2003:22), "Managers of participating NGOs note that they have strengthened their systems for planning, financial monitoring, and impact evaluation." This is accomplished through two primary actions in their contracts:[18] First an "award fee"—10 percent of the operational budget—that is only given if the NGO successfully attains performance measures (if not, the NGO loses 5 percent of its original budget). In addition, clauses are written into the contracts that permit the donor to withhold reimbursements if they deem costs excessive. According to the report, these "created an incentive for managers to control costs and monitor the utility of expenditures and to use this monitoring data to identify problems and inefficiencies in their operating systems."

Another of Sove Lavi's donors, the Global Fund, was founded in January 2002 with a mandate to go beyond "business as usual." Results-based management was a central plank in this platform. According to its first self-assessment, the Global Fund's (2004) performance-based funding was a success. Both models, USAID and the Global Fund, emphasize ownership, participation, and innovation. A significant difference is in their structure: whereas USAID manages their health program through private, U.S. contractors such as Management Sciences for Health, the Global Fund requires countries to assemble a Country Coordinating Mechanism (CCM). The CCM is envisioned as a public/private partnership, with foreign and national representatives from both governmental and nongovernmental agencies. The CCM reviews proposals, selects the "primary recipient" agency that will disburse funds and manage the program, sends a single proposal to the Global Fund, and is responsible for oversight of the process. In Haiti, the minister of public health heads the CCM, which signed a contract with the Global Fund in December 2002.

Sove Lavi developed a series of measures responding to the results-based management. First, staff developed numerical performance outcomes for every quarter. In the Global Fund program, these are called "milestones" (in English). These include having an active distance-learning program with thirty local schools, securing partnerships with two new radio stations per quarter, establishing the website by March 2003, followed by attracting 50 hits in the following quarter, 150 the next, and finally 250 in the last quarter of 2003 and 5 links from other pages. These milestones form the basis for performance review: in their reports, Sove Lavi lists a percentage of each milestone's completion. Sove Lavi faces one of the central challenges to nonprofit work: how to measure progress. This Midas touch, turning abstract processes and "social change" into numbers, is difficult to achieve, and perhaps even insidious, recalling Audre Lorde's (1984:6) caution that "the master's tools will never dismantle the master's house." Under the new performance-based management regime, Sove Lavi was suddenly expected to attain all these milestones, and risked not receiving full funding if they failed to do so. Sove Lavi hired a person whose job description was to manage the database for the reports. In practice, this person's job also included overseeing written pre- and post-tests, evaluating knowledge of HIV/AIDS transmission and prevention from program participants (CAC members, schoolchildren, and parents). At each site, nineteen people were chosen to take the test, consisting of about twenty true/false, open-ended, and multiple-choice questions. Three staff were also hired for evaluation purposes. Mme Lejeune, the technical director, also spent most of her time writing proposals and grant reports. As is evident, Sove Lavi became more top-heavy.

There has been little independent evaluation of performance-based contracting's on-the-ground impacts. Sove Lavi's experience, and staff analysis, suggests that several consequences of this approach are not uniformly positive. First, Sove Lavi was hamstrung during much of the period during this study. Like people who worked for the Aristide government who went months without pay, Sove Lavi employees endured periods when travel expenses were not reimbursed. Staff were unaware whether Mme Versailles failed to submit a report on time listing the "results," or donors were not satisfied with said results. There was an accounting of these "arrears," some of which were more than eight months old. In addition, regular salaries were held for a period of almost two months beginning in December 2004. The lack of available funds exacerbated the structural problems noted above, including the check-signing procedures. In addition, the lack of available money was behind the shortage of paper and why they could not repair or upgrade their copier. Instead, a staff person—the "gopher" on shift—had to walk five minutes down the block to pay for copies at a much higher rate, on credit, rendering this situation less cost-effective than before.[19] More important, the lack of funds resulted in an inability to plan.

Financial procedures implied by results-based management hampered planning efforts, and in turn hurting outcomes. In at least two technical team meetings, the staff responsible for coordinating missions to the provinces requested an additional day in the field for planning. The donors' reluctance to spend money on planning created a situation in which "we are always running behind." The World AIDS Day experience mentioned in chapter 2, when no one came to the training, was hampered by their *prese-prese* (rush-rush) approach to the communities. Sove Lavi staff do not have adequate time to get to know their volunteers, or to find out when church services or local markets are held, for example.

Local autonomy might be more cost-effective than centralized planning, especially in light of these travel expenses. But results-based management constricts local autonomy as well. At the same local center discussed in chapter 2, youth and staff had taken the initiative to organize a series of activities for the 2005 Kanaval, traditionally a big affair in the community. The plan included participating in the parade, utilizing cultural programming similar to the World AIDS Day events. They planned to have a Kanaval stand where volunteers would pass out materials, and staff would counsel youth on STIs and provide youth-oriented alcohol-free festivities in the center of an open-house environment. Having learned lessons about planning, they had made a collective effort to organize things on their own and not wait for direction from Pòtoprens. According to a satellite office staff, they had been told that they were supposed to take responsibility for their own programming. So they did, e-mailing their plan, which included a realistic budget, to the central office. There was no response for two weeks. Frustrated, one of the provincial staff traveled to Pòtoprens on her own dime to hear word about their plans. Josue told her that he hadn't replied because they were waiting for Global Fund's response, and Sove Lavi did not have their own money for requisite expenses like printing T-shirts. Lobbying on behalf of the local center, a couple of Pòtoprens staff finally went around Josue and met directly with Mme Versailles a week before Kanaval. The response was the same: this activity was not planned in the budget, so Sove Lavi would not receive reimbursement for it. That was the last time any local staff took initiative to plan their own events, despite attempts by Pòtoprens staff to break this dependency. "We know there is a problem," said Mme Lejeune. "This is what occupies all of my time."

According to Mme Versailles, another difficulty in making the changes she alluded to in her interview was a lack of qualified staff. Mme Versailles outlined the need for more money, to be able to hire qualified staff. This raises questions about the sustainability and purpose of fund-raising: many NGOs always look for more funding, some citing the corporate principle, "if you're not growing, you're dying." Mme Versailles continued to push for organizational expansion after the 2003 scale-up. Both the Global Fund and USAID refused. The Global Fund required Sove Lavi to focus their energies on attaining their objectives in the locations where they had already worked. USAID had changed their strategic focus altogether. Both highlight the concern with "turf" that began this section, about which donor was on which province's T-shirt.

The Global Fund decided to freeze funds to Sove Lavi for a period of three months, beginning in December 2004. According to the oversight staff at Fondation Sogebank, "If [these problems] do not change, we can stop financing the NGO for a period. For all of these cases, all of the programs—to my knowledge—there are two we did this to. Sove Lavi was one of them." Few staff had a direct working relationship with the foundation. During this period when people did not receive their paychecks, one of them theorized that it was because Sogebank—also a commercial bank—was earning interest on the money that the Global Fund invested. This staff had spoken with people working at other NGOs, who shared similar experiences of habitually being paid two weeks late, which also happened to Sove Lavi leading up to the funding freeze. At the beginning of 2005, three Sove Lavi staff had a meeting with foundation staff. According to two of the staff, and a follow-up memo, the foundation had just notified Sove Lavi of a funding cut at noon the day of the meeting, also requiring substantial changes to Sove Lavi's proposed action plan. According to foundation staff, "There were many problems with financial management, and they did not accept the course [we gave them]. Concerning verification, there would be things that did not happen, [or] suggested actions in the budget. In general, there were things that needed to improve." According to their own annual reports, Sove Lavi was not attaining 100 percent of their performance measures as early as 2003. A written exchange between Sove Lavi and Global Fund outlined several measures. Sove Lavi's response to Global Fund's concern (written in English) that there were "too many milestones. To regroup similar ones . . . an annex could detail the figures per site," triggered a defensive reaction (written in French), defending the need to include intermediary goals. Another concern concerned rapid growth in expenses without being clear about their purpose: "Infrastructure line item increased from $61,000 to $127,000." Mme Versailles's written response was to argue that "these observations appear not to reflect the reality because in addition to Caravans, the infrastructure expenses are also divided [into] for example community and social mobilization. I think that there is a confusion because we did not arrive at the cited amounts."

During the summer of 2004, funds from Sove Lavi's other major donor, USAID, suddenly stopped. As mentioned in chapter 2, Sove Lavi staff set up meetings for the following month and even organized new CACs in July 2004, the month that the project was terminated. According to Mme Auguste, "Very simply, Josue told us that the HS-2004 project stopped!" upon their return.

USAID had done away entirely with the CAC as a strategy, preferring to fund something like the Caravan, which USAID staff deemed more cost-effective. Sove Lavi's sudden departure was shocking to CAC members and Sove Lavi; four staff mentioned it in their interview. In their focus group interviews for USAID's report, CAC members in two locations expressed their frustration at Sove Lavi's unexplained departure and ensuing silence for the eight previous months.

While it could simply be that the donors were using Sove Lavi as an example to scare other Haitian NGOs to perform better—as word travels quickly in the relatively small NGO world, and certainly in the HIV/AIDS community—there are difficult questions that remain unanswered about the timing and the abruptness of the changes. First, representatives from both the foundation and the Global Fund in Geneva said that they do not think of themselves as "police," that it is in their interests to work with the NGOs to improve their performance. In the world of international development, unspent funds are an embarrassment. According to staff in Geneva, this is particularly embarrassing for a group such as the Global Fund that is promising new approaches, true participation, and partnership. The USAID representatives—during both the Aristide and interim governments—spoke very highly of Sove Lavi. One Sove Lavi veteran guessed that donors' abrupt actions were about putting them in their place, literally keeping them assigned to a particular geographic area.

Partners? Relationships between Fanm Tèt Ansanm and Donors

Fanm Tèt Ansanm's situation is quite different. First, Fanm Tèt Ansanm donors call themselves "partners," referring to Fanm Tèt Ansanm as one of their "Haitian partners." In contrast to Sove Lavi, Fanm Tèt Ansanm has been able to defend their own vision and policies to their donors. In short, Fanm Tèt Ansanm enjoys a certain amount of organizational autonomy that Sove Lavi lacks. According to Fanm Tèt Ansanm staff, a couple of factors explain this.

Northern NGO representatives in Pòtoprens and in Europe told me that they have "partnerships" with the Southern NGOs they finance. This language reflects a social democratic ideology of cooperation and egalitarianism, in sharp contrast to the capitalist "results"- or "performance"-based management models of USAID and the Global Fund. Is this only a semantic distinction, reflecting current fads in development jargon papering over vast inequalities between North and South? (Eriksson Baaz 2005). For answers we must analyze actual interactions between Fanm Tèt Ansanm and their donors. While there was no question in anyone's mind about Fanm Tèt Ansanm being financially dependent on their donors, several staff, especially those whose jobs entailed regular interaction with donors, argued that Fanm Tèt Ansanm was reasonably autonomous. The two phrases I heard most often were that Fanm Tèt Ansanm *konn jere tèt li* (knows how to manage itself) and is an institution with *granmoun tèt li* (literally "elders in its head," people who are responsible and treated as autonomous). To illustrate this point, I will discuss two examples most cited by Fanm Tèt Ansanm staff.

"We Know How to Defend Ourselves"

Fanm Tèt Ansanm, like Sove Lavi, was a recipient of Global Fund support. Unlike Sove Lavi, however, the initial "principal recipient" was not Fondation Sogebank but the UNDP. Noted above, the foundation took over the entire Global Fund portfolio midstream, which included Fanm Tèt Ansanm. During their first meeting with Fanm Tèt Ansanm, foundation staff made several demands for new specific milestones to be added. Among these, the foundation demanded that Fanm Tèt Ansanm have specific targets for number of women who receive family planning methods such as the pill or Norplant. Mme Dominique, Giselle, and Jonette flatly refused. As I entered the office, the meeting had just ended, and these three were debriefing. As with most aspects of work at Fanm Tèt Ansanm, this conversation was held out in the open. Several staff had gathered to listen in and give their opinion. Jonette, a program director, was flustered, critical of the foundation's "dictatorial approach," arguing that it was wrong to just show up and to make demands like that. Other women voiced their support for this concern. Director Mme Dominique did not seem fazed, smiling as she said that it was the first meeting, and that the foundation was trying to be firm, to mark its territory. Giselle, the clinic director, repeated what she had said in the meeting to the foundation representative: "We know you are a medical doctor and that you are good at what you do. But I direct the clinic, supervising three doctors. I know the area of public health." Again this triggered assenting titters from the small crowd. Mme Dominique repeated her response, saying, "We are not arguing with your science, and have no objection in principle to the idea, but we know the terrain. We have been working here for almost twenty years. We know what will work here and what will not work here." This line drew applause from the other staff. Variations of the three arguments were repeated the rest of the afternoon, especially to staff in the afternoon shift as they reported to work.

The foundation sent Fanm Tèt Ansanm a letter the following week, welcoming the NGO to their portfolio, approving their milestones and budget without revision. In other words, they backed off. Giselle recalled, "When we present one of our projects with a donor, we discuss it with them. The donor tells us to do something specific. We say that we can't because we are on the ground. We know the value of the field: we know the weaknesses in the field, we know the field. We know what they're asking can't happen. And if it can't happen, don't finance it. Yes! Marie [Mme Dominique] is very clear. We have gone to meetings when Marie says, 'I'm sorry that this can't happen.' You understand?" Fanm Tèt Ansanm has a long history of defending their *politik* (Kreyòl for both "politics" as well as "policies")[20] to donor groups. Several staff said in interviews, "We know how to defend ourselves." A few years prior, USAID made a similar request. As Catherine Maternowska (2006) argues, family planning has been a consistent point of contention between donor groups, Haitian feminists, and public health professionals. Fanm Tèt Ansanm public health promoters—paid staff as well as volunteers—often talk about the importance of family planning. Paulette, a very religious Protestant, said that the medanm, the women who frequent Fanm Tèt Ansanm, "like family planning, because they have too many children. When you have too many children, you can't fully take care of them. The women are happy; they come so that they can take their health in their own hands."

Behind this concern of donors wanting to increase the number of family-planning methods was the only way this would be possible: for Leonie and her coworkers to hand them out on factory workers' lunch break. I have seen this "feeding frenzy" many times, the ravenous consumption of any and all materials that Fanm Tèt Ansanm hands out during World AIDS Day, during a lunch break, or inside the factories at the end of workers' shift, whether they be pamphlets, booklets, journals, or condoms. Workers who do not have time to stay and talk with Leonie or the other motivator (this is to say, nearly all of them) literally swarm the NGO representatives and grab what they can, while they can. One time when I went along, within less than a minute five boxes of condoms, each containing 144 packets of three condoms, were gone. A stack of five hundred journals was gone within five minutes as well. In fact, Fanm Tèt Ansanm maxed out their allocation of condoms that they were allowed to distribute. In addition to giving them out in the clinic and in visits to the industrial park or individual factories, public health "promoters" like Lisette, Beatrice, or Carlene received a box per month to give away to their neighbors, their coworkers, or their religious community. Staff and volunteers gave out 103,956 condoms in 2003. The HIV-prevention staff told the volunteer motivators in one of their monthly meetings that Fanm Tèt Ansanm could not even buy additional condoms, a frequent suggestion the motivators made to deal with the condom shortage. There was a limited supply of this brand of condom manufactured in India, only a certain number are sent to Haiti on a monthly basis, and Fanm Tèt Ansanm already received the lion's share. During the summer of 2006, Fanm Tèt Ansanm was reduced to a distribution every other month instead of every month, stirring up discussion and discontent among the volunteer promoters.

While there is a very broad support base for family planning in Haiti, and certainly among Fanm Tèt Ansanm's service population of working women, at times donor approaches are heavy-handed and coercive, bound up in politics (Maternowska 2006). Some years ago, USAID demanded that, just like the informational materials and the condoms they cannot have enough of to give away, Fanm Tèt Ansanm hand out other family planning methods, like Norplant or

Depo-Provera during the "feeding frenzy." In fact, the Fanm Tèt Ansanm clinic has boxes of these two methods to give to people upon consultation. But USAID wanted to establish greater numbers, giving out ten thousand in a month. Again Fanm Tèt Ansanm flatly refused. Several people discussed this. Giselle recalled, "Ourselves, we don't look for quantity. We have quality of service." Sometimes, such as with Fanm Tèt Ansanm's current donors, a couple of whom have supported them for almost twenty years, the donor's and the NGO's interest and politik are shared. Other times, donors have a different agenda. In this situation, Giselle advises, "To begin with, you need to be clear with the person, clear that we don't have adequate time to give individuals because here we are not an industry. It's not a factory, it's a . . . Because if you take in ten people in a [medical] consultation—there are places that take in more than one hundred people in a consultation—the person comes like an animal, you understand? We, we do not seek out this kind of thing."

Mme Dominique explained several public health reasons why they refused to give out the pill in the factories the same way they distribute condoms, notably the concern about appropriateness and the more severe side effects. "We said that we, for a worker to take for example the pill, they need to first come here to see a doctor, to see if she doesn't have a problem. If she has a problem, an STD, she could have others. People with high blood pressure shouldn't take the pill. [USAID] didn't accept. For them, we should go to the factories directly to distribute the pill." Moreover, this coercive approach "ran counter to our institutional policies, against the same work we're doing with the women. We can't explain to women how to take their health into their hands only to do something contrary to what we say."

Unlike the Global Fund, USAID did not back down in their request. In response, Mme Dominique wrote a letter to the USAID mission and their health contractor, thanking them for their years of support for their programs, but refusing the offer for funding because they did not accept the conditions stipulated. Even in the United States, it is rare that an organization refuses funding from a donor. As Mme Dominique said, "There are other institutions that would do it, but we said that we'll never do it. So I believe that it's a very large form of autonomy." While some organizations in Haiti—feminist women's groups, global justice advocates, or grassroots foundations—told me they will never apply for U.S. government money, I know of only one other NGO making such a refusal of funds offered. This is a rare decision, especially from an NGO that had been a recipient of USAID funding. This decision was mentioned in several interviews with staff, but also in interviews with other donor groups, as an example of the importance that Fanm Tèt Ansanm attaches to their principles. They value their mission of women's empowerment over funding and are willing to defend it and even refuse money if a donor offers funding that violates these principles. Besides this forceful approach to imposing its politik on NGOs,

Mme Dominique describes coercive management practices: "I almost signed a contract with them for three years. I was interested, but in the contract terms underneath the signature I saw that at any moment they could decide to cancel it. I didn't sign it like that."

"We Know What We're Doing"

Especially in light of the myriad ways that donors maintain control, as outlined in this chapter, this decision requires explanation. How was Fanm Tèt Ansanm able to stand up to their new Global Fund administrator and refuse USAID funding? Fanm Tèt Ansanm staff provided several explanations. First, according to Mme Dominique, "We know what we're doing." As noted above, Fanm Tèt Ansanm had been "in the field" for almost twenty years. The most frequent staff response to the question of what was Fanm Tèt Ansanm's strength was its longevity. Mme Laurent argued, "Fanm Tèt Ansanm's first strength is its stability in the area, because Fanm Tèt Ansanm will be twenty years old, the stability of our employees, and the quality of services that Fanm Tèt Ansanm offers everyone." Edele said, "I am a quitter. I don't stay long at any job. But I've been here for what is it, ten years? Wow. That says a lot about Fanm Tèt Ansanm." To the institutional stability and the longevity of staff's tenure at Fanm Tèt Ansanm, Giselle added recurrent training: "Fanm Tèt Ansanm has strength beginning with the employees who work for Fanm Tèt Ansanm, employees who have been here for a long time, and the recurrent training done for employees, a way to be up-to-date."

Besides the years of on-the-ground experience, the other element of "knowing what we're doing" is the shared understanding of Fanm Tèt Ansanm's mission. Unlike Sove Lavi staff, many of whom could not answer this question, the responses about Fanm Tèt Ansanm's mission were very similar. The simplest response was "We exist to empower the factory workers." This focus on the mission was the second most common staff response to the question of Fanm Tèt Ansanm's strength. As proof, staff referred to the fact that factory workers continue coming. Giselle put the argument simply: "If they didn't come, Fanm Tèt Ansanm wouldn't need to be here." Note the double negative, "voting with one's feet."

Partnership, Not "Results"

An additional reason staff cited for their ability to stand up for themselves was that Fanm Tèt Ansanm had five donors. None individually had the veto power that it would if it was their only donor, or one of two. Said Mme Dominique, "It might be more work to keep track of everyone, but in the end it's better that we have many donors because every so often they change their politik and finance other programs instead. This way we aren't dependent on any one individual where we would be destroyed should they choose to leave."

Finally, Fanm Tèt Ansanm's donors were primarily NGOs themselves, generating most of their revenue from individual donations and not the government. According to Mme Dominique, "We have truly exceptional donors, certainly the European donors. They give us all the latitude we need to do our work. They come, they inspect, they do everything. And I believe that the rapport we have with them is very tight. We believe it is because Fanm Tèt Ansanm never lies, you understand?" While she could have elaborated this point about not lying, she chose to focus on the positive. As she and many others said, "We know what we do, and then we do what we say." In at least three reports for different funding agencies, Fanm Tèt Ansanm exceeded its numerical service targets for two-thirds of the milestones. A donor representative said, "Happily, Fanm Tèt Ansanm is in the top rung of institutions in terms of organizational capacity, management and governance, and giving reports on time." This donor representative divided the field of forty "partners" into three rungs, with only two other NGOs on the top rung with Fanm Tèt Ansanm.

These European NGOs that fund Fanm Tèt Ansanm use the language of "partners" to describe their relationships with the Haitian NGOs they support. While this might be a rhetorical flourish, the European NGO representatives I interviewed did employ different management practices than the U.S. NGOs that are USAID contractors. Two significant differences are the length of "partnership" and the oversight/evaluation relationship. One European NGO in particular has funded Fanm Tèt Ansanm for almost its entire twenty years of existence, with two others for around fifteen years. At least until late 2005, part of the reason for maintaining long-term relationships might have been because these European NGOs did not have a Haiti office and officer. Travel to and from Europe is not as easy as it is to and from the United States, representing a significant institutional barrier to meeting new Haitian partners. But the donor representatives in Europe as well as their Haitian management contractor argued that these long-term relationships are explicitly part of their organizational philosophy. Said a European NGO employee, "We all know that lasting social change, not to mention development, is a long-term process. The project cycle does not work for us." She also mentioned that they had the freedom to engage in long-term relationships with Southern partners in part because they themselves generated the majority of their own revenue from individual donations, particularly churches and trade unions. This is in direct contrast with most U.S. NGOs whose budgets are almost entirely financed by the U.S. government. Other anthropologists and NGO researchers have also noted this difference between NGOs financed by European and North American donors (Edelman 2005:31; Macdonald 1997).

Fanm Tèt Ansanm staff identified several areas for improvement, especially concerning donors. While some argued that they should raise only what they need, others—including Mme Dominique—argued that they could do better at attracting other donors. Giselle argued, "When we discuss a project we don't ever ask for a lot of money. That is, we ask for the amount that people can see that is really needed for an activity." By 2009 they had much more money and seemed able to spend it, and this came with many other changes described in the book's conclusion. Partially explaining why they don't do as well as other NGOs in attracting funding, in direct contrast to Mme Versailles's strength, Mme Dominique decried that Fanm Tèt Ansanm suffered from a lack of "openness": "I believe that Fanm Tèt Ansanm, one of its problems is a lack of openness because of a lack of publicity that we do for ourselves. We don't have a person to sell Fanm Tèt Ansanm. While we have technicians, we don't have a technician who sells, who lobbies, for Fanm Tèt Ansanm. I believe that it's important, because I can't do it myself at the same time, because I am participating in much of the administration, management, and direction. I know directors who are never in the office: they're outside, lobbying everywhere." Mme Dominique could have spent less time on management and administration and more on lobbying, but decided not to. This has consequences, as Mme Dominique outlined: "There are things done outside that Fanm Tèt Ansanm is not aware of because we don't have someone there to hear of it. It's not because they don't want to give you funds, but because you don't have someone there, maybe they forget you, you understand?" While Fanm Tèt Ansanm does comparatively well, and has a certain stability vis-à-vis donors, staff are aware that the donor world is constantly changing, as Mme Dominique explained: "You know that from time to time, donors change. For example the Inter-American Foundation financed us for a long time but what happened, they changed their politik."

"*Grès kochon kwit kochon*": Autonomy

As mentioned in the book's introduction, autonomy, like participation, is a key concept within NGOs, yet is similarly difficult to define. One scholar defines an NGO as autonomous if it can "devise its own policies, determine its own structures and relies upon its own efforts to raise money. It is thus independent from the Party/state" (Howell 1997:205). Note the focus on the state, which is shared by other researchers (e.g., Biggs and Neame 1996; Blair 1997; Dicklitch 1998; Morton 1997; Ray 1999; Riordan and Sarkar 1998; Thomas-Slayter 1992). Kamat (2003:93) argued that it is important for NGOs to keep their distance from donors in addition to states. Biggs and Neame (1996:40), however, refocus this preoccupation with autonomy as a question of "how to strengthen multiple accountabilities and 'room for manoeuvre' so that they can negotiate more effectively." The "multiple accountabilities" to which they refer are the various "stakeholder" groups or "constituencies"—including members, service recipients, state agencies, multilateral donor groups, and individual supporters. Edwards and Hulme (1996b:254–255) note that "downward accountability is nearly always weaker than upward accountability."

While Sove Lavi is a classic donor-led organization, Fanm Tèt Ansanm has certain autonomy. Since both are working with poor communities, and they are not engaged in income-generating activities like micro-credit or craft sales, neither NGO can ever be financially autonomous. A Haitian proverb quoted to me several times defines this form of financial autonomy: "grès kochon kwit kochon," which literally translates as "the pig cooks in its own fat." In other words, nothing outside is required.[21] If this was the only operable standard of autonomy in Haiti, very few NGOs could be considered autonomous: I can count those NGOs for whom this is even possible on one hand. Most of these are associations that organize a professional constituency, like the Haitian American Chamber of Commerce, the Association des Industrialists d'Haïti, or Femmes en Démocratie.[22]

There is a second relevant definition of autonomy expressed in the phrase *gran moun tèt li*, that an institution (or Haiti) has adults at its head. This means that the person or institution is capable of making decisions on her/his/its own. In the NGO context, this means that the NGO can defend their politik, like Fanm Tèt Ansanm has continued to do. More broadly, an autonomous NGO can decide its own politics and policies, choose strategies and projects by an internal process, and not simply "follow the money" as do many NGOs, particularly in Haiti.

Like the differences in participation explained in chapter 2 and the differences in organizational management discussed in the previous chapter, the two NGOs in the present study offer a rich and clear comparison regarding autonomy. While neither Fanm Tèt Ansanm nor Sove Lavi is autonomous in the first financial sense, grès kochon kwit kochon, Fanm Tèt Ansanm has high levels of programmatic autonomy, gran moun tèt li, whereas Sove Lavi is far from anything like that. Fanm Tèt Ansanm defended their politik by turning down USAID funding. By contrast, Sove Lavi changed its entire focus with the shifts in USAID's politik from Clinton's WID to Bush's youth HIV/AIDS-prevention orientation, and then suddenly dropping CACs when USAID stopped funding them in favor of the Caravan—all in an effort to follow the money. This chapter has provided some examples of how donors took control of Sove Lavi. Mme Versailles, the director, declared openness to be a virtue. Coupled with this favorable orientation are windows of opportunity for donor control when Sove Lavi failed to meet its specified objectives, such as the Caravan meeting described. In other words, the relationship is codependent (Vincent 2006).

Structurally, the two NGOs are in very different positions. Whereas Sove Lavi is entirely dependent on only two public development agencies, and their logic and cycles of projects (Sampson 1996; Schade 2005), Fanm Tèt Ansanm has a diverse array of support, most of them European NGOs. Because Fanm Tèt

Ansanm has five donors, no single individual donor has veto power over the organization. As I have shown in this chapter, public funding and directions can change rapidly and fundamentally. For example, USAID suddenly dropped Sove Lavi and the strategy of CACs altogether. More broadly, development aid is contracted through short-term projects. This chapter has also shown that both the brusqueness of funding shifts and the constant shortfall of funding that hampered local planning and participation can be traced to a new donor practice, results- or performance-based management. In contrast, European NGOs—at least those that fund Fanm Tèt Ansanm—which are not contractors of their government and are not executing projects defined by its development arm, are not constrained by the logic and rhythm of the project with short-term "deliverables" and outcomes. The European NGOs engaged in long-term partnerships, which offered Southern organizations more latitude to define how the work is to be done, respecting their position in the field.

So far, the analysis of the two women's NGOs' civic infrastructure has shown that, indeed, there appear to be some correlations in the different spheres of relationships between NGO stakeholder groups. Sove Lavi had low levels of participation, developed and reproduced vertical relationships with target populations, and had low levels of individual staff autonomy and similarly low levels of organizational autonomy. Sove Lavi's clientelist relationship with its donors was reproduced in the field. By contrast, Fanm Tèt Ansanm had much higher levels of community participation, attempted to construct and support horizontal relationships, and had high levels of staff autonomy and organizational programmatic autonomy. My research has shown that these two NGOs might be so different because of the differences in dependency on public aid to development. This chapter has highlighted specific public donor policies, including results-based management and abstinence promotion.

The remaining question is why? What explains the genesis of these two recent policies? More generally, what accounts for the vast differences in USAID's and European NGOs' politik? The following chapter provides an istwa, a historical account, to answer these questions.

5

Tectonic Shifts and
the Political Tsunami

USAID and the Disaster of Haiti

We are trying to juggle multiple constituencies–multiple issues involved.
If it was just poverty, there would not be as much money. There's the boat
people issue, the drugs issue, the Congressional Black Caucus. Here's a
new issue–Haiti is a failed state at the U.S. borders.

–Jillian, USAID veteran

Wednesday, October 12, 2005, 7:47 P.M.
Today I met with Jillian, a USAID "retiree" who is now working with the agency
as a "contractor," making more money but taking fewer benefits (e.g., she has to
pay her own health care and retirement). Since she was a retiree I was thinking
she could talk more freely, which she further signaled by meeting me at the
lobby to go downstairs to the food court.

This was my third visit to USAID's headquarters, in the public–private
Ronald Reagan Building, and so I was getting used to the metal detector. It struck
me how the security culture is made to feel normal, everyday.

After about ten minutes, Jillian came down to meet me and take me to
lunch. We had to pass metal detectors on our way out. We passed the bank of
elevators in favor of the escalator. We went down two flights, chatting along the
way about how she was busier since retirement. There were several large corporate chains offering familiarly overpriced fare: Chinese, pizza, Italian, Mexican,
a couple of burger joints, and a "healthy" option.

Jillian was a bit wistful as she discussed her career as an anthropologist in
a development agency. She outlined the many changes, frustrations, and missed
opportunities in her job. As one of the first noneconomists to be hired by USAID
and as a woman, Jillian was often frustrated by the prevailing order, "but now
there is much more space for other voices." (She did not mention race, though
she is white and may not have noticed the overrepresentation of white staff.)

Do these voices get listened to?, I wondered. "It depends," she began, "on where you are in the food chain." When I was able to assess that she indeed climbed up the food chain to the point where she actually had some "budgeting authority" and "agenda setting" ability, I repeated what the U.S. ambassador said about Haiti, that we needed to "get Haiti right this time." At this point, she clammed up, intoning, "We can't help Haiti. Haiti needs to help Haiti."

Following this, Jillian offered a lesson to this new anthropologist, a story about her own PhD thesis. She was all set to write a scathing critique of the Bureau of Indian Affairs, about how they screwed up life on this particular reservation she studied. She shared her conclusions with the tribal elders, and one in particular shook his head and told her that she got it all wrong, that the tribe itself was to blame for its problems. That was the end of her story, her analysis, and the interview.

Structure or Agency within the Food Chain?

Jillian's story highlights a central debate within social theory, that of structure versus agency. Are human beings agents acting with free will, or are our actions and our place determined wholly by our social structure? If her own *istwa* is to be read literally, Jillian took this as an "either–or" situation and dropped her social analysis altogether following this comment by a single tribal elder—so much so that years later she pins all of Haiti's problems on "Haiti." In this, Jillian was far from unique; this was a similar refrain in my discussions in Washington. I have seen other young activists with a similar binary framework in their heads about a singular, essentialized Haiti being victimized by U.S. imperialism and globalization turn cynical when they observe behaviors that don't fit their romanticized ideal. One young man in particular, climbing up the food chain as it were, was a good case in point: my sporadic contact with him revealed an increasing cynicism. He now works for USAID. Another lesson Jillian offers for the structure/agency debate is that it matters where one is in the food chain.

This chapter explores these questions, uncovering clues to understand the very different outcomes at Fanm Tèt Ansanm and Sove Lavi. Development policies like the focus on abstinence and "results" discussed in the previous chapter can represent different realities to people depending on their place in the food chain. And as products of human action and decision, policies have a "social life" (Appadurai 1986). This chapter analyzes the social life of these two policies, abstinence promotion and performance- or results-based contracting. Both policies began in a particular milieu, the post-9/11 security apparatus and its impact on development institutions and the ongoing political battleground surrounding "development" within the two-party U.S. political system. This chapter outlines this political dimension to aid in general, and particularly Haiti and these policies.

Chapters 2 through 4 presented a comparison between the civic infrastructure of the two NGOs, Sove Lavi and Fanm Tèt Ansanm. Comparing the two NGOs is instructive: the donor–NGO relationship seems to shape the levels and quality of beneficiaries' participation and the NGOs' autonomy. The previous chapter argued that Sove Lavi's low level and quality of participation stems from a rapidly shifting approach in which their donors—especially USAID—impose their *politik* on Sove Lavi, including performance-based management approaches and an "ABC" method of HIV/AIDS prevention with an emphasis on abstinence. What accounts for the difference in the two NGOs' donors' approaches?

Answering this question is the focus of this chapter. To do so requires attention to the internal dynamics and structures of the donor agencies, as well as organizational constraints. With public aid to development in the United States tied to foreign policy, there is also always a political element to debates, policies, and institutional structures. While Haiti was experiencing its own crisis, in the United States following 9/11 these processes and structures were in flux, as the legitimating discourses and institutional structures underwent radical shifts. Understanding them requires a nuanced interpretation of geopolitical shifts.

I use the term "tectonic shifts" because of their vast scope and global scale, as well as their relative invisibility. Like continental plates, these shifts appear underground. Movement within and between them causes friction, transforming the visible landscape through processes generating earthquakes or volcanic activity, which Anna Tsing (2005) points out can be productive as well as destructive. If these plates—say, the North American and the Eurasian—are sitting beneath an ocean, the rumblings as one pushes atop the other generates a tsunami. The friction as the interest groups and constituencies are bumping into one another likewise causes rumblings that, as in the case of the 2004 East Indian Ocean tsunami, cause massive and potentially dangerous tidal waves on foreign shores. While the shift may be subtle and unnoticeable at its epicenter, the effect is magnified and disastrous as it reaches Southern shores. I use the language of disaster consciously, since the post-Aristide period is a clear example of "disaster capitalism" (Klein 2007). These tectonic shifts are often subterranean, escaping notice of many scholars, NGOs, and even social movements.

I selected USAID as the focus of this analysis because, first and foremost, it is the largest international development agency that dispenses grant aid. Overall, the United States gave more than $23 billion in FY 2004; by way of comparison, the European Commission gave more than $9 billion (Riddell 2007:56). In Haiti, this general pattern holds, as the United States gave $400 million during the two years that followed Aristide's departure, compared to $250 million from the European Commission (International Monetary Fund 2006). At least until the HOPE Act offering tax incentives for offshore apparel factories, private direct investment in Haiti has traditionally been a fraction of official development aid, $4.7 and 7.8 million in fiscal years 2002 and 2003 (International Monetary Fund 2005b:24).

This chapter begins with a brief discussion of USAID, outlining its history, its structure, and finally its position within the U.S. government. Following this is a thumbnail sketch of the process of "national interest" through which USAID emerged and within which it works as an institution. Following this "static" portrait, I discuss the tectonic shifts, the political vacuum following the end of the Cold War, and the rise of a corporatist model of governance. The bulk of this chapter discusses USAID's institutional responses during the 2001–2009 Bush administration, including a results orientation, a shift in focus toward HIV/AIDS, and the promotion of abstinence and the empowerment of faith-based groups. Institutional/structural changes also include the creation of the global AIDS coordinator, the Millennium Challenge Corporation, and the Office of Stabilization and Reconstruction, and an increase in Office of Transition Initiatives (OTI) funding. All these changes triggered a complete overhaul of international assistance in January 2006.

USAID

The Ronald Reagan Building housing USAID is a big, glassy, modernist, mall-like "public-private" building containing U.S. federal government, NGO, and corporate office suites, which Mary Hancock (2006) describes as a reflection of neoliberal ethos of privatization and erosion of public space. It would look and feel no different than other downtown office-building lobbies in the United States except for one detail; people are metal-detected when they enter. Every time I visited, three black women (or two black women and one black man) working security stopped me and asked for my ID. Behind a glass door with a modest USAID sign in white block letters was another reception area, looking very much like a hotel or bank lobby—with two separate lines, one for visitors and one for staff. Two black women and a black man who staffed security gave visitors badges and told them to wait.

The waiting room was made of faux marble and glass, without couches, and without even a set of periodicals to leaf through, as is common at other donor institutions such as the Global Fund or the European Union. Visitors have to stand, with nothing to do except look at the posters discussing USAID's various "pillars." In fact, they were posted on the outer walls of the building: democracy, humanitarian assistance, agricultural development, infrastructure, health, education, and so forth. On the far wall, separating the USAID office from the rest of the Ronald Reagan Building, was a likeness of George Marshall, of the Marshall Plan, whose 1947 speech at Harvard's graduation kicked off the era of international development assistance.

History of USAID

USAID's origin myth continues with a bust of John F. Kennedy in their waiting area, skipping over the controversial Mutual Security Program of 1952 that cost $39.8 billion. According to USAID, the youthful President Kennedy, robbed of even a full term of office, raised the spirits and hopes of a generation, giving confidence that the world's problems, as well as "America's," can be solved. Rather than establish it as its own cabinet-level position like the United Kingdom, or place it under the jurisdiction of the Health and Human Services or Treasury Departments, Kennedy placed USAID under the auspices of the State Department. Its founding principles, also expressed in the spacious, well-lit reception area, are simple: Do well by doing good. That is, promote U.S. (foreign) interests by giving out humanitarian assistance to peoples of "developing countries."

Unlike the Marshall Plan before it, USAID began with a divided popular will. In a coordinated bipartisan public relations effort, USAID was sold as a good strategic investment. Representative Morris K. Udall of Arizona published an open letter during the 1961 vote authorizing the new agency, citing his testimony to the House Committee on Foreign Affairs that "the whole southern hemisphere of our world is in ferment. New nations are emerging. Peoples are seeking a voice in their affairs and higher living standards. The siren call of Communism is being heard in nearly every land" (Udall 1961:4). Arguing for the controversial (and now defunct) Alliance for Progress, targeting "America's back yard" of the Western Hemisphere, Udall wrote, "Here is a program that sets out to combat the forces of extreme poverty and political oppression which are the best possible breeding ground for Communism." Kennedy himself argued that "widespread poverty and chaos lead to a collapse of existing political and social structures which would inevitably invite the advance of totalitarianism into every weak and unstable area. Thus our own security would be endangered and our prosperity imperiled" (USAID 2006b). This was the beginnings of Kennedy's "American century" wherein the United States assumed leadership of the "free world," paying any price and making every sacrifice in the defense of liberty. W. W. Rostow's (1952, 1960) theory of stages of growth and development provided USAID's conceptual model.[1]

By this very public celebration of George Marshall, representing an "ancestor" to USAID, the institution deliberately skips its own controversial beginnings. Nostalgically highlighting icons such as Marshall and Kennedy, USAID thus represents its best ideals to the public that developing the "third world" is good policy for the United States, highlighting a defensive legacy of insisting that U.S. foreign interests should naturally guide an institution dedicated to international development. The ancestor shrine, indeed the entire origin myth, represents a symbolic attempt to naturalize the linkage between development and foreign policy and preclude the imagination or articulation of alternative conceptions of international assistance that are not bound with strategic interests.

This grafting of foreign policy objectives onto aid programs lends foreign aid a political character, making it a space for contests over how the national interest is defined.

Structure of USAID

During my first visit, long after I finished reading about USAID's history and while I was reading about USAID's pillars, a white woman in her mid-fifties who had twenty-seven years with the agency met me, and I again went through security, my briefcase searched. We went up the elevator into a third-floor office. The elevator opened to a small, unadorned hallway leading to a large room with several rows of five-foot-tall gray cubicle dividers. Nothing distinguished this office from corporate offices where I had temped, except for fewer signs of individual personality on the cubicle dividers (a street sign saying "Elvis Presley Rd." and a huge stuffed M&M doll were all that were visible). Three glass-walled offices looked out onto the field of cubicles for people in supervisory positions. The first interview was conducted in such an office, so we could close the door and "talk without interruptions." My interviewee's superior was apparently out for the day, "on the Hill," but there were few telltale signs of its use: no family pictures or piles of paper on the desk.

Making and setting policy at USAID, at least in theory, is a relatively small group of social scientists[2] working as development specialists in the Washington office. They sift through evaluations, quarterly grantee reports, annual mission reports, and executive summaries of special "field visits." They particularly look for policy recommendations that arise from these prepared documents, looking for "best practices" or success stories that can be pulled out of the local context and be replicated elsewhere. Policymakers are entirely dependent on open and honest lines of communication from report authors—NGO directors, contractors, and mission staff—who ideally engage in open dialogue with their beneficiaries. After a draft policy has been written, it is circulated to all the geographic "bureaus" and the relevant issue "pillars" for comments. At this stage, potential exemptions or contradictions are invited by people who ostensibly have more "on the ground" experience working for in-country "missions." Sometimes commentary is made and the policy rewritten. Intra-agency communication is of the utmost importance during this process because once a policy is in place, every USAID employee, contractor, and grantee in every part of the world is accountable to uphold it. It becomes "auditable."

Gradual shifts to USAID policies have been made over time, for example with Women in Development, begun in 1974 to implement the 1973 Percy Amendment (named after the sponsoring congressperson, and called an "amendment" because it amends the 1961 Foreign Assistance Act) calling on the agency to address women's issues. According to a policy specialist, WID had full-time staff only in the 1980s, and it had only "budgeting authority" in the 1990s.

It never attained the status of a "pillar" but remained a relatively marginal "cross-cutting" issue that had the ability only to recommend policies to the pillars, whose chiefs had direct access to the director. WID's justification "remained marginal; we always have to argue why paying attention to women pays off in a mainstream economic analysis," said a policy planner. "But at least we can shift policy through our data analysis. It's slowgoing but some progress." The nominal process for policy change at USAID is slow and deliberate. How well this process is followed under normal circumstances is an open question. The conditions for finding best practices in the field and then communicating them upward leave much room for human error, at the least, not to mention politics. Regardless of whether the policymaking process is actually followed, its existence and dissemination (to USAID staff people at least) plays a symbolic function, shaping normative discourses and practices (Hilhorst 2003:123).

Actual practice does not often match the official process for policy formation. According to a USAID veteran, policy is "smuggled into" the process from "on high" through the use of earmarks, congressional directives attached to an authorizing legislation or appropriation. According to a policy specialist, these earmarks usually arise from an amendment to a bill proposed by an individual member of Congress, responding to a particular constituency or interest group. Complicating this, there are at least twenty-three laws governing U.S. foreign aid (Oxfam America 2008:11). The 1988 Hamilton-Gilmon Report from House Committee on Foreign Affairs was critical of USAID's confusing structure: "Foreign aid legislation and administration impede the effectiveness of the program thereby confirming the public's view of the value of these programs: there are too many objectives in the FAA [Foreign Assistance Act], so numerous in fact that they 'cannot provide meaningful direction or be effectively implemented'" (USAID 2006b). One example of a congressional earmark that this USAID planner found particularly unhelpful was the removal of user fees in education in southern Africa attached to an appropriations bill when they had already been done away with.[3] Said a USAID planner, "We lose our credibility when we do things like that, imposing policies, directing a pilot project in the wrong area." Sometimes this process of earmarks was linked to an organized movement for social change, such as WID. Because Congress is the site for political contestation, the process of USAID earmarks is inseparable from the political process. Most frustrating for USAID staff is family planning, what a policy staff called a "hornet's nest," wherein different political pressure groups advocate for directly opposing policy options.

Decisions about funding and "strategic objectives" (SOs) are made through a hierarchical process initiated by in-country mission staff. These SO supervisors propose a budget to the mission director, who compiles them and makes a report and a request to the bureau through a process called "R4"—the Resource Request and Results Review. These R4s are not technically "public"—meaning that to obtain access to them, an outsider would have to initiate a formal written request through the Freedom of Information Act (FOIA). FOIA requests are notoriously slow and expensive, and requesters are charged twenty cents per page for copies. The bureaus compile the country reports and submit a budget request to the central administration. The names of grantees and budget line items are removed at this level. USAID bureau and pillar chiefs hammer out an agreement about the budget that is finally submitted to Congress, then publishing a "budget justification" that is available for public inspection, review, and comment. In recent years the document has been available on USAID's website. Only once did Congress formally reject USAID's budget, in 1971, at the nadir of the Vietnam War, an expression of the widespread mistrust in Washington at the time (USAID 2006b). As with other federal agencies, final amounts are set by a process of negotiation between the president, the House of Representatives, and the Senate.

Two specialized units within USAID have been exempt from the process of earmarks and have been granted "notwithstanding" authority to set and monitor their own policies. Ostensibly because of the need for rapid response, the Office of Transition Initiatives and the Office of Disaster Response were exempted from these time-consuming and often burdensome set of requirements, such as the need to acquire a competitive bid for contracts through USAID's procurement office.

The National Interest

This system was sent into flux following the end of the Cold War (Enloe 1993), and different interest groups collided over the struggle to define the national interest. Central to USAID's existence and mission is the promotion of the U.S. national interest. Founded in 1961 during the height of the Cold War, two years after the Cuban Revolution, USAID's legitimating discourse focused on the threat posed by communism. The October 1989 fall of the Berlin Wall, heralding the end of the Soviet empire and hence the Cold War, presented a legitimation crisis at USAID. According to a thirty-year USAID veteran, the "public core constituency" that supported international development evaporated following the end of the Cold War. This change generated significant ripples that were felt in Haiti. An institutional response was the results-oriented approach discussed in the previous chapter, a defensive posture to show that money is not wasted. Particular interest constituencies took the opportunity to fill the void. Under the Bush-Rice team beginning in 2005, more recent structural changes took root.

Under President Clinton, famous for his description of political maneuvering against what he perceived to be the conservative political winds as "tacking," USAID continued to function but its policies were unstable, constantly changing. In this legitimacy crisis, the Clinton USAID was more aggressive in its public relations, in effect selling the national interest to specific constituencies. One of the last publications of the Clinton USAID (2001:21) argued that the agency "return[s] substantial dividends to this country in expanded trade opportunities . . . [and] contribute[s] a great deal to our domestic prosperity and demonstrate[s] to the American people that foreign assistance is really an investment in America." This article cites an executive of a U.S. corporation who thanked USAID for helping him secure a $750,000 satellite contract in Cameroon. Thus with the end of the Cold War, economic interests began to overshadow security interests in the formulation of the U.S. national interest. An expression of this privileging of economic interest is that in 2005, fully 93 percent of USAID funds in Haiti came back to the United States through U.S. providers of goods and services (OECD 2006). In development discourse, this is called "tied aid." USAID's focus on U.S. business interests explains the relative similarities—with the exception of approach to Aristide, described below—between Democratic and Republican administrations regarding Haiti.

USAID's post–Cold War institutional identity struggles also occurred within an ascendant neoliberal ideology. The belief that free-market capitalism—unfettered by any government regulation—is the best engine for growth and the fairest system for its distribution became dominant following a crusade led by the University of Chicago economist Milton Friedman. Known in the United States as Reaganomics, neoliberalism took root following the 1973 coup d'état in Chile (Harvey 2005; Klein 2007). IFIs such as the World Bank, previously dismissed as "statist," gradually were taken over by Chicago-trained neoliberal economists (Perkins 2006; Stiglitz 2002). Meanwhile, think tanks flooded the media—increasingly concentrated in fewer hands (Bagdikian 1993; Williams 1995)—and the political parties with a pro-business message. Since Reagan's and Thatcher's terms in office, these ideas came to dominate both domestic and foreign policy, to the point where the Democrat Bill Clinton was economically to the right of the Republican Richard Nixon. Flush with corporate sponsorship, Clinton's Democratic Leadership Council succeeded in bringing the party to what they called the "center," accomplishing a Republican, neoliberal, pro-business agenda, especially with the passage of the North American Free Trade Agreement and the radical restructuring (or destruction) of welfare.

In this unstable policy environment, a senior USAID planning official argued that "interest constituencies" define the U.S. national interest. In this list she included "Midwestern soy farmers" (she did not use the word "agribusiness") as well as NGOs that were created by the system of international aid, organized under a "foreign aid" lobby known as InterAction. InterAction, the colloquial name for a coalition of 160 NGOs called the American Council for Voluntary International Action, succeeded in creating constituent support for overseas health interventions. In addition, she certainly could have mentioned telecommunications industries and textiles manufacturers, as well as the oil industry.

While planning staff deplore the fact that "individual members [of Congress] sometimes act like we are accountable to them personally," it is nonetheless clear that USAID is supposed to be accountable to Congress as a whole. This congressional oversight could explain USAID's defensive posturing; however, there is evidence that such a position may be unnecessary. The University of Maryland's Program on International Policy Attitudes found that, if anything, U.S. public opinion is showing signs of strengthening support for foreign assistance since the mid-1990s following the end of USAID's Cold War public justification. In two polls, in 1995 and 2000, 80 and 79 percent (respectively) of people polled favored in principle the use of taxpayer funds for international aid (Program on International Policy Attitudes 2001:6). In 1995 a strong majority of people (64 percent) polled favored cutting foreign aid, while in 2000 a minority (40 percent) felt the same way. This minority was still significant, but the report's authors argued that it was because research participants extremely overestimated the actual aid given: the median estimate in the 2000 poll was 20 percent of the federal budget, more than thirty times the actual amount. A 2005 poll, PIPA's latest on the subject, shows that 65 percent of U.S. citizens support increasing U.S. development aid to 0.7 percent of the U.S. GDP, the goal of the ONE Campaign, and 70 percent support levying $50 per household to meet the Millennium Development Goals.

Since the 2008 financial meltdown this support may finally be evaporating. In my class, several inner-city students in New York, many of them immigrants to the United States and most of them the first in their families to go to college, have emphatically argued in class that we should not be sending foreign aid because there are many real problems here in the United States. People of decidedly different racial and economic backgrounds in the "Tea Party" movement among other groups advocate isolationism and a reduction in taxes, both heralding much lower support for international development aid. The Tea Party's organizing was well funded—by the oil industry scions the Koch brothers among others—and amplified by the press, so members of Congress, including those with whom my students and I have met, are again "jittery" about sending money overseas. Time will tell if the Occupy movement, which arguably drew inspiration from the "Arab Spring" in North Africa and which quickly went global after activists squatted on Zuccotti Park near Wall Street on September 17, 2011, will open up new political spaces for international development, as it did for ending tax cuts for the wealthiest U.S. citizens, reinstating the so-called millionaires' tax.

Interestingly, the people polled in PIPA's survey were less enthusiastic about the political/foreign policy role of U.S. foreign aid than about the humanitarian purposes, as almost twice as many people (63 percent compared to 34 percent) believe that aid should not be directed as a function of current security interests (Program on International Policy Attitudes 2001:13).[4] The authors conclude that "an abundance of evidence shows that Americans are quite unenthusiastic about the Cold War tradition of giving aid as a means of gaining influence over other countries" (30). Notwithstanding this trend in public attitudes, USAID's history web page cites the 1988 Hamilton-Gilmon Report, arguably the most thorough congressional investigation into the agency: "U.S. public support for helping poor people remains strong, but the public does not view the aid program as doing this effectively. The public has very little concept of the aid program as an instrument of foreign policy, used to advance U.S. interests."[5] Whereas the public is not enthused about the political aspects of aid, this idea of doing well by doing good is symbolically reinforced to staff as they walk past the plaque of George Marshall every day on their way to work, and serves as a reminder to visitors. With popular support for U.S. foreign aid increasing, and resistance partially based on faulty assumptions diminishing, why would USAID be on the defensive in the 1990s and early 2000s? A potential answer lies in what development agency staff refer to as their "constituency."

Constituency

Several current and former USAID staff discussed the issue of the institution's constituency. This discourse of constituencies had wide currency among the development institution staff that I interviewed in United States and Europe at a range of bilateral, multilateral, and private institutions. In its broadest usage, a constituency is a group of people to whom an institution or public official feels accountable. Elected officials' constituents are the voters in their district. In terms of organizations, constituents are the "stakeholders" in it, the groups or individuals who are concerned with the outcome. The quotations introducing this chapter outlined several constituencies for USAID's work in Haiti, clusters of foci based on such issues as drugs, anti-immigrant sentiment, and poverty. Of her list, only one—the Congressional Black Caucus—referred to a specific group of people. The others were presumably amorphous interest groups concerned with the clusters of issues. Her colleague noted that there can be competing constituencies on the same issue: "There are targeted constituencies for family planning. While it is shown that FP [family planning] has ancillary benefits to the health and education of both the child and the mother, as you know there are constituencies who want it gone."

These two examples gesture toward groups external to the institutions. Counterparts at other institutions use the word constituency to describe intra-organizational stakeholder groups. A European Union development officer decried the "situation in which we work for two constituencies: there is the service line and the commissioner line, the DG [Directorate General]. It's often difficult to discover how to serve these people. Each has to get briefs. We're constantly servicing two structures." To this staff, juggling two institutional structures—one ostensibly elected body, the European Council, and the permanent bureaucracies,

the Commissions—was weakening the focus on development: "With this structure in the Commission, we are doing both foreign affairs and development.
And I am not comfortable with that." Each of the institutional groups—the
constituencies—had different expectations of their development staff. A Global
Fund official argued that "when listing the constituencies, there is always donors,
recipients, and the multilaterals, and there's always a pause. And then NGOs.
That pause needs to go away. We're still an afterthought." The Global Fund's
work—as organized through their charter and oversight processes—is divided
into perceived common interest groups. Northern donor states are believed to
share common interests, as are Southern recipient states, and NGOs of every
size and from every country. This division, codified into their governance structure and charter, papers over real differences between NGOs: "The NGO representatives in the North tend to be policy or political people. They are very
experienced in the arena, as lobbyists and as activists. They have a lot of confi-
dence and experience conducting research, and can therefore pick apart others'—
they have the competence in the field." There is a difference in the level of
participation between Northern and Southern NGOs, as outlined by this Global
Fund official: "Participation in the board is written into the Northern NGO representatives' job descriptions. For the Southern NGOs it is something on top of
their work. Often it's hard to get a hold of them because they are in the field,
doing their jobs." Northern NGOs are also likely to have much larger travel
budgets. NGOs are not a monolithic entity, yet some donors such as the Global
Fund treat them as such, conflating multinational Northern NGOs with small
outfits within Southern countries.

While it is possible that these different conceptions of constituency are
idiosyncratic, or merely a semantic issue, I argue that this lack of precision is
symptomatic of a general problem within international development. During
one of the most candid interviews I had with a former USAID mission head, he
flatly stated, "We also talk to international NGOs. They are part of our constituency. If we don't get the support that we need in Washington, we need their
support." This statement—that international NGOs through InterAction are a
primary constituency for international aid in the United States—was corroborated by other interviews. While research has shown that the U.S. voting public
strongly supports international development in principle—and even supports
giving 10 percent of the U.S. budget to foreign aid, a much higher percentage
than is actually being allocated (Program on International Policy Attitudes
2001:8)[6]—there is no consistent, general lobby or pressure group making
international aid a visible priority in Washington, except for InterAction.

This provides one possible explanation for the comparatively low amount of
funds being allocated to international development, and also possibly accounts
for Congress members' defensiveness. Other federal programs—such as Social
Security, highway and infrastructure projects, or education—have constituent

group support through one of two processes. The first is direct lobbying support through organizations such as the American Association of Retired Persons, various building and trades' unions, the American Automobile Association, or the American Federation of Teachers. Alexis de Tocqueville ([1835] 2000), who wrote the first outsider ethnography of the United States in 1835—still read in political science courses—hails these voluntary associations as embodying the nation's democratic spirit. Second, these projects are seen as part of voting citizens' enlightened self-interest, a holdover from Enlightenment ideals of civil society.

International aid presents a challenge to both processes within the received understanding of the U.S. political system. Aside from NGOs that eventually receive USAID funding, there are no organized groups advocating for aid, presenting a situation of a conflict of interest or a cycle of patronage. If InterAction member NGOs weren't nonprofits, they would be roundly criticized for their self-serving lobbying efforts, since collectively these groups receive billions in U.S. aid annually. International development and poverty eradication are not often seen as part of citizens' direct self-interest, a problem shared by groups that advocate for "the environment"—just like trees or spotted owls, foreigners living abroad cannot vote in U.S. elections. As a consequence of this lack of a general constituency, USAID is particularly vulnerable to pressure groups and ever-changing perceptions of "public opinion," even and sometimes especially one that is misinformed.

Responses

According to senior USAID policy staff, the concept of results-oriented contracting arose to appease jittery Congress members who reluctantly supported U.S. health NGOs in the post–Cold War political vacuum: "As a result, we are directed toward easily measurable things that can be explained to the taxpayer: results, public goods, whatever." In part, this concept arose out of Clinton and Gore's "reinventing government," applying corporate-style management policies and practices to the U.S. federal government. An early example of this was "outcomes-based education" that, ramped up, has transformed into the No Child Left Behind legislation in education that threatens poorly performing school districts with financial penalties. Generally, because it is implemented on foreigners, foreign aid is often a site for field-testing corporate-style policies, what Susan George (1992) called the "boomerang" effect: policies such as privatization and state devolution are field-tested first in foreign development settings, where they are tried in the South and then implemented in the North, in donor countries. For example, the author of neoliberalism, Milton Friedman, began the experimentation in the dictator Augusto Pinochet's Chile. In the international development arena, this concept was first applied as a pilot program in the HIV-prevention sector. Interestingly, Haiti was selected as one of the pilot countries, managed by USAID/Haiti's HIV-prevention contractor, Management

Sciences for Health (Pollock 2003). This performance-based approach specifies financial incentives and punishments in contracts, solidifying an increasing push for numerical evaluation measures that every NGO director I interviewed noticed. In the Haiti pilot study, if all the performance targets were met, a 5 percent bonus was given to the NGO. If they were not met, a 5 percent penalty was withheld from the NGO. This pilot project was replicated with all HIV/AIDS-prevention funding, and possibly all health funding. And it has become more generalized, highlighted in the FY 2006 budget justification: "In this budget we propose a performance-based approach, comparing need and performance across regions, to allocate a share of the Development Assistance account based on standard criteria."[7]

Other institutions, including the Global Fund, are also employing results-oriented approaches. The Global Fund was founded in January 2002 with a mandate to go "beyond business as usual"—and results-oriented management was a key plank in that platform (Global Fund 2004). The European Union has also implemented a "Results-Oriented Monitoring" System. As Sove Lavi's experience shows, this policy has a potential consequence of centralizing NGO planning and undermining local participation. Other scholars of NGOs have noted this tension between accountability from "above" as well as "below" (Biggs and Neame 1996; Edwards and Hulme 1996a; Hilhorst 2003:125; Thayer 2001:254). This shift toward the Global Fund's results-based management and USAID's performance-based contracting tips the balance even further toward accountability from above (Hulme and Edwards 1997; Kamat 2003; Nelson 1995), further eroding local participation.

Defining the National Interest

This embattled USAID, still struggling to redefine itself, was also the fertile ground for another constituency. George W. Bush took office both terms following two close and contested presidential elections. Taking credit for his razor-thin margin of victory was a newly empowered evangelical movement, slowly built throughout the 1980s and 1990s through organizations such as the Christian Coalition. Playing highly visible roles within Bush's 2000 and 2004 campaigns, Rightist constituencies were given powerful and important, but relatively low-profile, positions within his administration. With the U.S. progressive movement focusing on defending abortion rights and to a lesser extent same-sex marriage, imploring Congress to carefully scrutinize cabinet-level appointments and Supreme Court nominations, attention in the U.S. public sphere was not directed toward foreign assistance. For example, in January 2006 there were two stories in the New York Times about Secretary of State Condoleezza Rice's reshuffling of U.S. foreign assistance and naming a new USAID administrator, compared to 177 stories about the nomination of Samuel Alito to the Supreme Court.[8]

This evangelical constituency was rewarded for their crucial role in Bush's rise to the presidency. In his 2003 State of the Union address, in which he made the case for war on Iraq, Bush also unveiled a $15 billion plan to combat AIDS. The President's Emergency Plan for AIDS Relief (PEPFAR) was created under the direction of the new, ambassador-level post of global AIDS coordinator. Named to this new post was the pharmaceutical executive Randall Tobias, former CEO of pharmaceutical giant Lilly. In addition to the performance-based contracting, the new PEPFAR entailed two significant, interrelated policy shifts: a focus on abstinence and a faith-based service delivery model.

The focus on abstinence, including a specific earmark for funding abstinence-related activities, did not come about through the slow, deliberative process described earlier in this chapter. "It was a political decision, handed down from above," recalled a USAID veteran. "It's just frustrating to be handed down these policy mandates that go against best practices and our own research or policy. Many of us have lamented it." According to an AIDS specialist, PEPFAR grants attention only toward health indicators, while "those of us in the field who have been doing development for years know about the social and economic aspects of AIDS transmission, why people get infected as well as how AIDS affects society and the economy. There are a lot of policy papers by people who know what they're talking about, arguing the need to simultaneously address the non-health aspects of HIV/AIDS." Several studies, including some by anthropologists, have shown that an abstinence-only prevention policy does not work, and in fact often triggers a backlash (Gayle 2006; Gootnick 2006). Further, as mentioned in the previous chapter, according to the USAID/Haiti AIDS specialist, 90 percent of Haitians know the three methods of HIV/AIDS prevention in USAID's "ABC" plan: *a*bstinence, *b*eing faithful, or *c*ondom use.

A recipient of USAID funding, Sove Lavi's message of AIDS prevention is focused on abstinence. Sove Lavi's aid recipients were "youth," despite the fact that many CAC members were over forty years old. As the line of reasoning of USAID/PEPFAR goes, abstinence is the most appropriate policy and message for youth, because prevention is more cost-effective than the expensive antiretroviral drug treatment. One agency representative cited the proverb, "an ounce of prevention is worth a pound of cure." For example, a Sove Lavi brochure jointly authored by USAID published in 2006 recommends that youth wait until they turn twenty-three for their first sexual encounter. No one at Sove Lavi could explain the significance of twenty-three. Further, while there are questions on Sove Lavi's pre- and post-tests about alcohol and drug use as a means for putting oneself at risk of contracting HIV,[9] there are no such questions about the link between discrimination against women or economic vulnerability and the rise of AIDS. Given this, and given that 90 percent of the population knows how AIDS is contracted and prevented, why do donors continue to promote Sove Lavi's high-cost Caravan? First is a focus on appearances. It serves as a backdrop for photos showing crowds of people or engaging cultural activities, to be shown on both Sove Lavi's and USAID's websites, one response to "jittery members of

Congress" to show that they are doing something. A closer look at the discourse suggests a hyper-individualist analysis and intervention. Sove Lavi's organizational motto is "changing behaviors." This USAID analysis necessarily erases social causes for the rise of HIV/AIDS transmission, such as economic and gender discrimination, which community members constantly brought up at meetings, as Gabrielle's istwa powerfully demonstrates (Farmer 1992; Farmer et al. 1996; Robins 2006; Susser 2009). As such, PEPFAR's abstinence promotion is the latest in the "blame the victim" tradition (Ryan 1971).

Further, a close inspection of PEPFAR reveals that USAID is openly and explicitly allowed to fund faith-based organizations (USAID 2004a). An October 4, 2004, press release announcing $100 million in abstinence-focused grants cites President Bush as saying, "I think our country needs a practical, effective and moral message." Tobias was also cited in the press release: "Faith-based and community-based organizations have a reach, authority and legitimacy that make them crucial partners in the fight against HIV/AIDS." Like performance-based contracting, faith-based groups also found their way into the general 2006 budget justification: "USAID is actively engaged in identifying and forging agreements with non-traditional partners, including faith-based organizations" (USAID 2006a). According to a USAID official, after this policy opening in Washington, an evangelical missionary organization called World Vision International applied for and received funding from USAID's AIDS-prevention program (see Bornstein's [2003] study for a history and analysis of World Vision).[10] In one province where Sove Lavi worked with thirty schools, only three were public, and two others were Catholic. The remaining twenty-five were Protestant, and judging from their names (e.g., Maranatha, Eben-Ezer), the majority were Pentecostal.[11] This is significant in the context of Haiti's religious field,which was still predominantly Catholic, at least nominally (Hefferan 2007; Rey 1999).[12] Most Protestant churches in Haiti have direct links to U.S.-based missionary organizations, whereas most Catholic groups eschew direct proselytizing (Hefferan 2007:150). Many Sove Lavi trainings I observed began with a prayer, a symbol of this effective religious mobilization. Since the January 12 earthquake, these mission organizations and their Haitian partners are much more empowered and on the offensive. Protestant groups killed forty-five traditional Vodou leaders in December 2010, on the pretext that this "Devil worship" caused the cholera outbreak (Delva 2010).

Competition: The Global Fund

Some people who work at development agencies in Washington, Haiti, and Europe also see PEPFAR as a response to the Global Fund. It is multilateral, a public–private partnership that within three years amassed a $10 billion annual budget, according to its 2005 annual report. According to staff in Washington and Geneva, other reasons explained the Bush administration's jealousy of the

Global Fund. It received substantial support from the Bill and Melinda Gates Foundation—$150 million in its first two years—and was seen as a Clinton endeavor. The conversations and institutional support began with Clinton's support and leadership, and the Global Fund counts the Clinton Global Initiative as one of its major in-kind donors. Additionally, the Global Fund promotes "harm reduction" strategies that acknowledge that people engage in behaviors that cause them to be at risk for contracting HIV/AIDS. The goal is to provide safer alternatives rather than, according to staff, promote a "social engineering" model whereby they "finger-wag" and expect that youth will stop having sex, or that intravenous drug users will suddenly quit, simply because a community elder told them to. The finger-wagging, abstinence-only message "is a death sentence," said a Global Fund staff member who was, incidentally, HIV positive. Highlighting the differences between the two agencies, the Global Fund's 2004 annual report contains a photograph of an urban, Eastern European needle-exchange program prominently placed on page 6, across from the introduction.

In addition to policy differences, the organization's decision-making structure is quite different. Funding decisions for the Global Fund are made through Country Coordinating Mechanisms (CCMs), constituting national government agencies, NGOs, and international organizations. According to staff, "People can be critical of the CCMs. But it is imperative that we keep the CCM system. No other funding structure offers NGOs a seat at the table. Only in the Global Fund do we have that kind of input."[13] Beginning with the third round of funding, in 2004, the Global Fund made requirements that the CCMs include organizations that represent people living with HIV/AIDS and fund more ARV treatment, but according to their materials and staff, the Global Fund operates with few other directives about CCM composition or funding stream. Finally, instead of setting up country offices (akin to USAID "missions"), the Global Fund contracts with national funding agencies, like Fondation Sogebank, which in the logic of the Global Fund is more desirable because it is both "indigenous" (headquartered in Haiti) and in "the private sector."

These specific policy differences aside, the Global Fund and PEPFAR have many similarities. Staff at both USAID and the Global Fund state that there is a good working relationship. In his role as global AIDS coordinator, Randall Tobias was on the Global Fund's board, chaired by U.S. Secretary of Health and Human Services Tommy Thompson.[14] Both promote a form of results-based management. Both streamline assistance toward HIV/AIDS-specific service delivery, away from policy or general health care sector infrastructure. According to Global Fund staff, funding other programs like basic health care infrastructure or reinforcing women's economic capacity takes the "bang" out of their results orientation.

These shared approaches from both new titans of HIV-prevention work impact recipient NGOs in many ways. This "scale-up" has exponentially increased "local" institutional capacity to combat the disease. And the combined efforts of many institutions investing resources in governments and NGOs for HIV prevention do appear to be slowing HIV transmission rates in Haiti, down from 6.2 to 3.1 percent over a decade (Cohen 2006). But specific donor policies are also increasing existing hierarchies and imbalances. Local participation and autonomy are being eroded. When Mme Versailles brought up CAC members' concerns and suggestions for a small projects fund, she was told to apply to USAID's micro-credit program. Since Sove Lavi was not a bank and the program was not *rentable* (in English, something between "profitable" and "solvent"), her request was denied, and CAC suggestions fell through the cracks. As mentioned in the previous chapter, Mme Versailles is no stranger to the world of donors, and generally successful at securing resources. Unfortunately for CAC members and their communities, Sove Lavi did not communicate USAID's decision to not support a small project fund to them. Sove Lavi also missed an opportunity for community advocacy and lobby efforts by marginalizing space for member discussion at the symposium discussed in chapter 2. As both Mme Versailles and Mme Dominique recall, this segmentation within development aid is not new. USAID's "cross-cutting themes" such as WID or OTI have been attempts to break down these barriers and encourage cross-sectoral dialogue and coordination. But results-based management is forcing even more rigid separation between programmatic lines, weakening member participation in the process.

Institutional Shifts

Since September 11, 2001, security again topped the U.S. foreign agenda, waged as a "war on terror." President Bush quickly created a new cabinet-level position and department, Homeland Security. This discursive and institutional shift has significant consequences for foreign development. In his 2002 National Security Strategy, President Bush named "development" as one of the three key pillars, joining defense and diplomacy. Some senior USAID staff welcomed this rhetorical move because they hoped it would signal the end of the "special interest" control and the regaining of a general "popular support." While there has not been follow-up research, this staff person pointed to an increase in USAID's budget, as well as fewer earmarks. Not counting "supplementals" like Iraq reconstruction,[15] USAID's budget saw a steady increase, from $7 billion in FY 2001 to $9 billion in FY 2006 (see table 5.1). This budget increase coupled with a decrease in congressional mandates may also be a result of Republican control of both houses of Congress and the executive branch until the 2006 election, but for several USAID staff this is a sign of a decrease of "heat" on the agency, "allowing us to do our job of development." Others are more skeptical, arguing that the politicization and privatization of the national interest cannot be easily reversed: "Once the flood gates have been opened, it's hard to close them again."

TABLE 5.1

USAID Allocation in Millions of Dollars, 2001–2007

Year	Allocation
2001	$7,050
2002	$7,517
2003	$8,638
2004	$8,837[a]
2005	$8,971
2006	$9,068
2007	$9,300[b]

Source: Congressional budget justifications for fiscal years 2004 and 2007.

[a]Figure does not include "supplementals," such as Iraq reconstruction.

[b]Budget request. Since the reorganization, the line item for USAID has been changed, and it is no longer possible for citizens to track USAID funding specifically.

Two significant discursive shifts accompanied the 2002 National Security Strategy that arguably bolstered support for USAID. The first concept is "transformational" development and diplomacy, and the second is a renewed focus on "failed states." New institutions accompanied both discursive shifts. At its most basic level, transformational development arose from development agencies' concern and self-critique of development-generated dependency,[16] including the "sustainable" development in vogue under Clinton. Said a former USAID mission director, "We failed to develop countries, but we did a lot. We provided good careers to people here in the United States with great travel opportunities. It was like feeding the horse to feed the fly." A particular recommendation was that aid be developed in such a way as to "graduate" countries from aid dependency. This staff person lamented that after sixty years of development, the development system was able to "graduate" only four countries: Thailand, Costa Rica, South Korea, and Taiwan.[17] According to this person, who worked for the Millennium Challenge Corporation (MCC) at the time of the interview, lessons about development success and failure have been taken up by this new U.S. development agency. The MCC was set up in 2003 by Bush as the U.S. response to the Millennium Development Goals, unanimously approved by the UN General Assembly in 2000. The MCC explicitly works with low-income or "IDA-eligible" countries (referring to the division within the World Bank)[18] that score above average in three general criteria: human development, good governance, and institutions. The most important of the sixteen specific indicators is that countries score above median in corruption, measured by Transparency International's Corruption Perception Index.[19] MCC's assistance is explicitly focused on building private-sector development. In the context of Central America (e.g., Honduras and Guatemala), this signifies the development of foreign tourism and export-processing industries. Other general lessons acknowledged by self-critiques in the late 1990s,[20] including that Southern countries (governments as well as "civil society") need to "own" the process of development, did not affect funding decisions (Farmer 2011a). The MCC enjoyed the additional benefit of being in line with the interests of the transnational business class.

The National Security Strategy refocused attention on "weak states" as vectors of the "dark side of globalization" (USAID 2005b:v). This focus on fragile states portends a significant shift in development discourse, not unlike Truman's organizing the world into "developed" and "underdeveloped" or "developing" nations (Escobar 1995). The National Security Strategy, codified by a 2004 USAID white paper, now divides the world into "stable states" and "fragile states" (USAID 2004b:13).[21] Weak states have become the new target of U.S. foreign assistance in the war on terror, because they "provide the most permissive environments and the least resistance for threats" of terrorism, weapons of mass destruction, and international criminal networks (USAID 2005b:7). Secretary of State Rice (2006) argued that "in today's world, America's security is linked to the capacity of foreign states to govern justly and effectively." By way of definition, USAID (2005b:13) declares that fragile states "include those on a downward spiral toward crisis and chaos, some that are recovering from conflict and crisis, and others that are essentially failed states." According to USAID, there are thirty-four such fragile states. While all fragile states are poor, not all poor states are fragile, and these non-fragile states are eligible for MCC assistance. The rest become targets for other funding, such as OTI or other post-conflict funding. Not even considering the $3 billion to Iraq that was separately accounted for in USAID's FY 2006 congressional budget justification, post-conflict states constitute a quarter of USAID's budget (2005a). The post-conflict budget of the World Bank (1998:13) went up from just under 8 percent in 1980, to 16 percent in 1998, to almost a third in 2005 by the time of my interviews with staff. Since there wasn't a rise in conflicts, the increase in post-conflict budgets suggests their strategic importance, or some additional benefit to the IFIs and donor agencies.

In order to manage and coordinate the multiple government agencies involved in a post-conflict country such as Haiti or Iraq, Bush created the coordinator for reconstruction and stabilization (S/CRS) at the Department of State on August 5, 2004. This office assumes control and coordinates all activities, including the military, diplomatic corps, and USAID. Reception to this idea was lukewarm in some quarters of USAID. Said one representative, "It's basically saying that the U.S. government didn't listen to itself. If we had, we wouldn't have gone to Iraq. But of course we know why we went to Iraq." However positive, this new institutional layer added bureaucratic responsibilities: "The practical effect of all this 'coordination' is that they are taking people away from what they're doing. There is only so much time that we have." The S/CRS works very closely with OTI, especially in Haiti. Interestingly, the OTI budget request increased six-fold in one year, from $48.6 million in FY 2005 to $325 million in FY 2006 (USAID 2005a).[22] This far outpaced USAID's incremental growth over the past seven years. Of this, $30 million was allocated to Haiti. Countries that have an OTI program are not eligible for "Development Assistance" funding, which is earmarked for states with good governance.

With the institutional "shock and awe" creation of the three new agencies mentioned in this chapter, the global AIDS coordinator, the MCC, and the S/CRS, not to mention quick and radical policy shifts and OTI's growth, U.S. Secretary of State Condoleezza Rice reorganized the entire system of development assistance. On January 19, 2006, Rice created the post of director of foreign assistance, simultaneously appointed as the USAID administrator. Rice named Randall Tobias, administrator of PEPFAR, to this new position. The director of foreign assistance works directly under the secretary of state. According to Rice (2006), "This reform will create a more unified and rational leadership structure. It will enhance accountability from both the donors and recipients of assistance. And it will focus our foreign assistance on promoting greater ownership and responsibility on the part of host nations and their citizens." Any institutional autonomy or flexibility that USAID had to insulate "sustainable development" (Clinton's buzzword, now replaced with "transformational development") from the political process described above was rendered much more difficult; USAID has become more directly linked with the State Department, with not even a separate line item that citizens can identify. Oxfam America (2008) has argued that this is the wrong direction for "smart development," which requires a long-term vision and a focus on poverty reduction for its own sake. The case of Haiti highlights the problems when foreign development aid is tied to political processes such as the two-party conflict and the formulation of national interests in foreign policy. As the different interest groups rub up against one another, the ripple effects of these tectonic shifts are magnified in an aid-dependent country such as Haiti.

Effects in Haiti

USAID's mandate is to promote U.S. interests abroad; its primary function has been U.S. security, first against communism, and in the George W. Bush years against terrorism and "weak states." This geopolitical interest explains why Iraq received $6 billion in USAID funding for the first two years following the U.S. Armed Forces' capture of Baghdad in June 2003. "Strategic states" also include Israel, consistently among the top three USAID recipient countries despite its many development indicators higher than even the United States. Haiti highlights the difficulties of an unclear and inconsistent political mandate. Wild vacillations in policies and funding in Haiti have their roots in the U.S. political system, as interest groups and political parties collide into one another in a bid for dominance. The effect on Haiti is disastrous.

Given Haiti's proximity to the United States and the imperialist "Monroe Doctrine," the U.S. government consistently explains its interest there in terms of stability, with the threat of a deluge of "boat people" washing up on Florida shores (USAID 2003). A first wave in the 1980s preceded the United States removing an unpopular dictator, Jean-Claude Duvalier, and replacing him with a military junta. Through the National Endowment for Democracy (NED), founded in 1982 by President Reagan, the U.S. government poured $12 million into the 1990 elections, backing the candidacy of the former World Bank official Marc Bazin (Clement 1997:21; Griffin 1992). Justifying the use of public money on foreign political campaigns, the World Bank argued that elections can be good for imposing changes, but only when they have the right outcomes: "Given the heavy short term costs entailed by economic liberalization policies, only democratically elected governments have the legitimacy to carry them out" (Dethier et al. 1999:23). The landslide election of a populist liberation theology priest seemed to threaten to dismantle the extreme racial and economic inequality buttressing low-wage export-processing zones, employing between seventy and eighty thousand Haitian workers at its peak in the 1980s (Ferguson 1987:83; Hachette 1981:23). On September 30, 1991, after eight months of whirlwind reforms, local and international elite groups united with U.S. backing to remove Aristide from power, again triggering a massive wave of migration to Florida and neighboring Caribbean countries.

George H. W. Bush imposed infamously leaky economic sanctions on the coup government, which was formally recognized by Pope Jean Paul II. In addition to worsening the economic situation for Haiti's people (Gibbons 1999; Griffin 1992), the sanctions served to strengthen the informal market to which only the wealthy had access, implicating Haiti in the international drug trade (Deibert 2005; Klarreich 2005). The crisis spiraled with a massive influx of migrants to the United States and other countries, spurring a passionate debate about the appropriate solution. This racialized "boat people" debate found its way into the 1992 presidential election, during which Clinton promised to restore democratic order to Haiti.[23] After a nearly lost budget vote during his first year of office, Clinton needed to thank loyal Democratic members of Congress. In order to appease the Congressional Black Caucus, Clinton stepped up the pressure to return Aristide, brokering the Governor's Island Accord under UN auspices and sending an invasion force.[24]

In addition to promoting a power-sharing agreement under which Aristide was forced to include opposition leaders, such as Bazin, into his government, the Governor's Island Accord and Paris Club agreement of Haiti's creditors called for economic reconstruction, including privatization (Clement 1997; Doyle 1994). With the coup government (and a new paramilitary organization, FRAPH) murdering tens of thousands of his supporters, Aristide signed, legitimizing structural adjustment. A year after a handful of paramilitary FRAPH forces quelled a U.S. invasion, Aristide was returned on October 15, 1994, with a thirty thousand–strong UN force, including twenty thousand U.S. Marines.

Within the month, Republicans took control of Congress under the banner of Newt Gingrich's "Contract with America." According to a former high-ranking USAID official, Republicans in this era were ideologically opposed to multilateralism and nation-building. A small minority, including the senior Senate Foreign Relations Committee member Jesse Helms, and especially his aide Roger Noriega,[25] were also personally opposed to Aristide. Under the Bush presidencies, Haiti policy was one of "estrangement," delegated to subordinates such as Noriega, whereas Clinton sent high-level administration officials to address Haiti, what the policy specialist Robert Maguire (2003) called "engagement." But generally, according to a former State Department official, the Republicans wanted to regain the White House and were looking to expose Clinton's inexperience in foreign policy—and Haiti, a ninety-minute plane ride from Miami, was their prime target.[26] Almost immediately, the Republican Congress regained control of USAID from the Clinton administration, imposing structural changes under the 1996 Helms Amendment. USAID was barred from directly funding the Haitian government; instead, USAID funded U.S. NGOs, using globalization-era legitimation strategies such as the ideology that NGOs are "closer to the people," more democratic, and less prone to corruption than nation-states. The legislation also secured U.S. control over development priorities in Haiti.

USAID was caught between opposing policy directives in Haiti, officially supporting the return of democratic order while rendering democracy irrelevant by setting Haiti's development agenda through NGOs. But at least until 2001, overall levels of USAID assistance remained high. Bush shifted the direction of USAID in Haiti, and Congress eased its control over USAID, according to a USAID/Haiti staff in January 2004: "The Republicans in Congress put some restrictions on USAID money, but that was under Clinton. They have now removed the restrictions [and] made it clear that they trust Bush wouldn't give money to this government." Instead, USAID worked with NGOs, as a chief of party outlined, also in January 2004: "The most significant evolution is that we used to work with the government. Now we don't. Now we work with NGOs. In 1999, after Préval dissolved Parliament and ruled by decree, that was the beginning of the shift in tides. Donor groups just have to come in to implement their own agenda." Following the May 2000 parliamentary elections, the results of which were contested by Aristide's opposition, all bilateral and multilateral donors boycotted the Haitian government, channeling their assistance directly through NGOs. A USAID Pòtoprens official critiqued what the Aristide government "disingenuously referred to as an embargo, which really only means that it's not going to them, when they know damn well that it's going to Haiti." Multilateral lending institutions—such as the World Bank and IDB—that according to their charters support governments, could not release approved loans until the electoral "crisis" was resolved. The United States used its permanent veto power in the Organization of American States to block IDB loans to Haiti and its plurality in the World Bank to follow suit, withholding a total of $535 million (Farmer 2003).[27]

As argued in chapter 1, there is good evidence that the international community, including the U.S. government, actively supported Aristide's 2004 removal. They cut funds to the government while funding his opposition. They demanded Aristide negotiate while encouraging the opposition to continue pressing for his removal, not cutting funds when they could have. In December 2003, or earlier, the U.S. military had begun preparing Guantanamo Bay for a massive influx of Haitian refugees (Elsner 2004). At each impasse on the "political" stage—including every time the "popular" student-led movement broke away from the bourgeois Group of 184's leadership—the supposedly independent "thugs and murderers," including CIA-trained military and FRAPH leaders, ratcheted up their activities. In an interview granted in late May 2007, Guy Philippe—whom an OTI staff had expressed admiration for in her October 2005 interview—said that despite words to the contrary at the time that the "political" opposition was distinct from Philippe and the "rebels," he was in daily contact with political opposition leaders and the United States (Jacklin 2007). They used hard-to-obtain, U.S.-made M16s that the U.S. government had just given to the Dominican Army to police the free trade zone (Darion Garcia 2003; San Martin 2002). Even granting that each of these situations could be coincidental, and granting one to one odds, when all added up together there is a one in one thousand chance that all of these are coincidental ($2^{10} = 1,024$). What explains the U.S. interest in "regime change" in Haiti? First is the issue of extralegal migration, a sensitive issue in Florida, pivotal in both the 2000 and 2004 presidential contests. According to Washington agency staff, the threat of migration to Florida drives development policy in Haiti. In addition to this issue, people from across the political spectrum in Haiti shared a different analysis.

Disaster Capitalism

Recall Yvette's quote in chapter 1, "If it wasn't in the UN's interests, they would have brought about peace already." At first blush, this passage, suggesting that the international community had interests in the violence, might seem to reflect paranoia, what some call the "Haitian mentality" (Gold 1991; Heinl and Heinl 1996). If not paranoia, then the passage might seem to reflect at the very least propaganda or ideological spin.[28] But Yvette's is a common perception among people in Haiti—and she was an outspoken critic of Aristide. Yvette continued, "Those bandits, where did they find their weapons? The police say that they don't have munitions, the country has an arms embargo. But the bandits, they find ammunition. Where do they find them? In Haiti do they produce them?" In this section I ask many questions, both difficult and compelling: How did the arms get in the hands of bandits?[29] What interests might the international community have in the violence? Naomi Klein coined the concept of "disaster capitalism" to describe how private corporations attempt to profit off disaster situations. In an edited volume, I elaborated on the term: "National and transnational governmental institutions' instrumental use of catastrophe (both so-called 'natural' and human-mediated disasters, including post-conflict situations) to promote and empower a range of private, neoliberal capitalist interests" (2008:20).

Regardless of his actions, including neoliberal policy advances, Aristide's forced departure provided international financial institutions with the opportunity to convene and coordinate their political and economic agenda for Haiti through a process called the Cadre de Coopération Intérimaire (CCI), adopted at a July 2004 donors' meeting in Washington (Interim Government of Haiti 2004). A USAID/Haiti official explained that "donors just have to come in and implement their agendas." The World Bank (1998:24–25) candidly argued that "the weakened capacity of government often found in post-conflict settings magnifies the need for an external aid coordination role." According to twenty-three of twenty-four of the donor representatives I interviewed in Pòtoprens, Brussels, and Washington, the CCI is an unparalleled success, a groundbreaking new era in cooperation, especially for a post-conflict situation. In addition to the coordinated plan and donor pledges—amounting to a billion dollars over a period originally specified as two years—the CCI also called for a collaborative, donor-led process of implementation with the interim government. Different donors led work groups based on their interests and expertise. For example, the World Bank led the team charged with economic governance, USAID with HIV/AIDS, and the EU with education. All the donor agency staff in Washington praised the interim government for its serious commitment to reform and development (reaction was mixed in Europe), despite such sagging indicators as GDP growth and Transparency International's Corruption Perception Index.

Seen from below, the CCI looks different: it has been severely criticized by Haitian NGOs as an attempt by foreign powers to take over. Interestingly, seven groups that were listed as participants also denounced the process as representing a loss of sovereignty, as an attempt by the international organizations to obtain greater control. At least one of the organizations listed as "participating" in the CCI process was sent only a single invitation letter for a meeting that staff did not attend. An ad hoc coalition of forty-four organizations pointed out that the process was rushed and coercive: "The CCI's approach concretely reflects the reality of the occupation of our territory by foreign military forces" (SOFA et al. 2004:3). Especially following the earthquake, the distinction between development and military agencies is blurred, as the aid distribution on the cover demonstrates. These groups considered "partners" subsequently critiqued the process for running roughshod, without meaningful dialogue and participation, no mechanisms in place for debate, not enough time for discussion, nothing in Kreyòl, the only language of 90 percent of Haiti's population, and a lack of real dissemination plan. Two years following the CCI's passage, a civil society coalition decried the process for continuing to lack transparency and true participation (CoHE and CoEH 2006). As a result, the process rubber-stamped and gave legitimacy to the interests of the international community, which spent almost $2 million employing 250 experts, the vast majority of whom were foreign. The plan itself is a vast assemblage of propositions that have been long promulgated by the international community, few of them specific to Haiti. The aforementioned coalition argued, "Haiti isn't Afghanistan, nor Liberia, and still less Iraq. One has to avoid the 'ready to wear' solutions and procedures that elsewhere in certain national contexts have led to relentless failures" (SOFA et al. 2004:3).

Privatization was mentioned several times in the CCI as paving the way to development (Interim Government of Haiti 2004:19, 23, 24, 28). This echoes Latortue's public promotions of privatization. At a Caribbean conference held in Miami on December 8, 2004, and again at a conference held in Haiti the following week, Latortue said that Haiti needs to get over this notion that privatization is a "mortal sin," and vowed to do better to privatize the Haitian government's industries, such as electricity, power, telecommunications, and water.[30] In 2000, state-owned enterprises in service provision generated more than eight million goud in revenue, or $476 million (International Monetary Fund 2002:42–47). Publicly owned enterprises are among the only productive resources remaining in Southern countries like Haiti, the only surplus value to extract from a country already devastated by environmental destruction and centuries of underdevelopment. Following the earthquake, the telephone company was finally privatized.

In addition to process and privatization, progressive Haitian NGOs have other criticisms of the CCI. While there were some positive aspects according to these groups, such as gestures toward women's equality and decentralization, two main pillars triggered heated criticism. The "economic governance" plan simply legitimated de facto World Bank and IMF control over the country's finances and planning. While some of the specifics, like tighter financial accounting measures, may prove helpful in the long run, the overall plan keeps more power in the hands of international organizations to set priorities through control of state finances.[31] According to Yvette, "They are just selling the country whole-sale to the *blan* [foreigners] . . . and our leaders accept." Edele argued, "You will find with every government that comes to power, they support the IMF's and World Bank's structural adjustment plan more and more."

The CCI also promises Haiti's cooperation in structural adjustment meas-ures: "The Government is also committed to developing a plan for the clearance of external arrears and ensuring regular debt service" (23). Haiti's external debt was estimated at $1.5 billion at the end of the transition period, with rising debt service projections: $56.3 million for FY 2005, and $58.3 million for FY 2009 (International Monetary Fund 2005b:27–28). While this figure seems small compared to some countries in sub-Saharan Africa, forcing Haiti to continue repaying the debt deprived Haiti's people of needed services. In 2003 Haiti's scheduled debt service was $57.4 million, whereas the entire scheduled grants for education, health care, environment, and transportation combined were $39.21 million (International Monetary Fund 2005a:88; World Bank 2002b:vii). A result is that five hundred thousand children have no access to school, and only 35 percent finish primary school (Interim Government of Haiti 2004:33). Structural adjustment measures include such direct, forced reductions in social spending. In 2000/2001, the IMF demanded that Haiti reduce its social spend-ing from 3 percent of the GDP to 2 percent (Duhaime 2002). In addition to direct cuts, international financial institutions have demanded user fees for services such as education and health care. As noted in chapter 1, education is one of the primary expenses for a family. The cost of registration and tuition even for a low-rung, *lekòl bòlèt* school in Pòtoprens is at least five or six thousand goud a year, about four months' salary working minimum wage. (Incidentally, follow-ing a long and collaborative mobilization, Haiti's debt was partially canceled in 2009, with more canceled since the earthquake.)

A third plan within the CCI is a traditional part of the "ready-to-wear" neoliberal program. Globalization was the model for agriculture and food secu-rity: high-value crops for exports, benefiting few Haitian farmers, and importa-tion of subsidized or monetized rice, draining Haitian peasants' productive capacity to feed themselves (Richardson 1997). U.S. "food security" policy has destroyed national production in two ways: by flooding the market with free or subsidized U.S. agricultural products, underselling the Haitian peasantry; and by the trade liberalization measures tied to the receipt of food aid, removing protective tariffs. Once an exporter of rice, Haiti now produces only 18 percent of the rice it consumes, importing $200 million worth per year (MOREPLA and PAPDA 2004). In addition, the interim government authorized a U.S. company, T&S Rice, to operate in Haiti and increase rice imports, further weakening Haiti's national production. According to a national campaign, this move will cost twenty-eight thousand jobs. Continuing and providing legitimation for these neoliberal policies for food security, an explicit goal in the CCI was to further integrate Haiti into regional markets such as the Free Trade Area of the Americas (Interim Government of Haiti 2004:25). The plan for agriculture in the CCI promoted specialty items for consumption in the U.S. market, a long-standing USAID platform (e.g., USAID 1997), instead of for national production and consumption. This export orientation in formal development policy did not begin in the 1980s with USAID, but at the beginning of the "Development Encounter" (Escobar 1995). The first UN mission to Haiti in 1948 outlined coffee export as a primary motor of Haiti's development (United Nations 1949). As the ad hoc group of progressive NGOs argued, the best produce gets shipped out, benefiting the United States with cheaper exotic produce, and benefiting a small group of relatively well-off Haitian farmers. Over time, this globalization of agriculture has destroyed national production. Edele expressed the frustration of many others: "We used to have Creole pigs—they destroyed that. We used to have factories that used to make tomato paste—they destroyed that. We had factories that processed milk—they destroyed that. Well, we used to have factories to refine sugar—they destroyed that. Let me ask you a question, Mark. If they are truly helping us, if it's aid they give us, why don't they support our national production instead, so they can assure that the money goes toward production?" Monetization further accelerates both capital flow out of the country and a growing imbalance between rich and poor within Haiti. Neoliberal agricultural measures were a primary "push" factor in the massive urbanization in the 1980s, creating in Marxist terms a "reserve army" of unemployed, the lumpenproletariat, justifying low-wage industrial jobs as beneficial to this desperate and vulnerable population (DeWind and Kinley 1988; Trouillot 1994b). The interim period provided the finishing touches on this form of exploitation, as chapter 1 details—and Haiti's food crisis, which led to the April 2008 "riots," is a direct result.

Intermediaries

The situation of disaster capitalism is an expression of this political tug-of-war. It is a highly visible manifestation of the damage caused by the political tsunami, the ripple effects of the competition of interest groups behind international development. But the geopolitical forces—the tectonic shifts—are operating in other, less visible contexts. By themselves the tectonic shifts do not cause the disaster; they are magnified as the rumblings travel through the water, like swells gaining momentum and eventually crashing as waves. As noted above, in the case of public aid to development, there are many intermediaries between the ultimate donors—taxpayers of Northern countries—and the ultimate recipients of this aid—residents of Southern communities. Taking the example of USAID, Congress appropriates taxes and plays an oversight role. Once the funds have been approved, the State Department oversees the strategic lines, and the USAID administrator (since January 2006, in a concurrent post as the director of foreign assistance, reporting to the secretary of state) oversees the work of the issue-focused pillars and geographic bureaus, each of which supervises in-country missions. The missions craft a long-term plan and an annual R4, outlining the priorities and identifying contractors, almost invariably international NGOs. These NGOs manage the contracts, subcontracting with international and Southern NGOs. Often these NGOs in turn support and supervise the work of local associations.

I argued above that USAID's defensive posture arose in part because USAID lacks a public constituency. This system of intermediaries provides the rest of the explanation. If the USAID administration felt directly accountable to U.S. taxpayers and not jittery members of Congress, it might have heard the message that citizens overwhelmingly support international aid, and even at higher levels than spent at present, and are more interested in the humanitarian rather than the foreign policy justifications. As an institution with accountability to both Congress and the State Department, USAID can be the site for inter-branch tension and sometimes open conflict, especially in a situation of "divided government" such as in 2007–2009, whereby each branch was controlled by opposing political parties. USAID's work in Haiti was a good example of how this political tug-of-war affects how development was done. With Obama's election this constraint was lifted. Since Republicans regained the House in the 2010 elections, with Democrats still in control of the Senate and White House, USAID is likely going to be another arena for the political contest—certainly with a large minority of vocal Tea Party candidates who favor lower taxes and diplomatic isolationism.

Institutional levels—local and international NGOs, USAID mission and Washington staff—mediate contact between donors and recipients. As mentioned in the previous chapter, the Global Fund's new (to Fanm Tèt Ansanm) "primary recipient" wanted to mark territory. Noted above, USAID policy formation and implementation ("best practices") presuppose open lines of communication within the "food chain." In this ideal situation, policy is made by accurate, complete, and open consultation with local aid recipients, communicated through reports up to Washington planning staff. Also ideally, subordinates implement these directives in a complete, unbiased, and participatory manner without applying personal interests.

Even in non-charged contexts, the communication lines are not open, giving staff in Pòtoprens, both NGOs and international agencies, an important "translator" role (Bending and Rosendo 2006; Hefferan 2007:86; Salemink 2006). Development staff in Washington and Brussels rely on the mission reports to find out about the needs of the community. One person in Europe said that they hear about what's going on in Haiti "the same as you . . . through the media." Another in Washington relied on the *Nuevo Herald* or the *Economist Intelligence Unit*. A USAID policy analyst I met with deplored the fact that she did not get "out to the field" as often as she would have liked (it had been three years at the time of the October 2005 interview). A relatively new employee of a multilateral institution lamented the fact that while she has been "to the field" several times, she knew she wasn't "seeing the real Haiti" because she was confined to a Petyonvil hotel. The only Haitian people she regularly interacted with worked for her international agency or others: "If it weren't for my driver I wouldn't even hear Haitian music."

As shown, local development staff play a central mediating role. Said a U.S. agency employee, "We have an in-country consultant who helps the flow of communication. It's often very difficult. We receive proposals, and sometimes we have questions about the proposals. Sometimes they just drop off the face of the earth. There's no electricity, no phones, or they change their phone numbers." Being "stuck in Washington," staff at USAID headquarters argued that mission staff have more power. Said one, "Most missions have annual reporting, where they are aware of what the grantees are doing, on their own, but the most that we here at headquarters [in Washington] can do is recommend nonrenewal." A former USAID mission director was more direct: "I decided the priorities from my office." At times, mission staff feel that the mandates "coming down" are too complex. To dramatize this during an interview, a World Bank staff person threw down a dog-eared three-ring binder four inches thick, which he identified as the "operational policies . . . all 170 of them." Mission staff occasionally identified problems working within a branch of the U.S. government: "Sometimes Washington shoves something down your throat and you have to decide whether to fight it or accept it," but at the end of the day, as this staff acknowledged, "We're a government agency. We are them. [laughs] We are one. Like it or not, there it is."

Complicating this role of "translator" is a language barrier. As mentioned several times in this book, the first and only language of the vast majority of Haitian people is Kreyòl. The de facto official language of the government and business is French, the second language of the 10 percent of the population that is literate. While French is one of the UN's official languages, preferred in diplomatic circles, especially in the European Union, Kreyòl is much less commonly taught outside of Haiti. At the time I was looking (summer 2001), only two U.S. universities offered a summer language school, and only two others offered courses on Haitian Kreyòl.[32] Of the twenty-one foreign development staff I interviewed in Pòtoprens, Brussels, and Washington whose job implied regular interaction in Haiti, only three were fluent in Kreyòl. I was able to assess this easily by clearly speaking a common greeting in Haiti, something like "Sa k pase? Kijan tout bagay w ap mache?" (What's up? How's everything going for you?), or

"Ki moun ou yè?" (Who are you?). The grammar and many of the staple words in these phrases do not have French cognates. While some Francophone staff—particularly in Europe—mistook this as yet another American speaking bad French, rolling their eyes and switching to English, most people just stared back at me blankly. Said one USAID veteran with over twenty years of experience, "I was too busy being a bureaucrat to learn Kreyòl."[33] Language—specifically the use of French—is a central means of excluding Haiti's poor majority, and so the only people who could speak with donors not fluent in Kreyòl are middle-class NGO directors and managers, who have their own perspectives and biases.

For several reasons but especially because of the language barrier, NGO directors who mediate contact between the service population and the aid agencies serve as powerful brokers (Mosse and Lewis 2006; Nagar 2006; Richard 2009). As argued in chapter 2, socioeconomic differences divide NGO staff and their aid recipients, and these divisions color perceptions of participation. It would not be unreasonable to question whether these differences also shape priorities. Noted in chapter 1, Mme Laurent critiqued mainstream feminist organizations for not including the agendas and priorities of low-income women: "Peasant women's demands are, first, education: she would like to go to school. Health care is another necessity. These demands are shared by urban underprivileged classes as well. But for me in the middle class, my demands don't include health care because I can go to the hospital in the U.S. I can go to Martinique. I can go to Cuba." Recall in chapter 2 that aid recipients have different views on their participation within the NGOs as staff. These are some of the many manifestations of Haiti's entrenched class divisions.

Effects "on the Shore": Sove Lavi

So far the discussion has focused on macro-, state-level effects of development funding. Since the mid-1990s, NGOs have been the direct beneficiaries of Northern development aid in Haiti. The tectonic shifts discussed in this chapter have ripple effects on recipient NGOs as well. Employees of recipient NGOs critique the national interest component of bilateral development aid for several reasons. First is their understanding of the differences in priorities, what the CAC member Maxime outlined as "common interests" required for "frank participation." Answering Edele's question about investment in national production, Georges critiqued the barriers to participatory development: "The donor, when he gives some money, he does not give it to support your priorities that you defined. He gives the money in his vision, in his perceptions." Other NGO veterans see the economic interest behind international aid in more direct, concrete terms as literal exchanges: donors say, "'You need to buy this car from me.' You understand? True, you need to buy a car, but they make you buy a certain brand of car. In other words, the money comes but it returns to the same place again because they impose something on you." As noted above, 93 percent of USAID funds return to the United States. A former USAID employee offered an explanation: "That's our nod to 'buy American.'"

The various layers of NGOs between donors and recipient communities—that is, the intermediaries—leave their imprint on the process, as several front-line staff at Sove Lavi identified. To some, these intermediaries appear as a black box. "Maybe HS-2004 gives money to distribute, so it's an intermediary. In other words, it received $50 million to distribute to give us organizations for our projects. So, when we account for our work, we are accountable to HS-2004, but we don't know if they themselves have to be accountable to the donors. It's the same with Global Fund and the European Union." To others, these intermediaries appear to get in the way of benefiting local communities, taking their "cut" of donors' aid: "Often, community members, they don't receive anything at all because they invade with a group of consultants. And the money stays blocked somewhere, and truly, at times, the community doesn't really benefit." Of all the funds NGOs receive, members of the Haitian elite and transnational companies receive a significant portion, in rent for office space, cars, computers, genera-tors, and gas. On top of this, the personnel—mostly middle class—accounts for the majority of the budget, with most of the salaries going toward "upstairs" or "central office" staff.[34] Therefore very few funds are spent on the recipients. Recall the CAC member Djoni imploring that with all the money spent, at least Sove Lavi could bring along boxes of condoms.

As I argued above, in addition to the material benefits attached as condi-tions to development aid, the national interest is codified in program design. Sove Lavi staff hired to implement the project of HIV/AIDS prevention are forced to abide by the contract's terms, regardless of whether they support the ideol-ogy or logic behind it: "Donors make decisions; they chose the terms: absti-nence, fidelity, or else condom. I don't believe in this, but it wasn't my choice. I don't know if [the donor] said that or else if it was a choice here [at Sove Lavi]. I wasn't involved, I don't know." Interestingly, this staff person could not iden-tify whether decisions were made by Mme Versailles or imposed from above. In addition to disagreeing with the donors' politik, staff have critiques of the man-agement style, and different understandings of the central theme in the approach: "When they tell you 'results-based management,' it isn't true. For me, it's the name only, the title, but it isn't true. At least you can say it's badly applied. They don't give you autonomy. They outline your work that they impose on you, and after this you give a result. So, that's not 'results-based management.' Pretty words." As noted in chapter 2, CAC members also believe in results.

Predictably, staff who have more direct contact with donors, or their inter-mediary Northern NGO contractors, have a more complex understanding. Tacitly accepting the logic of the results orientation, Mme Lejeune offered an alternative interpretation that Mme Versailles could have used to defend Sove Lavi. Mme Lejeune wondered, "Is it really true that they can penalize you for this, or don't you have a tool to defend yourself? You could say that they didn't give the money on time, that the project finished in March, but I can only conduct the training during vacation?" Mme Lejeune's interpretation gives agency to recipient NGOs. She argued that rather than being passive consumers of donor discourses, including results-based management, they should have the ability to use this tool for their own interests (Gupta and Sharma 2006; Rossi 2006; Sharma 2008). Later in the interview, explicitly drawing parallels with Haiti's political situation, Mme Lejeune offered her own analysis of the crisis at Sove Lavi: "We are ultimately responsible for what we do with what we're told." This analysis offers a solution to the bind presented by a binary, either–or understanding of structure versus agency—one that is useful to Jillian and other neophytes, one that also gets away from a romanticized or victimhood discourse, one that can acknowledge Aristide's responsibility without losing sight of the foreign domination.

Higher Ground: Fanm Tèt Ansanm

Northern NGOs that do not apply for official public aid (ODA) are insulated from these constraints and political pressures that public development agencies, certainly bilateral agencies, confront. Fanm Tèt Ansanm is primarily financed by four private European NGOs that—as they each raise at least half their funds outside their governments—are not constrained from supporting long-term "partner" relationships, and are able to support Southern NGOs' infrastructure and basic administrative costs. This long-term, stable partnership might explain Fanm Tèt Ansanm's ability to defend itself, its high level of *gran moun tèt li* autonomy. Fanm Tèt Ansanm has been a partner of one Northern NGO for almost its entire existence (over twenty years). And two other donors supported Fanm Tèt Ansanm for about fifteen years until then. Mme Dominique, with almost two decades of experience with different donors, explained a difference between European NGOs and USAID in their approach to working with Southern NGOs (see also Edelman 2005:31; Macdonald 1997): "European donors are more open to the problems you encounter on the ground and also open to you as well, what you can tell them. They give you a certain latitude to change things once you alert them that you're having a problem. That is, you have a participative management with them. And they understand the problems that present themselves. On the other hand, USAID has another approach." The tectonic shifts mentioned in this chapter, the privatization of the national interest that generated the results orientation as well as the abstinence-only policy, are felt on the ground in the recipient NGOs. As mentioned in chapter 4, and explained in the present chapter, USAID's management style is more brusque than Fanm Tèt Ansanm's other donors. Instead of partnership relationships, USAID practices results-based management whereby it retains more control of defining priorities, for example shaping Sove Lavi's Caravan and attempting to control Fanm Tèt Ansanm. This new management tool has effectively cut off local planning, initiative, and innovation from Sove Lavi programs by centralizing decisionmaking and by not providing adequate funds for planning. Changes or other specific policy suggestions—such as the provincial Kanaval celebration mentioned in the previous chapter, and the CAC recommendations for combating discrimination against women and low economic capacity discussed in chapter 2—are unable to be accommodated in this centralized planning and funding process. An NGO director also noted that the new management style is less favorable: "When there was another NGO that managed USAID funds, they managed them much more openly. They defended the NGOs who received aid. So, when USAID went with [name withheld], we did one, two years with them. This branch of [name withheld], I have come not to like their approach too much." These tectonic shifts can explain why Fanm Tèt Ansanm, largely protected from them, has higher levels of both participation and autonomy than does Sove Lavi, which is entirely dependent on public aid to development.

But Northern NGOs, such as those that finance Fanm Tèt Ansanm, are not completely isolated from these external pressures. For one thing, as Mme Dominique recalled, they are following the Goliath Global Fund and PEPFAR by working in the AIDS arena:

> In '88 [AIDS] was already à la mode. And then suddenly, [international donors] decided that AIDS didn't exist anymore. So they stopped financing AIDS for a long time, while it continued to ravage. . . . And now, suddenly, AIDS is the great craze. Everyone needs to finance AIDS. And we have the impression that the day may come when there is too much money in AIDS, considering that all the rest, we are neglecting everything else, the human [development] element, other social problems, and this is not good. Because now you have the Global Fund giving a whole lot of money in AIDS, and now you have [name withheld] that has entered into the AIDS field, [name withheld] that entered AIDS. Everything is pointing toward AIDS.

Fanm Tèt Ansanm's donors are all supporting the AIDS program. This shift cuts the *medanm* off from addressing other current realities, which may explain why current recipients felt they only participated in implementation. Ideas to subsidize transportation, provide leadership development, create a *sòl* for medical expenses, or support neighborhood associations do not fit with current donor priorities, and therefore Fanm Tèt Ansanm lacks the financial resources to support these initiatives. In addition, the "project" logic, with numerical accounting of both finances and measurable outcomes, has spread to Northern NGOs, including Fanm Tèt Ansanm's partners.

A function of the logic of partnership, these European NGOs, especially those that do not have staff in Haiti, are more dependent on Southern NGO directors for their analysis and understanding. NGO staff in Europe whom I interviewed outlined travel to Haiti as a major undertaking, longer and much more expensive than travel from the United States. While this gives partners more freedom to not worry so much about the quarterly or semiannual project cycle and its brusque changes, it places more power in the hands of NGO directors, who may have very different perspectives from aid recipients. Additionally, local conditions can change over time, and there are some risks in too much stability. One progressive NGO in the United States, Grassroots International, shared the European donors' longevity of contracts. Over time, local partners became more and more involved in politics, notably Chavannes Jean-Baptiste and the MPP, leading the push against Aristide. This became a source of tension. Further, while their institutional autonomy provides some insulation from the political tsunami, European NGOs' roles and relationships with their national governments are changing. A couple have mentioned that while they were initially outsider advocates, they gradually moved into "consultancy" roles. In fact, some European NGOs in this study gradually began to receive funding from their government or from the EU.[35] And the rules for European development funding have changed, from the various Lomé Conventions to the current Cotonou Agreement, solidifying the neoliberal "race to the bottom" that several European solidarity activists attribute to European expansion. Finally, with EU enlargement, there was a perceived need to address concerns of European residents, especially new member states with lower development indicators, lessening the support for foreign development for its own sake that had been justified by historical colonial ties.

This completes the comparison of Fanm Tèt Ansanm and Sove Lavi. I have shown and then explained differences in the spheres of relationships through a "civic infrastructure" framework. There are correlations in the relationships between different sets of actors, with hierarchies in NGOs' relationship with donors reproduced in their relationship with aid recipients, and different donors and their policies constraining local participation at different levels (Butler 2008). This chapter explained the social life of two of these donor policies, suggesting that there is some room for people's capacity for individual action despite the institutional constraints. These constraints are obviously felt differently depending on where one is in the food chain. Still needed, however, is a coherent understanding of how these processes work, and how power and inequality operate within the system of international development.

Conclusion

Killing with Kindness?

NGOs are such a force multiplier for us, such an important part of our combat team.

—U.S. Secretary of State Colin Powell, September 2001

Wednesday, January 12, 2011 4:53 P.M.
It is a year—to the minute—since the earthquake that killed at least 230,000 people. A wave of silence has passed through the city. Like the immediate lead-up to the coup, the streets are empty. Roosters crowing in the distance are the only sound. It seemed that even the dogs, following the lead of their human caretakers, are honoring the moment of silence. This is how people chose to commemorate the loss of their loved ones: at home or at church, with their families, quietly and dignified.

I had to move out of my house because although it is still standing, a crack several inches wide traverses an entire wall on the first floor. My immediate neighbors like Lise weren't so lucky. Except for a small two-room wing carefully rescued and restored, the house collapsed on top of her father. Lise had to pull her father out from the rubble. Up the hill, Samuel lost both his parents as his house collapsed. Pascal lost his daughter. Julie lost her "best" son. "He was going to school, always studying when the other neighbor boys were playing football. He always told me that he would become a doctor and support his mother, to move us into a real house," Julie said, for the first time since the *goudougoudou* (what people call the earthquake, mimicking the sound of the earth shaking, not wanting to actually say the word, *tranblemanntè a*) able to shed a little tear in front of me and her neighbors. The two houses on top of the hill were totally destroyed, killing all members of both families. My street has become a *katye popilè* (low-income neighborhood) because in addition to these deaths, nearly all the middle-class survivors like Lise abandoned their damaged homes.

Despite this quiet reflection, foreigners marked the first anniversary of the quake with much fanfare: media-staged events, celebrations, crusades, protests, press conferences, and annual reports being sent on the Internet as either press releases or as "news," since many humanitarian actors have become bloggers.

Despite its sixty thousand residents, a far-flung camp called Kanaran did not officially exist according to the International Organization for Migration (IOM), and as such very little NGO aid arrived. In this abandoned, dusty, wind-swept camp, there is not one but two camp committees. In one "turf" was the camp's only water supply and toilets. On the other sat an empty and ripped UNICEF tent, on which graffiti denouncing the other committee representative was written. In the neutral zone, dwarfing everything around it, including the tents, toilets, and the wood structures that were to replace a makeshift school made on one side of the camp, people were building a soundstage using profes-sional building materials. "We're going to have a big crusade," boasted this committee member. While not wanting to be too direct, I asked who was going to come. He said that international organizations, the government, and NGOs were going to be there to commemorate their work. Of course journalists were invited, he said, probably thinking I was one.

A barber whose shop sat across from the sound stage said what was inevitably on many minds: "Instead of spending thousands of dollars driving people here, building the stage, renting the equipment and all this, they could just give us food. We're starving."

This morning, thousands of faithful were bused to Channmas, where tens of thousands of people lived among the ruins of the National Palace, to attend a "crusade" led by a foreign pastor. Because of the stand built, he was positioned higher than the statues of Haitian revolutionary heroes. Echoing Pat Robertson, and bolstered by a year of a veritable invasion by mission groups and Protestant NGOs doling out food aid, this pastor said to the crowd, in English, "You used to think playing with witchcraft was just a game. Now you know after January 12 that this is serious." A much smaller demonstration of people living under tents and grassroots organizations to accompany them, who had put aside their dif-ferences over Aristide that ripped the country apart in 2004, snaked through the plaza, protesting the many injustices still faced by what the IOM declared to be 810,000 people living in internally displaced people (IDP) camps.

The IOM declared this exodus of almost half the population of officially recognized IDP camps the "light at the end of the tunnel," dutifully repeated by UN Special Envoy Bill Clinton, claiming it as a success of international aid during many a press conference today.

The realities on the ground look quite different. In a camp in Kafou (Carrefour), at an Adventist Church, there were still no toilets when the cholera outbreak began in late October, ten months after the earthquake. Church lead-ers had been giving verbal warnings for people to leave. People stayed until one day in November, when eight cases of cholera were recorded in the camp. The next day, all 546 people fled the camp. Levi, a camp in Taba (Tabarre), is a shell of its former self: only 30 of 486 people remain following the cholera outbreak. The camp never had a toilet, so people went to a neighbor's house. Neighbors' generosity has limits, however, especially after the outbreak of the fecal-borne disease.

Where did they go? Some went to another camp. Others pitched what was left of their tent after ten months of tropical weather in front of a friend's house. Some may have squatted on an empty house slated for demolition.[1] Some may have gone to unofficial camps like Kanaran. Others may have created a whole new camp recently "discovered" by aid officials.

In short, no one knows.

So rather than the rapid depopulation being the light at the end of the tunnel, it may be an oncoming train.

NGOs and Cholera

Cholera is a clear symptom of the failures of the post-quake aid, and of NGOs in particular. Before the outbreak, a July/August 2010 study of a random sample of 108 IDP camps—one in eight in the metro area—found that 40.5 percent of camps did not have water, and 30.3 percent of camps did not have a single toilet. Overall in the Pòtoprens area, toilets were on average shared by 273 people (Schuller 2010b). These were prime conditions for the spread of cholera, a fecal-borne disease spread by contaminated water. And spread it did. The minister of health reported on January 24, 2011, that the disease claimed more than four thousand lives (AFP 2011). By January 2011, after two and a half months and hundreds of millions in newly pledged aid, there was a minimum of progress: 37.6 percent instead of 40.5 percent still lacked water, and 25.8 instead of 30.3 percent of camps were still without a toilet (Schuller 2011). What little progress was made was concentrated in Sitesolèy because of a coordinated process meeting in local government offices led by the Haitian government.

Haiti's earthquake thrust the international aid system, particularly NGOs, into the public spotlight. In addition to increased public scrutiny, the earthquake provided a "teachable moment" for the international aid system. For example, at a March 2010 congressional hearing, Bill Clinton apologized for destroying Haitian rice production under his presidency through the delivery of USAID food aid (discussed in chapters 1 and 5), calling it a "Devil's bargain." He and Secretary of State Hillary Clinton also publicly questioned donors' overdependence on NGOs and their circumventing elected governments. A discourse critical of the humanitarian response has proliferated following this exposure, particularly among aid workers and journalists (e.g., Disaster Accountability Project 2011; Humanitarian Accountability Project 2010; Oxfam International 2011). Even the representative for the Organization of American States, Ricardo Seitenfus of Brazil, said in a December 20, 2010, interview with the Swiss newspaper

Le Temps that "Haiti is the proof of the failure of international aid" (Robert 2010). Haiti may well become the Waterloo of the NGO system. What accounts for this collective failure, despite billions in aid being given, NGOs' efforts, and even some remarkable individual successes?[2]

It should first be acknowledged that the earthquake presented challenges because it struck an urban area, and the country's nerve center at that. According to IOM staff, "In rural disaster situations, it's easy to find land to relocate people. In Port-au-Prince, that was simply not the case." Another reason was the slowness of aid actually delivered. Of the $5.6 billion official development aid pledged for the period through the end of September 2011, only 37 percent was sent by January 2011, nine months after the pledges (Interim Haiti Recovery Commission 2011). This was up from 15 percent at the end of September 2010 (Katz 2010). According to the *Chronicle of Philanthropy* (Preston and Wallace 2011), NGOs only spent 38 percent of the private donations collected a year following the earthquake, but this is difficult to assess because most NGOs have poor transparency, according to the Disaster Accountability Project (2011). In any event, this lack of funding and opaque financial procedures cannot possibly account for the persistent gaps in aid. At the root, the problems are structural.

Understanding NGOs

Despite the increased attention, most success and failure stories focus on individual people and NGOs. Almost all accounts by aid workers understandably highlight their success, given that they are always looking for funding. The anthropologist Tim Schwartz (2008) was a notable exception. He published an exposé from his experience of the most reprehensible, shortsighted, self-serving actions of people within aid agencies. We have seen in the pages of this book similarly enraging actions, particularly by Sove Lavi but also in Fanm Tèt Ansanm. However, missing from even Schwartz's account is an analysis of why well-intentioned individuals end up reproducing inequality.

The experience of Sove Lavi and Fanm Tèt Ansanm highlight several structural problems even before the earthquake. People associated with them are, in fact, human, trying to make the best of a situation they were handed and responding to external reward structures. Good people, very well educated at that, work for Sove Lavi. Why is it, then, that they continue to fail? This book shows similar processes that cut off local participation also silence frontline staff with experience in the field and erode organizational autonomy. Post-cholera progress was stifled for the same reasons that Sove Lavi was stifled: instrumentalism eroding participation, communication, collaboration, and coordination.

NGOs have become instrumentalized—used for ends other than humanitarian—as they have become more attractive to donors. As many scholars noted, NGOs as a structure began as private, voluntary associations tied to faith-based communities that raised the majority of funds for their work them-selves (e.g., Bornstein 2003; Fisher 1997; Hefferan 2007; Mathurin et al. 1989). Many practitioners recall that these nonprofit associations were close-knit, self-sacrificing, and focused on a shared mission. It is arguably still true for grassroots organizations that raise most of their money from members. The system was remade following shifts in donor discourses, policies, and practices. Following the end of the Cold War, donors like USAID and the World Bank did not need strong centralized states to compete against the Soviet bloc. In fact, they discovered that states were too strong, centralized, corrupt, and removed from the people. So they began directly financing NGOs instead; the 1990s were often described as a "golden age" for NGOs (Agg 2006). During the decade before 1996, the number of NGOs working in more than one country more than doubled to thirty-eight thousand (Scholte and Schnabel, 2002:250). Currently, there are so many NGOs that we can't even guess at their number (Riddell 2007:53). This distrust of states reflects not only the ascendency of neoliberalism but also geopolitical struggles, such as in Haiti in 1995: Republicans who just took over Congress wanted to expose President Clinton's inexperience in foreign policy. Haiti was his only "success" story to date, unlike Rwanda or Somalia. So Congress forbade USAID—within the executive branch, under the State Department—to fund Aristide. NGOs were the (sometimes unwitting) beneficiaries, and their budgets exploded.

As NGOs became increasingly powerful, many were corrupted by the process, which affected participation. Policies like results- or performance-based man-agement have had the effect of centralizing decision-making authority and closing off avenues for meaningful local participation, dramatized by Sove Lavi. Rather than an open, participatory, democratic process, NGOs are increasingly rewarded for a "bean counting" approach that reduces people to statistics. Corrections and changes made from on-the-ground experience are increasingly difficult, as Sove Lavi's experience shows ("We are prisoners!"). Even at Fanm Tèt Ansanm, donor priorities are increasingly edging out those of their service recipients as AIDS became "the great craze."

These byzantine reporting requirements also cut off intra-NGO communica-tion. Staff who work "in the field" and who are the direct points of contact with aid recipients are increasingly removed from decision-making authority. Local needs deliberation has become increasingly irrelevant, as NGOs have to follow the "project" cycle and do exactly as they're told, implementing donor priorities, or risk their funding being pulled (as was the case at Sove Lavi). The reporting requirements create top-heavy NGOs with bloated administrations, usually with at least one full-time accountant versed in USAID reporting requirements and software (as with Sove Lavi's upstairs staff). Job ads—often in English—explicitly ask for these competencies. These difficulties only increased following the earthquake, with foreign, non-Kreyòl-speaking staff representing NGOs at cluster meetings while monolingual Kreyòl speakers were going to the camps.

The reporting and other requirements imposed by donors reorient NGOs to be more concerned with accountability from above, not from below. If, as in the case of the World AIDS Day activities or the CACs, an NGO like Sove Lavi fails a community, the community has no recourse. They have no direct contact with the donors or even the NGO directors. If a state-sponsored development project failed or merely lined the pockets of insiders, citizens would be in the streets protesting, because there is at least in theory some accountability, some responsibility, to the citizenry. NGOs cannot be compelled to work better, or work in underserved areas, because they are first and foremost private, voluntary initiatives. This is why any NGO can point to individual successes post-earthquake, while close to 40 percent of camps still lacked water a year following the quake. Compounding this, NGOs working in Haiti are funded and usually headquartered abroad. "Haitian" NGOs like Sove Lavi and Fanm Tèt Ansanm may have Haitian decision-making structures, but foreign funders still wield powerful influence, recalling the old saying that "the one who pays the piper calls the tune."

Since donors' relationships with NGOs trump others through ever-powerful reporting and management regimes, there is little incentive to work together. NGOs are in fact, structurally speaking, competitors with one another and even the Haitian government itself. Why share information or coordinate among entities that are competing for the same resources? Often these relationships erupt in hostilities, but given this, and donors' systematic undermining of the state's oversight and coordination capacity, only a fraction of NGOs in Haiti submit the bare minimum, annual reports, to the Haitian government. In many cases, donors' policies actually encourage NGOs to disregard the authority of the state. Recall that NGOs pay employees far more than do the government ministries (Morton 1997; Pierre-Louis 2011).

All the above are reflections of donors' policies and reward structures. Therefore, far from representing individual moral failures—a "Haitian mentality," as the majority of coverage, including Schwartz's, would suggest—actors within the system are behaving in an understandable fashion, responding to the power structure, inequality, and the reward system, what I call "trickle-down imperialism." Donors' reward structures work against collaboration, coordination, communication, and participation. This not only explains Sove Lavi's repeated failures despite its wealth of human capital, but also why gaping holes in the IDP camp coverage persisted despite millions in aid and the urgency following the cholera outbreak.

Theoretical Contributions

Notwithstanding the barrage of PR written by NGO employees, from the point of view of recipients of NGO aid—be it Sove Lavi's CACs, or IDPs who fled the camps for an even more precarious existence because of the failure to protect against cholera—the "results" are not being attained. This is not only true of Haiti. Aside from a handful of countries, six decades of development interventions have made only minimal progress, while poverty and inequality often deepened. The anthropologist James Ferguson (1990) described two kinds of explanations: "functional" critiques that seek technical solutions within mainstream development ideology, and "foundational" critiques arguing that the structure and premise need to be critically rethought, overhauled, or done away with entirely.

A similar divergence exists in the critical scholarship on NGOs. On the one hand, scholar/practitioners critique "instrumentalization"—the idea that humanitarian action is used for purposes other than humanitarianism, notably the promotion of foreign economic or geopolitical interests (e.g., Atmar 2001; Donini 2012). Scholars that are more radical argue that NGOs are tools of imperialism, primarily used to integrate the capitalist market economy into local communities (e.g., Lwijis 2009; Petras 1997). This distinction is primarily one of degree or interpretation, discussing the same structural reality. NGOs are structures that glue together local communities from countries across the globe: they are intermediaries.

As value-neutral structures, NGOs can be used to accomplish different ends. How NGOs are used and in the service of what ends requires attention to human agency and relationships. What NGO staff do, how they respond to the various relationships, actors, and pressures, can have great impact, but such actions are constrained by the social field surrounding the NGOs. With genuine space for beneficiary participation and sufficient *gran moun tèt li* autonomy to be able to defend local priorities, an NGO can be used by the community to meet their needs. Absent participation and autonomy, the NGO can be used by international agencies to implement foreign agendas. Therefore the human relationships, especially participation and autonomy surrounding the NGOs, are pivotal to understanding and evaluating their impact. Following a frame understanding these relationships and highlighting the structural position NGOs inhabit as intermediaries, this book concludes with an interrogation of the power that these intermediaries wield.

Civic Infrastructure

This book draws on some of the theoretical insights by anthropologists problematizing NGOs as a single entity (Hilhorst 2003; Kaag 2008; Kamat 2002). Different constituencies, including aid recipients, are actors with agency (Luetchford 2006; Rossi 2006; Salemink 2006). Thus the most appropriate way to study NGOs is as an interconnected sphere of relationships within the various constituencies: civic infrastructure. Civic infrastructure is the interrelated set of relationships between and among various stakeholder groups of a given social grouping (even temporary "assemblages"),[3] in this case women's NGOs. This book has explored the relationships "below," between the NGOs and beneficiaries; "inside," among NGO staff; and "above," among the NGO, their donors, and the Haitian government. Understood as a total system because each relationship affects the others (Schuller 2006b), we can nonetheless tease apart individual relationships, such as participation and autonomy.

The experiences at Sove Lavi in particular forcefully highlight that participation is understood differently across a series of divides, notably aid recipients and directors or donors (Eriksson Baaz 2005; Hilhorst 2003). This admittedly intuitive point still has yet to be implemented within development. This ethnography critiques simplistic ideas of participation that, while hardly new, are still important to mention. Despite their limitations, the snapshot tables in chapter 2 have some utility for scholars and practitioners. The form helps elaborate what participation means given the various stages of an NGO project, identifying which stakeholder groups participate in what part of the project. To NGOs like Sove Lavi and their donors, "participation" involves only execution, when in fact there are many more steps. Explaining why Sove Lavi didn't involve local communities in planning, two specific donor policies—abstinence-only granting, and results-based contracting—centralized authority in donors' favor, the first rendering local participation moot by imposing specific interventions, and the second by curtailing local consultation and reducing the flexibility needed to respond to local needs.

It is important to remember that inequalities and challenges to participation are occurring within a shared goal of eradicating HIV/AIDS, what CAC member Maxime called "common interest" within "frank participation." The dynamics discussed in these pages are only magnified when donors' national interest collides with that of recipient countries. This often occurs when donors promote their own technological, commercial, or agricultural commodities at the expense of national production, such as U.S. food aid in Haiti discussed earlier.

This book builds on critical ethnographic insights on autonomy. First, people identified two senses of autonomy, financial (*grès kochon kwit kochon*) and programmatic (*gran moun tèt li*). In addition to culturally meaningful distinctions in Haiti, this insight is useful for other low-income, heavily NGOized social spheres flush with aid money. Second, challenging the state-focused bias in development literature, this book highlights that NGOs need autonomy from donors as well (Auyero and Switsun 2009; Biggs and Neame 1996; Fisher 1997; Kamat 2003).

Moving beyond "social capital," a civic infrastructure analysis studies the modes of interaction between the stakeholder groups within a single analytic frame. As this book has shown, these relationships—for example, between an NGO and recipients, among NGO staff, and between NGO and donors—are interrelated, each bearing on other relationships. CACs were definitely affected by Sove Lavi's relationship with donors. In addition, by studying the modes of interaction and not the people themselves, civic infrastructure escapes a conceptual dilemma: individuals are studied but the "units of analysis" tend to be amorphous social groupings (cf. Putnam 2001). For example, "Haitians" are said to have low levels of social capital, erasing socially significant differences within a population—for example, gender, race/color, or class (Arneil 2006). Finally, civic infrastructure acknowledges the complexities of a social world that cannot easily be divided between "local" and "global," as they are interconnected by a series of intermediaries (Richard 2009).

NGOs as "Semi-elites"

Understanding the relationships as a total system—civic infrastructure—highlights the points of contact, or intermediaries. Mediating contact between Northern donors and agencies and local communities in the South, NGOs have been increasingly playing roles as intermediaries within the contemporary world system.

Critical globalization scholars focus on the transnational capitalist class (e.g., Robinson 2004; Sklair 2001). While a central actor within the world system, this class needs either hegemony or coercion to maintain control. Despite the growing rise in worldwide military expenditures and war-induced deaths, the imperial strategy of war is showing signs of faltering (Wallerstein 2003). Without a class of semi-elites, the capitalist class's rule is not possible. Neoliberal globalization, like imperialism, colonialism, and slavery before it, requires intermediaries, local people selected to receive some benefits of the system of exploitation, inequality, and exclusion, and who therefore identify with foreign interests. Many examples of such intermediaries—"semi-elites"—arose from Britain's strategy of "indirect rule" (Padmore 1969), like the Nuer's "government chief" (Evans-Pritchard [1940] 1969) and East India Company Brahmins. Southern NGOs are the contemporary inheritors of this structural position of intermediaries. These semi-elites are buttressing the contemporary neoliberal world system, "gluing globalization" (Schuller 2009).

Not merely institutional points of connection, NGOs tend to play important ideological functions. Even progressive Southern NGOs can provide institutional layers against grassroots social change movements and even undermine local development. Sove Lavi selected preexisting community organizations and community leaders as volunteer trainers in their HIV/AIDS-prevention program, shifting grassroots groups' priorities toward those of Sove Lavi and their donors. Sove Lavi ignored CAC members' series of recommendations for projects that identified poverty and gender-based discrimination as critical factors in HIV/AIDS transmission. Danielle expressed the frustration in economic terms: "They don't accept [our suggestions] because they are just doing business."

A more open, autonomous, and participative NGO, Fanm Tèt Ansanm had demonstrably more amicable relationships with aid recipients, who participated in more deliberation and decision-making processes and not simply implementation. Even at Fanm Tèt Ansanm, however, space for member discussion and decision-making were gradually, and then abruptly, eroded. This is connected to the changing landscape of aid financing, with ever-greater emphasis on numerical "results" (Oxfam America 2008). Consequently, in addition to closing the advocacy group, several ideas for projects arising from member participation, such as support for public transport, help for neighborhood associations, and a *sòl* for medical expenses remain unimplemented. Fanm Tèt Ansanm became increasingly known only for its HIV/AIDS-prevention work, ending their support for workers' rights and moving far away from their constituency because of their success at community education. Donors exerted indirect control of Fanm Tèt Ansanm's priorities, financing only what they agreed with, a subtler erosion of member participation undermining "bottom-up" initiatives. I have argued that internal social dynamics can shape NGOs' work, and the implantation of foreign-funded NGOs can support existing hierarchies and exclusions. Even NGOs like Fanm Tèt Ansanm with a history and desire for grassroots empowerment can centralize power and disempower communities.

Howard Zinn (1995:622) ended his *People's History of the United States* with a plea to the U.S. middle class, whom he called "guards of the system." He argued that when these intermediaries, uncertain of their position within the system, identify with "the people," change is possible. Ordinarily, the middle class identifies with the ruling class because of privileges granted. They become a stabilizing factor against class struggle or revolutionary change in a Keynesian/New Deal "class compromise." The self-identified "middle class" may be culturally and historically particular to the United States, and given recent policies adding fuel to the global financial crisis, may soon be a memory. But Zinn's idea of "guards of the system" is useful beyond this particular context. Even more so than a middle class in a postindustrial economy, the "NGO class" is dependent on the transnational ruling class. NGOs exist and employ professionals at current high levels because of donor policies. If and when these policies or financial flows change, this entire class could cease to exist. But as intermediaries, NGOs hold the keys for change. In Zinn's words, "The Establishment cannot survive without the obedience and loyalty of millions of people who are given small rewards to keep the system going. . . . If they stop obeying, the system falls." So why don't they disobey? Why do NGOs continue their roles as guards of the system? For answers we need to examine the inequalities and hierarchies inherent in the system of international aid.

Trickle-Down Imperialism

Finally, with attention to spheres of interrelationships and the roles of intermediaries, this book offers contextualized ethnographic detail with which to evaluate theories of power and how it operates, especially in international development. Building on Marxist analyses of inequality, much good work has been done uncovering the power IFIs wield, either as "economic hit men" (Perkins 2006) or simply through what used to be called "structural adjustment programs" (Bello 1996).

Parallel to the theoretical dismissing of intermediaries, however, most world systems approaches are limited in their understanding of power. Most focus their attention on institutions that are explicitly coercive in their application of sovereign power wrested from states—particularly the World Trade Organization, the IMF, and the World Bank. Donor institutions and NGOs are not the same, structurally, as IFIs like the World Bank and the IMF: in theory, recipient countries can refuse aid while not being able to default on IFI loans. IFIs have triggered a growing and vocal opposition social movement because of the coercive power they wield. This transnational movement's critique of structural adjustment programs forced IFIs to adopt new language. Interestingly, given the wave of protests in the first decade of the twenty-first century targeting the World Bank, IMF, and the World Trade Organization (e.g., Danaher 2004; Mertes 2004; Notes from Nowhere 2003; Starr 2005), the UN and bilateral donors—to say the least of NGOs—have escaped this criticism. This is in part because of donors' and NGOs' different mission and approach, namely humanitarianism. How are people to understand the obvious failures in the post-earthquake reconstruction, while granting that many humanitarian actors have a sincere desire to help? How are citizens able to critique the postmodern forms of power operating within donor institutions and the ostensibly apolitical armada of NGOs implementing USAID and other official donors' development agendas?

Critical globalization scholars tend to either ignore other institutional actors, notably humanitarian and development agencies, or paint them with a broad brush as collaborators of Empire; Michael Hardt and Antonio Negri (2001:36) called NGOs "mendicant orders." This moralistic, binary framework is far too simplistic to be useful. In fact, many critical globalization scholars share a tendency with humanitarians and solidarity activists to reserve a class of some "good" NGOs, such as those who fund activists' travel to the World Social Forum and other regional gatherings. This idealism may be behind an exhaustive array of classificatory schemas: "local" or "progressive" or "grassroots" or "membership-based" is a way to exempt some NGOs from the criticism of the system. It has become cliché to point out that NGOs are defined only by what they are not. Getting around this endlessly circular discussion, we should focus our attention on NGOs' actions, and the social impacts of these actions. To understand and evaluate we need a theoretical tool grounded in the realities of NGOs, as institutions that mediate relationships from local through global levels.

Arising from a Marxist tradition, world systems analysis inherits its theoretical limitations regarding power.[4] Except for organized transnational social movements (relying on "good" NGOs) noted above, there is no room in the analytic calculus for human agency, notably to change the system. In addition, the mainstream Marxian theoretical current fails to interrogate—and therefore ultimately be able to intervene in—what Zinn criticized, the alliances that intermediaries make with powerful groups, simply dismissing them as evidence of "false consciousness." Putting aside the paternalism inherent in this belief that only a revolutionary party—or a Soviet state—knows the "correct" consciousness for "its" working class, Marxian theory cannot understand how people become agents in their own oppression.

This is the starting point of Michel Foucault's work. The French theorist exploded our understandings of power, calling attention to processes of self-censorship through "discipline" (1979), critiquing the "repressive hypothesis" (1978) by outlining the generative aspects of power, and sketching a sociology of how modernist governments increasingly focus on the "conduct of conduct," perfecting a governmental rationality or "governmentality" (1991).

Basing his theorizing on a critical historiography of his native France, Foucault's theories are hampered by his own Eurocentrism, his inattention to the colonialist/imperialist dimensions of France, and his silence on the questions of race or even class inequality. His *istwa* of the evolution of "modern" power notably leaves out the brutality of slavery in the Caribbean, particularly in what was to become Haiti, and the centrality of this institution to the rising bourgeoisie that was ostensibly less "violent" or "barbaric" in their application of power, at least in the imperial center with non-slaves. This theoretical blind spot aside, Foucault's conceptualizations of power, whether "Panopticon," "means of correct training," "confession," or "biopower," are both individualizing/individuating and totalizing. Power is at once everywhere and nowhere, operating in and on individuals by amorphous institutions and ideologies and citizen-subjects' internalization of the above. Missing is an analysis of relevant social groupings, particularly the inequalities among these groups: racism, patriarchy, and class inequality.

Whereas Marxian analyses of power offers an incomplete picture of the functioning of power, approaches stemming solely from Foucault are devoid of important social realities, including hierarchy and inequality. One creative synthesis is "neoliberal governmentality," elaborated by the anthropologist Aradhana Sharma, who studied with Akhil Gupta (2006) an institution for women's empowerment that straddled the social space between the Indian government and an NGO. Through NGO actions and their regimes of "participation," aid recipients internalize and put into practice the logic of neoliberal capitalism. In addition, echoing Lenin (1922) and Michels (1949), bureaucratic inertia stifles social change (see also Nagar 2006). This is a productive grafting of Marx and Foucault that renders visible the underlying structure of a constellation of organizations addressing gender inequality. This analysis invites further inquiry into the structural mechanisms by which a range of intermediary actors produce and exert power. This is precisely the starting point of the process I call "trickle-down imperialism."

Trickle-Down Imperialism Defined

Given ambiguous or vague policy mandates, subordinates often assert a conservative interpretation with a view to please their supervisors, using the implicit power relationship as justification. Such an interpretation also increases their power vis-à-vis their subordinates, people "lower on the food chain," thus legitimating their authority. This inequality and conservative interpretation trickles down the system—for example, in a USAID context, from Congress to political appointees to mid-level bureaucrats in Washington, to mission directors, to Northern NGO contractors, to Southern NGO partners, to the implementation level. This is more effective than overt control by memos, directives, and formal policies because it is harder to identify and critique. Also, policies and aid packages tend to look good on paper in Congress or the World Bank, such as Bill Clinton's slogan of "building back better" following Haiti's earthquake. How do these well-intentioned policies translate into disastrous on-the-ground realities, and how can we analyze and critique the resulting failures?

Looking at how intentionally vague, positive-sounding development mandates translate into on-the-ground NGO practices, we need to interrogate the roles that intermediaries play in service delivery. They are at once constrained and empowered by the structure, with human action and agency paired in a balancing act. As highlighted above, in the case of Sove Lavi, several institutions mediate contact between donors (in this case, U.S. residents as taxpayers) and aid recipients (in this case, peasants association leaders, and by extension rural communities): Congress, the State Department, USAID management and other Washington staff, USAID/Haiti staff, contracting Northern NGOs, and then Sove Lavi administration and "downstairs" staff. Direct contact with either donors or people "on the ground" is thus very limited, which cuts off open communication and limits effectiveness.

The aid system requires the ideology of autonomous, self-governing units and a system of accountability that is by definition hierarchical. Intermediaries are supposed to be responsible managers tasked with implementing superiors' mandates and supervising subordinates. Given such a vague mandate, a USAID-Washington middle manager, USAID mission director, or NGO director can choose either a "conservative" or "liberal" interpretation (not in the political but the epistemological sense). Consistently at Sove Lavi, it was the former; at each step, an intermediary made more conservative, cautious interpretations. So by the time the policy is implemented with Sove Lavi CAC members, it cannot address local participation and hence it exacerbates conflict. NGO directors like Mme Versailles who are loath to admit they are not autonomous act more conservatively than their donors want or need, because their funding could be cut. This is partially why Mme Versailles and Sove Lavi don't even think to question or challenge, let alone imagine alternatives. There is often very little room in which NGOs can negotiate (Bebbington and Thiele 1993; Biggs and Neame 1996; Edwards and Hulme 1996a; Pearce 1997). As long as they act within a small sphere with a pretense of autonomy, practicing "good governance," a balance is maintained. But the moment an NGO director steps out of the sphere of allowable actions, the organization can be disciplined. The threat of power, in the pulling of funding, is not only internalized akin to Foucault's "discipline" but is also real and imminent, as described in chapter 4's discussion of Sove Lavi.

This trickle-down imperialism is also a means by which intermediaries assert their power over subordinates. Mediating direct contact between groups, one of the only powers that intermediaries—middle managers, contracting Northern NGOs, or Southern NGO directors—have within this system is to interpret mandates within a contract. These "conservative" interpretations are then sent down the chain of command as mandates, since subordinates are unable to question or challenge them because they are not in contact with higher-ups. Recall how Fondation Sogebank attempted to force its new sub-grantee Fanm Tèt Ansanm under its thumb. Fanm Tèt Ansanm was able to hold its ground with the Global Fund's new "primary recipient" because it already had a Global Fund grant and its leaders knew that the new "mandates" Sogebank attempted to impose were their own creation, and not from the Global Fund. But this is an exceptional case. Structurally speaking, intermediaries block contact, which is the source of their only bureaucratic power. Whether someone applying for food stamps is told that her request can't be accommodated because the usually underpaid frontline civil servant is afraid to ask her supervisor or is simply exerting power on someone below, the frustrated and dejected person in need will never know because she has no direct contact with people vested with decision-making authority.

A correlate to this analysis, which could also account for the difference between Sove Lavi's and Fanm Tèt Ansanm's participation and donors, involves the number of intermediaries. Greater social distance—not just national difference or socioeconomic status but the institutional layers noted above—between a client and a financial contributor thus is more likely to trigger a defensive, "trickle-down imperialist" response. There are at least two additional intermediaries at Sove Lavi, and these involve the political process. In the ideal type of a cooperative, the beneficiaries as members are structurally the same group as donors, so in theory members have more power and the director's power is held in check. In reality, elected leadership and sometimes paid staff do sometimes mediate contact, and sometimes abuse this power, as in Haiti in 2004 when the cooperatives went bankrupt when the pyramid scheme went bust.

Update on the NGOs

Trickle-down imperialism explains how the two NGOs have evolved since I studied them between 2003 and 2005. By most measures, Fanm Tèt Ansanm has been doing extremely well. In late fall 2007 they opened a second clinic, and began to offer "depistage"—confidential AIDS testing. Two of the *medanm*—both quoted in the book—joined the staff. But the Women's Committee is now only a memory. At the end of 2007, its leaders proposed a series of recommendations, the same ones they had always mentioned: transportation stipends for committee meetings in addition to those of the prevention program, the sòl for personal needs such as health care, support for neighborhood associations, and so forth. In response, Fanm Tèt Ansanm disbanded the group with a thank-you celebration. By summer 2009 even the AIDS-prevention program ceased, with staff telling the medanm, "We'll call you when we need you." Individuals are invited to "participate" in trainings, usually to pass out materials. Meanwhile staff are acting very much like Sove Lavi, going to visits in the provinces, far away from the industrial park. The front and middle office formally merged, air-conditioned and all wired with new computers. Meanwhile the new clinic in SONAPI—where the medanm most frequented—did not have electricity the times I visited, a sign of priorities in terms of directing resources. The "message" posters are now off the walls of the front/middle office. Following the earthquake, Fanm Tèt Ansanm garnered even more support than it had before.

As of summer 2009, Sove Lavi was limping along, down to only two new trainers. The whole of the downstairs office was transformed into a dusty storage area for the Caravan, since all but one of the downstairs staff who worked during 2005 were let go. Despite this, the majority of upstairs staff were still employed. A big truck—labeled "Education Sanitaire Mobile" (Mobil Health Education)—sat in front of the office most of the time, the loudspeakers locked inside. Despite this clear inaction, Mme Versailles's picture appeared in the paper every so often. A former employee who became third-in-command at a government ministry said, "Donors are just into showbiz [*chobiz*]. It's all about the beautiful photo [opportunity]." When asked why this was, he replied, "Everyone has to show something to their supervisor. Even the donors." This showbiz is only possible if the donors are gullible enough to buy it. He made a play on the Kreyòl words *enterè* (interests) and *egare* (a naif), how donors' naivite or ignorance is intentional; it is in their interest to remain ignorant. When asked if this explains the "results" orientation, after the laughter died out, he intoned, "Didn't I just call this showbiz?" Sove Lavi's focus on appearances thus worked, at least until January 12. The earthquake totally demolished their offices, and donors are obviously focused on other priorities at the moment. Mme Versailles took the opportunity to fire everyone, including her "*makout*" Josue, hire two children as program directors, and move the office into her home, which was luckily undamaged.

Other Applications

The theoretical insights gained from this case study of two NGOs in post-coup Haiti might prove useful to understanding local responses to the financial crisis increasingly engulfing the globe. Civil service intermediaries are already responding as Sove Lavi did. The global financial crisis has had a chilling effect on public education. Local governments are typically responsible for the K–12 schools, and state legislatures for public universities. Both city and state governments are strapped for cash, a problem exacerbated by dwindling federal dollars. My college has traditionally attracted a student population that couldn't get a university degree anywhere else because of the extreme financial hardship that comes hand in hand with educational disadvantages. Compounding this, many students come from outside the United States and do not have citizenship status. In other words, many depend on academic success programs in addition to low tuition.

The threats of state budget cuts are not being felt equally, and when they come they are not applied equally. Traditionally under-resourced units of the university, including programs for diversity and ethnic studies departments, including a Haitian Creole language program—one of only a handful across the country—saw their classes slashed. For example, there were no Haitian Creole classes offered a year following the earthquake, despite there being a growing strategic need for this program. While generally done because of low enrollment, there was no formula for class cancellations, granting deans and department chairs greater authority and leeway. Deals were made in private. Faculty, particularly part-time faculty, had no ability to even question the rubric under which these decisions were made. They have no direct contact with university administration, who for their part stayed out of the implementation discussions; when pressed by some courageous department chairs, university higher-ups intoned, "Read the news." Implicit in this threat is the expectation to be grateful we are not victim to more coercive approaches, such as in Arizona, whose legislature outlawed ethnic studies programs. There was no plan from the administration—to say the least about the legislature—to destroy Haitian Creole, cultural diversity, or African American studies, but these programs disproportionately felt the pinch, along with other nonacademic programs aimed at retention and success for traditionally disadvantaged students. Although there were no explicit directives such as in Arizona, conditions were set by the budget cuts and the hierarchical system of intermediaries to selectively apply these cuts, and faculty were powerless to respond because of their structural isolation and because of the overall context. At each step in the process, intermediaries gain power through their conservative interpretation and their ability to pass their decision onto subordinates. We recently heard that a "liberal arts" education may be too expensive and that our students need vocational training. Students saw their tuition increase 25 percent over the past two years, edging out the very people for whom our college was the only option for higher education. Meanwhile, executives from Wachovia and AIG received millions in golden parachutes from the federal bailout package, doing even better than before the October 2008 meltdown.

Concluding Reflections

As discussed in the previous chapter, this trickle-down imperialism begins at the top, with USAID maintaining a defensive posture to "jittery members of Congress," who themselves are worried about voters' concern about too much tax money being directed to foreign development. Research continues to point out a consensus position among citizens that the U.S. government should support development. Voting with their paychecks, over half of U.S. households contributed to an NGO following Haiti's earthquake. USAID's focus on foreign policy also is an act of interpretation that is an assertion of a mandate; data show that U.S. citizens care more about humanitarian than foreign policy goals. The policy of results- or performance-based contracting is thus a prime example of this trickle-down imperialism. As this book demonstrates, when this policy gets communicated down the system of intermediaries, an otherwise good idea, it can cut off local participation and erode NGOs' autonomy, and hence aid becomes less effective, what Oxfam America (2008) has called a "control paradox." As a result, HIV/AIDS is not being as effectively combated, and more people will needlessly continue to die, like Gabrielle.

That people are dying of starvation and of preventable diseases, and are being denied education, is not debatable. The question remains, is this trickle-down imperialism an act of kindness? A former USAID mission director had these parting words: "So why do we continue to pour our money there? The goal is to spend it all and say, 'See, we've done all we can for Haiti.' And nothing happens. And it's because of U.S. domestic politics." So the vicious cycle of bad press continues, adding to the stigma and fear, which scares investors. Does this system of trickle-down imperialism need to continue?

Yvette offers an answer:

> I would like to tell the American people that they should rise up and tell their government to stop destroying small countries. If the American people revolted and told their government to give small countries the chance to live, maybe [the U.S. government] could listen. Because I believe there are many Americans who do not know what is happening in the world, who do not know what the American government is doing in the world, because of the media. Because I know that many Americans have good hearts. This is what makes them send money. This aid, this generosity, is good.

Afterword

Some Policy Solutions

The solution begins with me.

–Danielle, Sove Lavi CAC leader

Since 2003, I have engaged in many conversations about the system of foreign aid and NGOs with colleagues, NGO professionals, students, and *ti pèp*. Below are a series of recommendations stemming from these conversations for ending this killing with kindness, once and for all. Following the structure of the book, these begin at the grassroots and move up the various constituencies within the civic infrastructure analysis.

For the Grassroots: *"Bay tèt nou vale"*

Danielle, Djoni, and Maxime learned from their experience at Sove Lavi. Maxon brought up the idea that grassroots groups should "recognize our own self-worth" or "value ourselves"—*bay tèt nou vale*. True, grassroots groups like theirs benefit from *èd* (NGO aid). But equally important, NGOs need local leaders such as themselves. Without grassroots groups, Sove Lavi and other NGOs would not be able to accomplish their work. Knowing this fact, local leaders can negotiate with outside NGOs on a more equal footing. Djoni added, "We should have asked Sove Lavi what they really wanted, who their donors were, and what exactly they wanted from us." Danielle was succinct: "We need them, they need us."

How can grassroots groups level the relationship with NGOs and donors? The CAC leader Marie-Ange was passionate in her response, from her experience with another NGO: "Father Vital showed us that rather than extend a hand in begging, we should show the donor what we can do on our own: look at the load on the ground. Let's lift it up on our own and set it on our knees. After it's already on our knees, we can show the donor. We can ask, it's already on our knees, please lend a hand to help us lift it on top of our heads." Neighborhood groups, peasants' associations, women's clubs, and cooperatives do have the ability to lift their burdens up to their knees. Simone discussed her women's group: "Every time we meet, everyone gives 5 goud. If we're 50 people, that is 250 goud. This money is available for when one of us is sick, so we can rush to the hospital with her." A peasants' association in Gwomòn (Gros-Morne) built a road and community school with no outside support. Despite persistent stereotypes about the capital, even when Pòtoprens was smoldering with the violence and kidnapping between 2003 and 2006, grassroots groups all over *katye popilè* (low-income neighborhoods) were engaged in small, sustainable activities such as trash cleanup and pothole repair. They would have a bucket and ask passersby to contribute what they could. One federation of neighborhood groups even opened free schools in their communities without any outside assistance at the start.

For NGOs: "*Vize anba*"

As should be obvious from this discussion, NGOs should provide more space for genuine participation, and do so during more phases of a project. In other words, NGOs should focus below, *vize anba*. Sove Lavi could have used their data collected from CACs and the symposium showing that more time to plan entails more successful outcomes. They could have stood firm with USAID and the Global Fund to demand they fund longer trips to the provinces. They could have argued that local initiatives like the Kanaval activities planned by the local center are both more effective and efficient, and they could have either planned ahead by sharing the responsibility to draft their work plans, or they could have planned a slush fund so that they wouldn't always be waiting for reimbursement. At least until the Global Fund started to predominate, Fanm Tèt Ansanm was able to offer more grassroots support because they had multiple sources of funding. As Maxime bottom-lined it, "They need to respect us, as equals." Recall Djoni's plea: "We're not asking for a big thing. All we're asking for is mutual respect."

Still better would be if NGOs had the interest and ability to support local initiatives—to have local partners who actually share their vision of priorities. As it stands, Sove Lavi takes preexisting groups, peasants' associations for the most part, and imposes its own priorities. The system would be more effective if local groups who had already defined HIV prevention as a priority sought Sove Lavi out for its technical support. This requires two things: a reorientation in NGOs' relationship with communities, and more transparency. Information about NGOs' strategies and projects is not generally available to the public, so local communities just take what they can get. Like anthropologists, NGOs are particular audiences for people's *istwa*, their stories constructed by reflexive people for a particular purpose, in this case receipt of *èd*. So people will gear their needs to those of the NGOs. This is part of what the Haitian anthropologist

Gina Ulysse (2008) calls "reflexive political economy." NGOs—and not just states—need to be accountable and transparent, especially to the people they are meant to serve. To CAC members like Djoni and Danielle, NGOs need to make their activities, geographical area served, and intervention domain public, which is a first step to inviting peasants' associations to propose particular projects. Given the importance of the radio in a country where the vast majority of people do not have reliable access to electricity, NGOs should consider using this medium to spread the word about their priorities, instead of just using it to advertise an imminent event. At the very least, the Haitian government wrote, "It is imperative that NGOs and donors *stop using peasants' organizations* to justify what they want to do or justify their projects" (Ministè Agrikilti 2000:21). In Mme Versailles' words, they should also "be open" to local communities and their priorities.

Another concrete suggestion would be to regularly share their information with the Haitian government, to publish their activities and priorities. UCAONG (Unité de Contrôle et d'Administration des ONG, Haiti's NGO regulatory agency) staff estimated that only 10–20 percent of NGOs in Haiti share such information regularly, despite Haitian law that requires them all to do so. If a U.S. charity failed to do this, they would lose their tax-exempt status. Why they would even attempt this in a foreign country can be explained only by feelings of superiority, contempt, or the habitus of imperialism. According to Bill Clinton, who does not share the Haitian government's narrow definition, there are ten thousand NGOs working in Haiti, conflating large international NGOs with community associations. This number has become sacrosanct. Only four hundred or so were officially registered before the quake. Since then, Clinton's office has published a website to help coordinate NGOs' activities,[1] which is definitely a step in the right direction, but it still relies on the willingness (and time) of NGO staff to input the information. Despite this, the data about strategies and choice of local partners, sources of funding, and their budgets, remain very difficult to find.

For Haiti's Government: Steer, Not Row

Several people in Haiti have called for decentralization, for Haiti's government to empower local initiatives, to release more funds to the local level through the ASEC (Assemblés des Sections Communales, akin to city councils for the lowest level, the Communal Section) and CASEC (Conseils d'Administration de Section Communale, a team of three mayors) (the local, elected community government structure). Nearly all donor funding goes through NGOs and not the government. But what little that does filter to the government—at least a portion thereof—might be most effectively used by local governments, where officials are in regular contact with citizens and grassroots groups and could be challenged if funds are not spent correctly and quickly, a function of what political anthropologists call informal social control. In fact, several Sove Lavi CAC leaders ran for local office. A high-ranking Préval government official told me, "We don't need to control everything, and we don't need all the money to come to us. But we are the elected government and need to be able to steer."

That would require a more active, hands-on approach from the government. Many studies of NGOs have concluded that the Haitian government should be establishing priorities and creating the framework for collaboration between NGOs, the government, and local populations (e.g., ARS Progretti 2005; Étienne 1997; Mangonès 1991; Mathurin et al. 1989; Morton 1997). Paul Farmer (2011a) offers post-genocide Rwanda as an example of such a government-led framework. An example of how not to collaborate is the CCI process described in chapter 5 (see Schuller [2008] for further discussion). The World Bank's Poverty Reduction Strategy Paper (PRSP) (2008) offered a little more space for discussion, including sectoral as well as geographic roundtables. But as this book has argued, participation is much more than consent: it involves debate, prioritization, and particular attention to Haitian trends of social exclusion that if not directly countered will continue to marginalize Haiti's poor majority. Time and again, national production is mentioned as a priority for the Haitian government, yet the PRSP did not mention this except in the vaguest terms. The Collier report (2009), not even making a pretense of local participation, dismisses this strategy. The earthquake and the reconstruction plan fully expose the Haitian government's impotence, as only 1 percent of funds are going through the state. Overseeing the reconstruction, Haiti's Parliament has been replaced by an appointed committee, the Interim Haitian Reconstruction Commission. The plan—the Post-Disaster Needs Assessment (PDNA)—was even openly acknowledged by the government to be a show for donors, and not arising from any participatory process.

For USAID and Other Donors: Accompany, Not Dictate

As the major donor in Haiti and across the world, USAID has a key role to play in any solution. Given the changing of the guard at the U.S. State Department, with President Obama and Secretary Clinton having made promises to reform aid, particularly following Haiti's earthquake, there's a window of opportunity that we need to crack all the way open. The ONE campaign argues that Northern countries—including the United States—should contribute 1 percent of its gross national income (GNI) toward development and humanitarian aid.[2] The United States lags far behind other OECD countries, contributing 0.16 percent in 2007.[3]

Especially given the current mood in the post–financial crisis world, many Americans—including not only the Tea Party but also many of my low-income, immigrant students—feel that we should be focusing our efforts "at home." USAID needs us, a strong "constituency," now more than ever. If ever there was a time of hope for real change, it is now. By and large, Haitian people aren't asking for more aid, they're asking for an equitable, effective distribution of the existing aid. In order to insure an equitable distribution, they're also asking for a say in how this aid is delivered and used.

Below is a list of suggestions to improve USAID policy and implementation in this spirit. Obviously the situation will evolve, and not all changes can be pressed at once. Readers can see updates or take action on this book's website, http://www.killingwithkindness.org.

1. USAID should be removed from the State Department and be given autonomy from the institution to develop policies and priorities that are not based on current foreign policy goals. This would reverse the January 2006 reorganization of foreign aid, whereby USAID does not even have a separate budget available to citizens for review. Other countries shield overseas development from foreign policy interests; for example, the United Kingdom has a separate ministry for international development.[4]

2. Almost twice as many Americans believe that we should be focusing on greatest need instead of directing funds toward countries based on current security interests.[5] Therefore, USAID should prioritize funding based on need, defined in terms of ability to meet the universally accepted Millennium Development Goals or the UN's Human Development Index.

3. USAID should require NGOs to always include space for true local participation, in more steps of the project process than simply implementation. Specifically, local groups organized within grassroots organizations and local governmental bodies need to be able to deliberate on problem identification, prioritization, conceptualization, planning, follow-through, and evaluation. A modified version of the "participation" table (table 2.1) could be a guide. We could require a local participation plan in contracts.

4. Similarly, USAID can shift the reward structure to require NGOs to coordinate with one another and collaborate with the elected governments. USAID could assume a performance-based approach, supporting government offices that are functioning, such as water and sanitation. USAID could also pay a "tax" to supervisory government agencies to help them fulfill their roles in coordinating private NGO actions.

5. USAID should reopen and sufficiently fund its suspended Small Grants Program that funded start-up, smaller, local, grassroots groups to address critical, emerging needs. Alternatively, Congress should revive and fully fund the more grassroots-oriented Inter-American Foundation, so that the small grants actually have an effect.

6. Since local realities are different from one another, and can shift over time, USAID should suspend the use of "earmarks," top-down directives of how funds should be spent, since the earthquake reconstruction called

"preferencing." Local people know best how to implement agreed-on programs, cognizant of what works, what doesn't, and why.

7. Untie aid. Currently 93 percent of USAID funds return to the United States. There should be enough common good to go around if Haiti is out of poverty, safe, peaceful, and democratic, without funds going back to the United States.

In sum, people have a right to development (Sen 1999), and as such we should have a rights-based approach to development (e.g., NYU School of Law et al. 2008). Haiti's earthquake highlights just how badly we need this framework of human rights. The framework of national interest is too narrow. Especially given that Haiti is a good case for it, a reparations framework would be more appropriate. Is this just pie in the sky? I don't think so. The experience of the George W. Bush years shows that radical structural reforms are not just possible, but they actually took place. What is required is a clear vision and the political will, from every level within USAID.

I know there are many people who work within USAID and other development institutions who are critical of the rightward drift of their employers, who understand the critical importance of genuine local participation within development efforts, who share a repugnance of using aid as a tool in a geopolitical game. I interviewed several such people in Washington and in Europe. To these individuals I say, Now is the time to speak up. Disrupt trickle-down imperialism by your courage to stick to your convictions rather than playing it safe. Don't lose your critical perspective as you get closer to power, higher up the food chain.

For Citizens: Occupy Government

These changes will get us closer to a solution for Haiti and elsewhere. But they will only take us so far, and these suggestions themselves will go nowhere without active citizen pressure. The citizen mobilization in Egypt that erupted in January 2011 and toppled a thirty-year strongman government showed the world that peaceful demonstration can change the world. Police in Wisconsin joined the protestors in shutting down the Capitol in response to draconian reforms stripping all public unions of their collective bargaining abilities. A group of protesters triggered a global movement when they occupied Zuccotti Park near Wall Street in September 2011. Yvette, like others, believes that if Americans knew what our government was doing to small countries like Haiti, we would demand change. Having toured the country while presenting the documentary *Poto Mitan*, I have to say I agree that people are simply not aware of what's happening, and many people who become aware decide to become involved. In a short time, more than 1,800 people signed up to receive our action alerts. As Yvette noted above, the problem goes deeper, with a general lack of knowledge coming from our media. We need to change that, not only for Haiti but also for ourselves.

Why should students who were forced to endure a 25 percent increase in their tuition over the past two years, all the while working one and sometimes two jobs to raise their families and send remittances overseas, or people facing furloughs and a 10 percent unemployment rate, care about Haiti? Why should we in the United States be sending our dwindling tax resources to international development aid? First, Grann, Gabrielle, Simone, Lisette, and Charlene are real people. As human beings, they have a right to the chance for a decent life. Second, as Paul Collier (2009:4) said, the stakes are higher than Haiti: if the international aid system doesn't work in Haiti, it's hard to imagine where else it could. The earthquake is exposing the weaknesses in the system of international aid. Since the quake, the general public and the mainstream media are thinking and talking about NGOs in a more realistic, critical light.

Third, we are in the same boat. These same neoliberal policies that destroyed Haiti are just beginning to be critiqued as the major culprits in the global financial crisis, and rightly so. Haiti is a canary in the coal mine, an early warning system we should pay attention to. The financial crisis has finally hit us here in the United States. Unsurprisingly, marginalized communities were hit first and most dramatically; unemployment is over 15 percent for African Americans as of November 2011, almost twice the national average. Black men in New York City face 50 percent unemployment. For those who were paying attention, the signs were there to be read. In addition to being behind the global financial crisis, over the past thirty years inequality within nations has increased in addition to between nations, also a direct result of neoliberalism. For example, according to the American Human Development Project (2008), in 1980 the average executive earned forty-two times the salary as the average worker. By 2007 this gap had increased more than tenfold: according to the International Labor Organization (2008), the CEOs of the fifteen largest companies earned 520 times the salary of the average worker, up from 360 times just four years prior.

To Everyone: *"Kenbe fem"*

We all need to *kenbe fem*, hold strong. Things are definitely bad. But we need to stay focused, organized, and know what we are worth as human beings. The question isn't, or shouldn't be, should we change, or even what needs to change? The question is, what are we as a humanity going to do about it? What am I, what are you, doing to bring about this change?

Truly, another world is possible. But only if we recognize that we are all in this together and we act in solidarity with one another.

Marie, a former factory worker and current *timachann*, offers these parting words for readers: "Before you can talk about helping Haiti, the best way you can help us in Haiti is to bring back democracy to Washington."

NOTES

FOREWORD

1. For more on accompaniment, see Farmer 2011a; 2011b.

2. The literature on foreign aid, what Philip Gourevitch has termed the "groaning bookshelf" is rueful but well worth plumbing. See especially Gourevitch 2010; Mbakwem and Smith 2009; Polman 2010; Schwartz 2008; and Terry 2002.

INTRODUCTION

1. In an effort to protect people's identity, I have changed names and if necessary omitted identifying information.

2. Boutiques are storefronts where people sold out of their homes, with doors that could lock.

3. In this book I will refer to place names using Kreyòl, the first language of all Haitians and the only language of the poor majority. Despite this, and despite the fact that it is an official language, it remains marginalized, a way to exclude Haiti's poor.

4. Notice the use of French, not Kreyòl, to signify that French was still the predominant language of the state.

5. In addition to all these establishments in Petyonvil, Haiti's wealthy and middle classes frequented these businesses.

6. Haiti is second only to Namibia in terms of income inequality (Jadotte 2006).

7. Most of my middle-class neighbors worked at either an NGO or at a branch of a government, but there were a couple of doctors, and a Dominican family whose business in Haiti eluded everyone I asked.

8. Restavèk children are indentured live-in servants. See Cadet's (1998) study for a detailed firsthand account.

9. Several people in Haiti would take issue with this ideological use of "the people" in the singular, erasing important social divisions. Nonetheless, it is the term that "the people" in my neighborhood used to describe themselves.

10. The government's estimate rose to 316,000 at the one-year anniversary. The USAID contractor Tim Schwartz estimated between 46,000 and 85,000 in an unpublished report in May 2011. Small Arms Survey estimated 158,000 (Muggah and Kolbe 2011).

11. A March 2011 report by NYU's Center for Global Justice and Human Rights documented a rise in transactional sex, whereby women agreed to have sex in order to gain access to food and other necessities.

12. For a fuller discussion of the issue of debt, consult Gaillard-Pourchet (2002), Schuller (2006a), and Weisbrot and Sandoval (2007).

13. "Global South" is coming to replace the term "third world" within some activist circles because of the latter's implicit hierarchy.

14. Like the individuals, I am concealing the name of the groups, since they are still active. The point is not to destroy their reputations or pull their funding, but to explain the processes that constrain NGO action.

15. "Blan" is Kreyòl for not only "white" but also "white person" *and* "foreigner"—solidifying the ideology that Haitian people are "black." See Schuller (2010a) for further discussion.

16. Readers are invited to read a more explicit methodological discussion in chapter 2 of my dissertation (Schuller 2007b).

17. I argue for grant aid as opposed to loan aid through banks like the World Bank and the Inter-American Development Bank, which poor countries have to pay back and which rack up debt.

CHAPTER 1   VIOLENCE AND VENEREAL DISEASE

1. Radyo Ginen is a local radio station, derided by some members of Haiti's upper classes as "Radio Lavalas," referring to the party of President Aristide, because it was the only one to give Lavalas activists—and poor people generally—the microphone.

2. Kafou Ayewopò is one of the main corners, the intersection of a busy street that connects downtown to Petyonvil, and the road to the airport.

3. This is a common story. There is an apparently growing nostalgia for the former president Jean-Claude Duvalier, because then, "at least you knew who the enemies were." This was also before neoliberal economic policies destroyed the economy.

4. That is, this journey from Pòtoprens to Tèryewouj took twelve hours until the road was rebuilt in 2007.

5. Jonette herself died in a car crash in Miami a year later.

6. For an anthropological account of this, see Harrison's (2008) book.

7. In a database I constructed of stories posted online about Haiti, I logged 422 stories in February and 226 stories in March until the Boca Raton resident and UN retiree Gérard Latortue was selected as prime minister on the ninth, followed by 47 the rest of that month and 92 for the next three months combined.

8. Only 10 percent of Haiti's people are fluent and literate in French.

9. Nonetheless, three years later France declared as groundless Aristide's request for reparations for this 1825 debt.

10. Often translated as "bogeymen," *tonton makout* literally means "Uncle Knapsack"—from the Haitian folklore about the bogeyman taking children away in the middle of the night to put in his knapsack.

11. People in Haiti understand this in racialized terms, because black Haitian pigs were replaced by pink U.S. pigs.

12. The University of Chicago Economics Department under Milton Freidman trained an entire generation of foreign economists, particularly in the Americas, to promote neoliberalism, a purer form of free market capitalism than the Keynesian/New Deal version it replaced (Harvey 2005; Klein 2007).

13. Calling the events of 2004 a "coup" is my interpretation. Many call it a "resignation" because truth in fact Aristide signed his name on the dotted line. Roxanne, an unemployed factory worker, qualified that it "wasn't a coup d'état. . . . During the first coup d'état [against Aristide] it wasn't like that. They went inside the palace and took him and put him in an airplane. The second time they went to his private house and pulled a gun on him. That's not a coup but disorder."

14. Haiti's imports were at $1.022 billion and exports at $479 million (World Bank 2002b).

15. These austerity measures included the imposition of user fees for education and health care, and the cutting of social expenditures from 3 to 2 percent of Haiti's GDP.

16. The Boulos received U.S. funding through both the USAID health partner Centres de Développement et de Santé (CDS) and the Haitian Chamber of Commerce.

17. The Group of 184 was so named because ostensibly 184 members were part of this coalition, though official membership in the group remains opaque.

18. The *leadership* of the Group of 184, as represented when negotiating with the Organization of American States and the Caribbean Community, did not include such groups.

19. The Channmas is the national heroes' plaza surrounding the National Palace, akin to the Mall in Washington.

20. Brazil was also angling for a permanent seat on the UN Security Council at the time.

21. This study has been challenged because of its methodology, but it is the only serious attempt at quantifying the terror in Pòtoprens.

22. The concept of the "Haitian dollar"—one dollar per five goud, Haiti's official currency—arose because the exchange rate was fixed (until Delatour floated the currency, as noted above).

23. At the time of my fieldwork, the value of the goud (gourd) fluctuated around forty goud per U.S. dollar.

24. Elite families continued to be spared until much later, when the wave was supposedly over (Ledan 2009).

25. On one occasion in August 2006, deportees never even reached prison as they were supposed to have.

26. In Haiti, *lamizè* refers to the poorest poverty, and *malere/malerèz* to the poorest people, distinguishing it from mere poverty (*povrete*), and poor people (*pòv*).

27. This istwa contrasts with that of rural women, who have traditionally been granted some control of financial resources within the family, largely owing to their role in the market (Mintz 2010:125).

28. In Kreyòl there is no word ending that turns singular nouns into plural, save the addition of the word *yo*. In keeping with the integrity of the Kreyòl, I am not distinguishing the singular from the plural form. There have been other attempts to correct this (e.g., Smith 2001), but journal editors have called this pretentious and demanded another solution. This departure of Kreyòl norms from those of English happens in only a couple of cases, so I apologize for the confusion.

29. Latortue's intervention was similar to that effected in Operation Bootstrap in Puerto Rico, where Latortue also worked.

30. Both houses of Parliament unanimously adopted a 200-goud ($5.00) minimum wage. Following pressure from Clinton, Préval rejected this and offered instead 125 goud ($3.12), with no constitutional backing.

31. The annual growth in the Consumer Price Index in 2003 was 39.3 percent (IHSI 2008b).

32. At that time, "Miami rice"—imported from the United States—sold for fifty goud.

33. And the original fares were themselves much higher than in the 1980s and 1990s.

34. This is most likely in "Haitian dollars," so multiply this by five to get Haitian goud. Given how quickly the goud lost its exchange value to the dollar, and my ignorance of when these figures were from, I do not offer U.S. dollar equivalents here.

35. According to people I have interviewed, rents even went up in more violence-prone areas, such as Kafou Fey and Kafou Ayewopò.

36. I have been told that some renters have an arrangement whereby they receive the title to the land after a period of ten years, but I did not know of a single person for whom this situation worked out.

37. This migration was itself caused by a complex array of push-and-pull factors, neoliberal policies pushed by international agencies and consented to by Jean-Claude Duvalier (DeWind and Kinley 1988; Maternowska 2006).

38. Many children do not, especially those living in the provinces. In addition, there is a legal category called "natural children," whereby the father is not recognized and responsible. Edele, a feminist-humanist activist, decries this practice as discriminatory. The Ministry of Women's Condition and Rights changed this law in 2006.

39. According to the anthropologist Jennie Smith-Pariola (personal communication), this practice of nicknaming may have been an African holdover, and in rural Haiti, at least until recently, ceremonies following birth were common—though not elaborate or formal.

40. This gendered activity was not an individual occurrence in my neighborhood; I noticed this after my colleague Mercedes Pichard made a similar observation about the neighborhood where she stayed (personal communication).

41. I sincerely apologize that more recent statistics have not been made available, in part because the Ministry of Women's Condition and Rightshas been underfunded and therefore unable to conduct research.

42. According to Jennie Smith-Pariola, the same is true in rural markets: high-ticket items that men sell include meat and *kleren* (moonshine).

43. People who can't buy a plate of food often eat plentiful sugarcane to fill their stomachs, thereby causing widespread diabetes.

CHAPTER 2   "THAT'S NOT PARTICIPATION!"

1. In 2000 the national contraceptive acceptance prevalence rate was 28.1 percent (Pan American Health Organization 2005).

2. This situation changed as of July 2009, when two, sometimes three, trainings were held at the same time.

3. I use this phrase instead of the other commonly used phrase, *andeyò* (literally "outside"; see Smith 2001), to refer to "not Pòtoprens" because I have found it to be the least confusing to non-Haitian readers.

4. I put this word in quotes because people used the English word for it—difficult for Kreyòl speakers to pronounce as there is no "ow" sound in the language—suggesting it was a term imposed by donors.

5. This was in part because I did not include underage subjects in my research protocol. But even had I attempted to sit in on conversations about intimate matters, my presence would have had a profound effect on people's frankness.

6. Given the spyware downloaded onto the hard drives, and the ever-present chiming of Yahoo! Messenger, computer use did not turn out as originally planned.

7. Of the 291 officially registered NGOs who gave this information to the government, 258 are headquartered in the *zone métropolitaine* (Pòtoprens and its suburbs), whereas only 45 of the NGOs said they provide services in the capital.

8. Incoming calls are free, but not outgoing calls.

9. The 1987 Haitian Constitution divides the territory into 565 communal sections, the smallest units of local governance. Many people introduced themselves by first giving their name, the name of their hamlet, and the number of their communal section.

10. As mentioned in the previous chapter, only one aid recipient I know from Fanm Tèt Ansanm owns her housing.

11. This is the price for untreated public water. For treated water, the cost is higher. Only 8.7 percent of Haitian households have a tap—a fifth (20.7 percent) visit a public fountain, and a fifth (19.4 percent) buy their water (IHSI 2003).

12. As noted in the prior chapter, People in Haiti have to pay for their schooling. Eighty percent of schoolchildren go to private schools, and public school children have to supply their own books and uniforms.

13. Given her meager finances, I don't know how the beans and rice are procured.

14. Traditionally Haiti did not have a bourgeoisie but a merchant class, rendering Marxist analytics difficult. In addition, since 80 percent of Haiti's people are "poor" by international standards, culturally meaningful distinctions like kouch sosyal—what Weber (1946) would call "subjective" status categories—are useful.

15. *Etranje* is the formal, polite form of the word *blan*.

16. *Motivasyon* is the term most used by NGOs to get the word out about an upcoming meeting or event. The term in U.S.-based community organizing most resembling it would be "outreach."

17. The fact that the *ti pèsonnèl* ("small personnel" like drivers or janitors, many of whom were former factory workers) tend to be the ones who serve refreshments deserves some attention. But to the factory worker who attends her first celebration, she cannot tell the difference, as everyone is either dressed up in formal business attire or in a Fanm Tèt Ansanm T-shirt.

18. This follows Daniel Miller's (1997) argument about local cultural meanings of capitalism and consumption proliferating, providing space for local expression while integrating the local into the transnational process.

19. In the Haitian provinces, even fewer people attend high school than in the cities.

20. Sove Lavi's paid staff also received a per diem, yet they also ate a lunch.

21. I do not have a large enough sample for rural schools.

22. All the speeches began with a several-minute introduction that saluted all other notables in the audience and ended with "my distinguished colleagues and all workshop

participants." Two such introductions lasted as long as the time slot that was allocated for those individuals. I was told several times that these formalities were "part of Haitian culture."

23. This is a variation on a theme that Rossi (2006) discussed, whereby NGO recipients creatively reinterpret and appropriate official developmentalist language.

24. He actually wanted his real name used, but using it would identify other people in the CAC and the organization.

25. Albeit as individuals, as OFATMA did not maintain a proactive stance to protect future workers from this same problem past this initial period of embarrassment.

CHAPTER 3   ALL IN THE FAMILY

1. Previously, the airport was named for François Duvalier, who had it built in 1965. The road was named after the Ethiopian emperor Halle Selassie I. Aristide had made other gestures to the revolutionary hero, building a memorial to his constitution and installing Toussaint's likeness in the Hall of the Heads of State in the National Palace.

2. Reflecting the tap-tap's cramped quarters, a common joke is, "How many people can fit in a tap-tap? One more."

3. I use the ethnographic present in this day-in-the life portrait, in contrast to the "crisis," which is already "history" (Maternowska 2006:18).

4. Often, local circuits are damaged by rain, fire, or political or gang violence. Given the government's finances, repairs can take a long time (days, weeks, even months). Most people of a certain means or cultural capital have cell phones, themselves dependent on whether the towers are in working order and have full electricity.

5. *Twipe* is the sound of sucking in the teeth to express annoyance, considered impolite but nonetheless a mainstay in social interactions, particularly between people from different status groups.

6. Electricity provision varied wildly during the twenty-month fieldwork period. Sometimes Pòtoprens endured several days on end without any electricity at all (the longest drought was eight days). Very occasionally, especially during important events such as the World Cup, the electricity was on all day. Most often, the city was divided into five different zones, each with a different ration of electricity. The zone where I lived also included other middle-class areas such as Delma and Kanape-Vèt; we averaged between six and eight hours of electricity per day, far greater than other zones.

7. This form of greeting was one of the customs of the French bourgeoisie that people in Haiti kept and passed down. An employee explained that they kept the "best" of French culture . . . for isn't it pleasant to do so?

8. All the phones can receive incoming calls, much like the cell phone plans that charge the user for placing but not receiving calls.

9. Ironwork is one of Haiti's relatively hidden artistic treasures, whereby artists hammer out used oil drums and carve intricate designs.

10. There was one person who was very shy; she was the only one whom I did not interview.

11. The clinic often ran out of condoms, and sometimes it could take up to two months to get more.

12. Like Clifford Geertz's (1973:7) "burlesque" wink, often "Madame" was mockingly used when subordinates were talking among themselves, especially when criticizing one particular individual's autocratic leadership style or differing political beliefs.

13. It should be noted women held several posts in the interim government. Anne-Marie Issa, owner of Signal FM, represented the business class in the Council of the Wise, which ostensibly served the role as executive council, overseeing the interim process. The industrialist sector was represented in the interim government by Danielle St. Lot as the minister of commerce and industry, and Josette Bijou was minister of public health.

14. This stated desire for foreign aid could also potentially be a reflection of their estimation of me and my purpose—as a (potential) donor for Fanm Tèt Ansanm.

15. These garments are called "rad Kenedi" because the first major shipments of used clothes that did not sell at U.S. thrift stores coincided with President John F. Kennedy's founding of USAID in 1961.

16. There were at least fifteen memos—all in French—posted by the administration during my field research at Sove Lavi.

17. Many of these staff people were replaced in the middle of my fieldwork, so I can't even use a pseudonym.

18. The offices were rearranged in 2005, following a first round of staff cuts.

19. In late 2005, when five top-level employees and "contractors" were let go and not replaced, Mme Versailles took this as her office, and I am told she did not have large meetings here.

20. In later times, the secretary would announce on the intercom that the power source would either switch or be turned off.

21. By late 2005 the database manager moved into the office formerly occupied by Mme Versailles.

22. But still not Kreyòl, only recognized by Google after the earthquake and still not Microsoft as a language, despite these companies recognizing other languages with fewer speakers.

23. Both tech workers could turn a box full of spare parts into a functional computer, for example.

24. I'm six feet two inches tall; three male staff were the same height, unusually tall in Haiti, suggesting adequate food and health care.

25. This soccer match was an early attempt by Brazil for good PR, as it had just taken the reins of the UN forces from the United States.

26. Pantè is the brand name of USAID-funded U.S. NGO Population Services International, translated in Haiti as Program Santé International "International Health Program," using the same acronym of PSI.

27. At a December 2005 tour of the Caravan that I attended, this act of throwing boxes of condoms in the air was repeated.

28. Strengths, weaknesses, opportunities, and threats—a management analysis tool in vogue in the United States in the 1980s. It was written in the English "SWOT."

29. By the end of 2006, an additional five people were let go from Sove Lavi.

30. She replaced a man in this post.

CHAPTER 4   "WE ARE PRISONERS!"

1. Others (e.g., Pierre-Louis 2011) estimate that NGO salaries are three times government salaries.

2. Some consider his "second" term as happening after his return in 1994.

3. KONAP and State University students, particularly the Federation of Haitian University Students, both claim to be the first to call for Aristide's resignation.

4. The planners of the event had actually preferred the prime minister, who had real power, but they had accepted the president. He never actually committed to come, however.

5. These community liaisons were all male.

6. This practice follows USAID's (2005a) protocol on branding.

7. Predictably, fewer than thirty people attended the grand opening, despite the projected three hundred.

8. Gabrielle hadn't finished writing her report until she had visited the office in January, when we met for the interview.

9. The three means of prevention are USAID and PEPFAR's "ABC" formula of *abstinence, being* faithful, or *condom* use.

10. This derision was possibly an expression of nationalism, often coming from the elite classes when reminded of Haiti's subjugation by foreign countries.

11. I translated this speaker's English into French, which was slightly better pronounced than my compatriot who worked at the CDC.

12. By this time I was considered one of the Sove Lavi staff, and so was served with the group.

13. They did not meet again before I left Haiti at the end of May 2005.

14. The number of master's degrees at Sove Lavi is particularly significant given that only 1 percent of Haiti's population has any college degree (Earth Trends 2006).

15. As an example of such cultivation of personal relationships, Mme. Versailles asked me to translate a personal e-mail written in English from a U.S government official.

16. There was a rather lengthy discussion about the concerns that individual staff raised in the first appendix to this contractor report—many of which did not end up in the conclusion.

17. See, for example, studies from Chambers (1992), Edwards and Hulme (1992), Morton (1997), Paul and Israel (1991), Thomas-Slayter (1992), Uvin (1996), and Wils (1996).

18. These are not grants, itself a significant difference. Contracts are more legally binding than grants.

19. This lack of funds also explained why the bathrooms never had toilet paper.

20. For example, *politik devlopman USAID [yo]* can read as "USAID's development policies" or "politics of USAID development," and *politik neyoliberal [yo]* can mean "neoliberal policies" or "politics of neoliberalism."

21. There are other uses/interpretations of *grès kochon kwit kochon* that are sometimes used, such as that a person provides the means to destroy her- or himself (e.g., through bad attitude or behavior). The interpretation used in the book is the more commonly held one, at least according to Haitian scholars and peasants I interviewed.

22. Colleagues have referred me to two other NGOs that they define as autonomous because of their own income generation: Matènwa sells crafts, and Fonkoze raises money through interest on micro-credit.

CHAPTER 5 TECTONIC SHIFTS AND THE POLITICAL TSUNAMI

1. Rostow's theory holds that all societies progress on a single evolutionary trajectory, with "the West" being most advanced, a continuation of earlier unilineal evolutionary thinking of the Victorian era.

2. "Social scientist" is the term for everyone who is not an economist, since the latter are by far the majority of USAID staff.

3. At least in public schools, for those who have access to public schools.

4. More people (57 percent compared to 39 percent) believed that aid should be directed toward multilateral rather than bilateral institutions (Program on International Policy Attitudes 2001:28). Disaster scholars have noted a rise in the "bilateralization" of foreign aid (Macrae and Leader 2001).

5. "USAID History," retrieved October 10, 2007, from http://www.usaid.gov/.

6. This situation may be changing since the Tea Party movement and the widespread critique of "Obamacare."

7. "USAID: Congressional Budget Justification FY 2006," retrieved October 10, 2007, from http://www.usaid.gov/.

8. LexisNexis search, retrieved September 24, 2007, from http://www.lexis.com/.

9. These messages about drugs and alcohol were mirrored by public service announcements, also funded by PEPFAR, aired on the radio in the summer of 2006.

10. Before being named USAID administrator, Andrew Natsios was director of World Vision International.

11. Data for schools were not broken down by religious affiliation.

12. Current estimates of Haiti's religious population put the proportion of Protestants at 25 percent, which is more than twice what it was a generation ago (Interim Government of Haiti 2004).

13. This individual also said, "We represent constituents that other donors can't or won't, like men who have sex with men, sex workers, and drug users. They are also a part of civil society."

14. As governor of Wisconsin, Thompson was known for his work toward ending "welfare" (particularly Aid to Families with Dependent Children, AFDC).

15. "Supplementals" include multibillion-dollar no-bid contracts given to for-profit companies such as Bechtel or Halliburton.

16. For an example of development agencies' self-assessment, see Dollar's (1998) study.

17. And the "graduation" of these countries had comparatively little to do with official development aid, said this person.

18. The World Bank is divided into the IDA (International Development Association) for low-income countries, and the IBRD (International Bank for Reconstruction and Development) for middle-income countries. Recall that the institution was first set up to rebuild western Europe after World War II.

19. This index is measured by asking business leaders if they perceive the state to be corrupt.

20. These self-critiques themselves responded to outside pressure, calling for the closure of institutions such as the World Bank.

21. The political scientist Robert Rotberg (2004) adds another definitional layer between "stable" and "failed" states, what he calls "hollowed-out" states, which are propped up only by a dictator, such as Iraq under Saddam Hussein.

22. While Congress allocated a lower level, the leap in the request nonetheless highlights OTI's centrality to USAID.

23. Clinton also promised to help Haitian refugees with more asylum applications, which he did not do as president.

24. One of Haiti's former ambassadors to the UN argued that Clinton had early connections with the Washington Office on Haiti, a think tank for progressive U.S. foreign policy toward Haiti, through election officials who were Kennedy staffers. A senior-level State Department staff person said, "It would have been surprising if Clinton did not make efforts to bring back Aristide because the Democratic Party symbolized human rights and a principled foreign policy."

25. Noriega was involved in many coups and other extralegal activities in the region, including playing a role with the CIA and the Contras in Nicaragua.

26. Several ideologically driven books critical of the Clinton-Aristide nexus have been published (e.g., Girard 2004; Rotberg 2003).

27. According to the World Bank (2002a:3), new loans to Haiti were suspended in 1997 because of the lack of a functioning government.

28. Interestingly, Yvette is *not* one of Aristide's supporters, proposing instead a return to the Haitian Army that Aristide dismantled.

29. In addition to the bandits I would add the former army and even police. How did all these groups arm themselves given the international arms embargo?

30. There was also an exploration of foreign governments collecting customs duties as ships left their ports, after the interim government shut down provincial ports, triggering a strike of dock workers.

31. During the years following the 1994 return of Aristide, 90 percent of Haiti's governmental budget was financed externally (Morton 1997:1).

32. Incidentally, my current institution is one of them, and it still offers courses.

33. I myself have been "tested" by native Kreyòl speakers, but the measure was whether I was familiar with one or another Kreyòl proverb. As often as not, I failed the test, once chided in front of NGO aid recipients by a journalist who "*soti pèp la*" (came from Haiti's impoverished majority).

34. Mme Versailles made twenty times more than the lowest-paid employee, for example.

35. At the highest end, however, these European NGOs received only 50 percent of their annual budget from government, far less than the vast majority of U.S.-based NGOs.

CONCLUSION

1. An unpublished USAID report (Schwartz 2011) released in May 2011 warned that 64 percent of houses tagged "red" for demolition were reoccupied.

2. Successes include Partners in Health/Zanmi Lasante rebuilding the state hospital and building a new teaching hospital, and Médecins Sans Frontières providing water treatment tools to IDPs and low-income neighborhoods.

3. This term, arising from Deleuze and Guattari's (1987) work, was elaborated by the anthropologists Aihwa Ong and Stephen Collier (2005) to describe the temporary, "rhizomatic" nature of groupings, in this case social groupings.

4. Marx himself moved beyond what was to become hegemonic Marxian interpretations of power, in the "Eighteenth Brumaire" ([1852] 1978) and the "Grundrisse" ([1857] 1978).

AFTERWORD

1. The website put together by Clinton's office can be found at http://www.csohaiti.org/.

2. Rich nations pledged 0.7 percent at the 1992 Rio Conference, including the United States.

3. "ODA by Donor," retrieved May 20, 2008, from http://stats.oecd.org/.

4. Oxfam America (2008:12) has made a similar reorganization recommendation.

5. Sixty-three percent, as opposed to 34 percent (Program on International Policy Attitudes 2001).

GLOSSARY

andeyò. "Outside," usually meaning living outside the capital city, but it can refer to being a marginalized outsider. See Smith (2001)

bidonvil. Shantytown

blan. Haitian term for "foreigner," also referring to the racial category of white people

blokis. Traffic jam

brase lide. Expression for a conversation to discuss ideas and problems, literally "stirring ideas"

chan pwen. "Pointing" songs, composed to make a point, often social commentary

dechoukaj. "Uprooting," referring to the volatile period in Haiti's history after the fall of Duvalier on February 7, 1986, and leading up to the first free election on December 16, 1990

dèlko. Gas-powered generator

èd. Foreign aid

goud. Haitian currency. Traditionally, the rate was five goud to the dollar, but the currency has floated since Haiti's liberalization in the 1980s. During the study, the value varied from thirty-five to forty-five goud to a dollar, usually around forty

goudougoudou. Earthquake, mimicking the sound of the earth shaking. The term is used instead of the official *tranblemanntè a* because people are afraid to speak its name

gran manjè. Fat cat, literally "big eater"

gran moun tèt li. Sovereign, autonomous, able to make one's own decisions

grès kochon kwit kochon. Haitian proverb. Literally "the pig cooks in its own fat." Used to describe financial autonomy

griyo. Storyteller, from African ancestral traditions

gwoupman katye. Neighborhood association

istwa. "History," as in national or life history, as well as "story"

Kanaval. Carnival

katye popilè. "Popular" or poor neighborhood

klas. "Class," in the Marxist sense

kouch. "Social layer," indigenous or Weberian "subjective" distinction between Marxist classes

lakou. A traditional rural family space, including common outdoor living space

Lavalas. Political party of Jean-Bertrand Aristide, also Fanmi Lavalas, translated as "landslide" or "cleansing flood"

lavi chè a. High cost of living

lekòl bòlèt. Literally "lottery school," of low or uncertain quality, usually a private enterprise, often run by the only literate person in the locality

medanm. "Women," referring to Fanm Tèt Ansanm's recipients

pèp la. "The people, "meaning Haiti's marginalized poor majority

politik. Same Kreyòl word for "politics" or "policies," used in this book to refer to the politics/policies of donors and NGOs

poto mitan. "Center posts," an expression—coming from traditional African ancestor worship—referring to women's central role in Haitian family, society, and economy

radyo trannde. "Radio of thirty-two [teeth]," rumor mill

responsab. Responsible party, person in charge

sòl. Organically organized solidarity lending, whereby a group of friends or coworkers regularly pool their resources; a zero-interest loan

tap-tap. Privately owned and operated "public" transport, often brightly colored converted pickup trucks or vans, organized into officially designated routes and fares

tèt ansanm. Literally "heads together," a brainstorming collaborative conversation or meeting, generating common solutions to problems

timachann. Street merchant, mostly women engaged in micro-commerce

ti pèsonnèl. "Small" personnel, cooks, janitors, logistical assistants

tonton makout. Duvalier's death squads, literally "Uncle Knapsack," referring to folktales wherein children were stolen at night

twipe. A gesture of sucking in the teeth, considered impolite but nonetheless a mainstay in social interactions

REFERENCES

Abramson, David M. 1999. "A Critical Look at NGOs and Civil Society as Means to an End in Uzbekistan." *Human Organization* 58:240–250.

Adams, Rebecca, Gayle Morris, Patricia Martin, and Hannah Baldwin. 1998. "Gender Analysis of USAID/Haiti's Strategic Objectives." WID Tech, Washington.

Afary, Janet. 1997. "The War Against Feminism in the Name of the Almighty: Making Sense of Gender and Muslim Fundamentalism." *New Left Review*:89–110.

Agence France-Presse (AFP). 2011. "Haiti Cholera Death Toll Tops 4,000." Agence France-Presse, January 28.

Agg, C. 2006. *Trends in Government Support for Non-Governmental Organizations: Is the "Golden Age" of NGO Behind Us?* Geneva: United Nations Research Institute on Social Development.

Alvaré, Bretton. 2010. "'Babylon Makes the Rules': Compliance, Fear, and Self-Discipline in the Quest for Official NGO Status." *Political and Legal Anthropology Review* 33:178–200.

Alvarez, Sonia E. 1999. "Advocating Feminism: The Latin American Feminist NGO 'Boom.'" *International Feminist Journal of Politics* 1:181–209.

Anglade, Georges. 1974. *L'espace haïtien.* Montreal: Presses de l'Université de Québec.

Anglade, Mirielle Neptune. 1995. *Fanm ayisyen an chif.* Port-au-Prince: Comité Interagences Femmes et Développement en Haïti.

Antrobus, Peggy. 2004. *The Global Women's Movement: Origins, Issues, and Strategies.* London: Zed.

Appadurai, Arjun. 1986. *The Social Life of Things: Commodities in Cultural Perspective.* Cambridge: Cambridge University Press.

Arneil, Barbara. 2006. *Diverse Communities: The Problem with Social Capital.* Cambridge: Cambridge University Press.

ARS Progretti. 2005. "Mission d'Assistance Technique à la Cartographie des Acteurs non-Étatiques en Haïti: Rapport Provisoire." Mission l'Union Européenne en Haïti, Port-au-Prince.

Atmar, Mohammed Haneef. 2001. "Politicisation of Humanitarian Aid and Its Consequences for Afghans." *Disasters* 25:321–330.

Auyero, Javier, and Déborah Alejandra Switsun. 2009. *Flammable: Environmental Suffering in an Argentine Shantytown.* New York: Oxford University Press.

Averill, Gage. 1997. *A Day for the Hunter, a Day for the Prey: Popular Music and Power in Haiti.* Chicago: University of Chicago Press.

Bachelet, Pablo. 2004. "Body Count in Morgue Suggests High Haiti Death Toll." *Reuters*, March 5.

Bagdikian, Ben H. 1993. *The Media Monopoly.* Boston: Beacon Press.

Bailey, Katherine M. 1998. *NGOs Take to Politics: The Role of Non-governmental Organizations in Mexico's Democratization Effort.* Pittsburgh: Latin American Studies Association.

Barthélémy, Gérard. 1990. *L'univers rural haïtien: Le pays en dehors*. Paris: L'Harmattan.

Bazin, Marc. 2008. *Des idées pour l'action*. Port-au-Prince: L'Imprimateur II.

Bebbington, Anthony, and Graham Thiele. 1993. *Non-governmental Organizations and the State in Latin America*. London: Routledge.

Behar, Ruth. 1993. *Translated Woman: Crossing the Border with Esperanza's Story*. Boston: Beacon Press.

———. 1996. *The Vulnerable Observer: Anthropology That Breaks Your Heart*. Boston: Beacon Press.

Bell, Beverly. 2001. *Walking on Fire: Haitian Women's Stories of Survival and Resistance*. Ithaca: Cornell University Press.

Bello, Walden. 1996. "Structural Adjustment Programs: 'Success' for Whom?" In *The Case Against the Local Economy*, edited by Jerry Mander and Edward Goldsmith, 285–294. London: Earthscan.

Bending, Tim, and Sergio Rosendo. 2006. "Rethinking the Mechanics of the 'Anti-politics Machine.'" In *Development Brokers and Translators: The Ethnography of Aid and Agencies*, edited by D. Lewis and D. Mosse, 217–237. Bloomfield, CT: Kumarian Press.

Benería, Lourdes, and Shelley Feldman. 1992. *Unequal Burden: Economic Crises, Persistent Poverty, and Women's Work*. Boulder: Westview Press.

Benoit, Olga. 1995. "Women's Popular Organizations." *Roots* 1:26–29.

Bergan, Renée, and Mark Schuller, directors. 2009. *Poto Mitan: Haitian Women, Pillars of the Global Economy*. Documentary Educational Resources.

Bergeron, Suzanne. 2001. "Political Economy Discourses of Globalization and Feminist Politics." *Signs* 26:983–1006.

Bernard, Jean Maxius, and Julio Desormeaux. 1996. *Culture, santé, sexualité à Cité Soleil*. Port-au-Prince: Centres pour le Développement et la Santé.

Bessis, Sophie. 2001. "The World Bank and Women: 'Institutional Feminism.'" In *Eye to Eye: Women Practising Development Across Cultures*, edited by S. Perry and C. Schenck, 10–24. London: Zed.

Besteman, Catherine, and Hugh Gusterson. 2005. *Why America's Top Pundits Are Wrong: Anthropologists Talk Back*. Berkeley: University of California Press.

Biggs, Stephen D., and Arthur D. Neame. 1996. "Negotiating Room to Maneuver: Reflections Concerning NGO Autonomy and Accountability Within the New Policy Agenda." In *Beyond the Magic Bullet: NGO Performance and Accountability in the Post–Cold War World*, edited by M. Edwards and D. Hulme, 31–41. West Hartford, CT: Kumarian Press.

Blair, Harry. 1997. "Donors, Democratisation, and Civil Society: Relating Theory to Practice." In *NGOs, States, and Donors: Too Close for Comfort?*, edited by D. Hulme and M. Edwards, 23–42. New York: St. Martin's Press.

Bogdanich, Walt, and Jenny Nordberg. 2006. "Mixed U.S. Signals Helped Tilt Haiti Toward Chaos." *New York Times*, January 29.

Bohning, Don. 2004. "An International Protectorate Could Bring Stability to Haiti: Nation in Chaos." *Miami Herald*, November 22.

Bornstein, Erica. 2003. *The Spirit of Development: Protestant NGOs, Morality, and Economics in Zimbabwe*. New York: Routledge.

Boserup, Ester. 1970. *Woman's Role in Economic Development*. London: Allen and Unwin.

Bourdieu, Pierre. 1980. *Le sens pratique*. Paris: Editions de Minuit.

———. 1990. *The Logic of Practice*. Translated by Richard Nice. Stanford: Stanford University Press.

———. 1998. *Practical Reason: On the Theory of Action*. Stanford: Stanford University Press.

Brenner, Johanna. 2000. *Women and the Politics of Class*. New York: Monthly Review Press.

Brown, David. 2004. "Participation in Poverty Reduction Strategies: Democracy Strengthened or Democracy Undermined?" In *Participation: From Tyranny to Transformation? Exploring New Approaches to Participation in Development*, edited by S. Hickey and G. Mohan, 237–251. London: Zed.

Brown, Wendy. 1992. "Finding the Man in the State." *Feminist Studies* 18:7–34.

Burd-Sharps, Sarah, Kristen Lewis, and Eduardo Borges Martins. 2007. *The Measure of America: American Human Development Report, 2008–2009*. New York: Columbia University Press.

Butler, Lynne Margaret. 2008. "Navigating the Aid World: Barriers to the Effective Participation of Local NGOs in the Post-conflict Environment of Timor-Leste." Master's diss., Curtin University of Technology.

Cadet, Jean-Robert. 1998. *Restavec: From Haitian Slave Child to Middle-Class American*. Austin: University of Texas Press.

Castells, Manuel. 1983. *The City and the Grassroots: A Cross-Cultural Theory of Urban Social Movements*. Berkeley: University of California Press.

Cayemittes, Michel, Marie Florence Placide, Bernard Barrière, Soumaïla Mariko, and Blaise Sévère. 2001. *Enquête Mortalité, Morbidité et Utilisation des Services (EMMUS III) Haiti 2000*. Port-au-Prince: Institut Haïtien de l'Enfance, Pan American Health Organization.

Chakrabarty, Dinesh. 1992. "Postcoloniality and the Artifice of History: Who Speaks for 'Indian' Pasts?" *Representations* 37:1–26.

de Certeau, Michel. 1984. *The Practice of Everyday Life*. Berkeley: University of California Press.

de Certeau, Michel, Pierre Mayol, and Luce Giard. 1998. *The Practice of Everyday Life*. Vol. 2: *Living and Cooking*. Minneapolis: University of Minnesota Press.

Chambers, Robert. 1992. "Spreading and Self-Improving: A Strategy for Scaling-Up." In *Making a Difference: NGOs and Development in a Changing World*, edited by M. Edwards and D. Hulme, 40–48. London: Earthscan.

Charles, Carolle. 1995. "Gender and Politics in Contemporary Haiti: The Duvalierist State, Transnationalism, and the Emergence of a New Feminism (1980–1990)." *Feminist Studies* 21:135–164.

Charles, Jacqueline. 2005. "Haiti: Aristide Stole Millions." *Miami Herald*, November 3.

Chatterjee, Piya. 2008. "Hungering for Power: Borders and Contradictions in Indian Tea Plantation Women's Organizing." *Signs* 33:497–505.

Chinchilla, Norma Stoltz. 1992. "Marxism, Feminism, and the Struggle for Democracy in Latin America." In *The Making of Social Movements in Latin America: Identity, Strategy, and Democracy*, edited by A. Escobar and S. E. Alvarez, 37–51. Boulder: Westview Press.

Chomsky, Noam, Paul Farmer, and Amy Goodman. 2004. *Getting Haiti Right This Time: The U.S. and the Coup*. Monroe, ME: Common Courage Press.

Churchill, Nancy. 2004. "Maquiladoras, Migration, and Daily Life." In *Women and Globalization*, edited by D. D. Aguilar and A. E. Lascamana, 120–153. Amherst, NY: Humanity.

Clark, John. 1991. "Democratising Development: NGOs and the State." *Development in Practice* 2:151–161.

Clarke, Edith. 1957. *My Mother Who Fathered Me: A Study of the Family in Three Selected Communities in Jamaica*. New York: G. Allen & Unwin.

Clement, Christopher. 1997. "Returning Aristide: The Contradictions of US Foreign Policy in Haiti." *Race and Class* 39:21–36.

Cohen, Jon. 2006. "Making Headway Under Hellacious Conditions." *Science* 313:470–473.

Collier, Jane, and Sylvia Yanagisako. 1987. "Theory in Anthropology Since Feminist Practice." *Critique of Anthropology* 9:27–37.

Collier, Paul. 2007. *The Bottom Billion: Why the Poorest Countries Are Failing and What Can Be Done About It*. New York: Oxford University Press.

———. 2009. "Haiti: From Natural Catastrophe to Economic Security." United Nations Secretary General, New York.

Collins, Jane L. 2003. *Threads: Gender, Labor, and Power in the Global Apparel Industry*. Chicago: University of Chicago Press.

Collins, Patricia Hill. 2000 [1990]. *Black Feminist Thought: Knowledge, Consciousness, and the Politics of Empowerment*. 2nd ed. New York: Routledge.

Comaroff, Jean. 1997. "The Empire's Old Clothes: Fashioning the Colonial Subject." In *Situated Lives: Gender and Culture in Everyday Life*, edited by L. Lamphere, H. Ragone, and P. Zavella, 400–419. New York: Routledge.

Cooke, Bill, and Uma Kothari, eds. 2001. *Participation: The New Tyranny?* New York: Zed.

Cooley, Alexander, and James Ron. 2002. "The NGO Scramble: Organizational Insecurity and the Political Economy of Transnational Action." *International Security* 27:5–39.

Coomaraswamy, Radhika. 2002. "Are Women's Rights Universal? Re-engaging the Local." *Meridians* 3:1–18.

Coordination Haïti-Europe (CoHE), and Coordination Europe-Haïti (CoEH). 2006. "Interim Cooperation Framework: What Needs to Change." Coordination Haïti-Europe and Coordination Europe-Haïti, Port-au-Prince and Brussels.

Corcoran-Nantes, Yvonne. 2000. "Female Consciousness or Feminist Consciousness? Women's Consciousness Raising in Community-Based Struggles in Brazil." In *Global Feminisms Since 1945*, edited by B. G. Smith, 81–100. London: Routledge.

Cornwall, Andrea. 2004. "Spaces for Transformation? Reflections on Issues of Power and Difference in Participation in Development." In *Participation: From Tyranny to Transformation? Exploring New Approaches to Participation in Development*, edited by S. Hickey and G. Mohan, 75–91. London: Zed.

Cravey, Altha J. 1998. *Women and Work in Mexico's Maquiladoras*. Lanham, MD: Rowman and Littlefield.

Crawford, David L. 2008. *Moroccan Households in the World Economy: Labor and Inequality in a Berber Village*. Baton Rouge: Louisiana State University Press.

Crenshaw, Kimberlé Williams. 1991. "Mapping the Margins: Intersectionality, Identity Politics, and Violence Against Women of Color." *Stanford Law Review* 43:1241–1299.

Crush, Jonathan. 1995. *Power of Development*. New York: Routledge.

Danaher, Kevin. 2004. *10 Reasons to Abolish the IMF and World Bank*. Foreword by Anuradha Mittal. New York: Seven Stories Press.

Danticat, Edwidge. 1994. *Breath, Eyes, Memory*. New York: Vintage.

Darion Garcia, Ruben. 2003. "6000+ US Troops in the Dominican Republic; Non-stop Imperialist Intervention in the Caribbean." *Turning the Tide* 16:2, 4.

Dash, J. Michael. 1997. *Haiti and the United States: National Stereotypes and the Literary Imagination*. New York: St. Martin's Press.

Davis, Angela Yvonne. 1983. *Women, Race, and Class*. New York: Vintage.

Davis, Coralynn. 2003. "Feminist Tigers and Patriarchal Lions: Rhetorical Strategies and Instrumental Effects in the Struggle for Definition and Control over Development in Nepal." *Meridians* 3:204–249.

Deibert, Michael. 2005. *Notes from the Last Testament: The Struggle for Haiti*. Introduction by Raoul Peck. New York: Seven Stories Press.

Deleuze, Gilles, and Félix Guattari. 1987. *A Thousand Plateaus: Capitalism and Schizophrenia*. Translated by B. Massaumi. Minneapolis: University of Minnesota Press.

Delva, Guyler. 2010. "Haiti Urged to Halt Cholera Anti-Voodoo Lynchings." Reuters, December 23.

Deshommes, Fritz. 1995. *Néo-libéralisme: Crise économique et alternative de développement*. Port-au-Prince: Imprimateur II.

———. 2006. *Haïti: Un Nation Écartelée: Entre "Plan Américain" et Projet National*. Port-au-Prince: Editions Cahiers Universitaires.

Dethier, Jean-Jacques, Hafez Ghanem, and Edda Zoli. 1999. "Does Democracy Facilitate the Economic Transition? An Empirical Study of Central and Eastern Europe and the Former Soviet Union." World Bank, Washington.

Development Initiatives. 2006. "Global Humanitarian Assistance, 2006." Development Initiatives, London.

DeWind, Josh, and David H. Kinley III. 1988. *Aiding Migration: The Impact of International Development Assistance on Haiti*. Boulder: Westview Press.

Dicklitch, Susan. 1998. *The Elusive Promise of NGOs in Africa: Lessons from Uganda*. New York: St. Martin's Press.

Diederich, Bernard. 1985. "Swine Fever Ironies: The Slaughter of the Haitian Black Pig." *Caribbean Review* 14:16–17, 41.

Diederich, Bernard, and Al Burt. (1970) 2005. *Papa Doc and the Tontons Macoutes*. Boulder: Marcus Wiener.

Disaster Accountability Project. 2011. "One Year Follow Up Report on the Transparency of Relief Organizations Responding to 2010 Haiti Earthquake." Disaster Accountability Project, Washington.

Dollar, David. 1998. "Assessing Aid: What Works, What Doesn't, and Why." World Bank, Washington.

Donini, Antonio, ed. 2012. *The Golden Fleece: Manipulation and Independence in Humanitarian Action*. Sterling, VA: Kumarian Press.

Doolittle, Amity. 2006. "Resources, Ideologies, and Nationalism: The Politics of Development in Malaysia." In *Development Brokers and Translators: The Ethnography of Aid and Agencies*, edited by D. Lewis and D. Mosse, 51–74. Bloomfield, CT: Kumarian Press.

Doyle, Kate. 1994. "Hollow Diplomacy in Haiti." *World Policy Journal* 11:50–58.

Duffield, Mark, Joanna Macrae, and Devon Curtis. 2001. "Editorial: Politics and Humanitarian Aid." *Disasters* 25:269–274.

Duhaime, Eric. 2002. "Haïti: Pourquoi payer la dette de Papa Doc?" Jubilé 2000 Haïti, Port-au-Prince.

Dumas, Reginald. 2008. *An Encounter with Haiti: Notes of a Special Advisor*. Port of Spain, Trinidad and Tobago: Medianet Limited.

Dupuy, Alex. 1989. *Haiti in the World Economy: Class, Race, and Underdevelopment Since 1700*. Boulder: Westview Press.

———. 1997. *Haiti in the New World Order: The Limits of the Democratic Revolution*. Boulder: Westview Press.

———. 2005. "From Jean-Bertrand Aristide to Gerard Latortue: The Unending Crisis of Democratization in Haiti." *Journal of Latin American Anthropology* 10:186–205.

———. 2007. *The Prophet and Power: Jean-Bertrand Aristide, Haiti, and the International Community*. Lanham, MD: Rowman and Littlefield.

Earth Trends. 2006. *Population, Health, and Well-Being: Haiti*. New York: Earth Trends.

Eckhardt, William, and Gernot Köhler. 1980. "Structural and Armed Violence in the 20th Century: Magnitudes and Trends." *International Interaction* 6:347–375.

Edelman, Marc. 2005. "When Networks Don't Work: The Rise and Fall and Rise of Civil Society Initiatives in Central America." In *Social Movements: An Anthropological Reader*, edited by J. C. Nash, 29–45. Malden, MA: Blackwell.

Edelman, Marc, and Angelique Haugerud. 2005. *The Anthropology of Development and Globalization: From Classical Political Economy to Contemporary Neoliberalism*. Oxford: Blackwell.

Edwards, Michael, and David Hulme. 1992. "Scaling-Up: The Development Impact of NGOs: Concepts and Experiences." In *Making a Difference: NGOs and Development in a Changing World*, edited by M. Edwards and D. Hulme, 13–27. London: Earthscan.

———, eds. 1996. *Beyond the Magic Bullet: NGO Performance and Accountability in the Post–Cold War World*. West Hartford, CT: Kumarian Press.

———. 1996b. "Beyond the Magic Bullet? Lessons and Conclusions." In *Beyond the Magic Bullet: NGO Performance and Accountability in the Post-Cold War World*, edited by M. Edwards and D. Hulme, 254–266. West Hartford, CT: Kumarian Press.

———. 1996c. "Too Close for Comfort? The Impact of Official Aid on Nongovernmental Organizations." *World Development* 24:961–973.

Ellis, Patricia. 2003. *Women, Gender and Development in the Caribbean: Reflections and Projections*. Kingston: Ian Randle.

Elsner, Alan. 2004. "Guantanamo Bay Prepared for Refugee Influx." Reuters, February 11.

Engels, Friedrich. (1884) 1986. *The Origin of the Family, Private Property, and the State*. New York: Penguin.

Engler, Yves, and Anthony Fenton. 2005. *Canada in Haiti: Waging War on the Poor Majority*. Vancouver: Red Publishing.

Enloe, Cynthia. 1993. *The Morning After: Sexual Politics at the End of the Cold War*. Berkeley: University of California Press.

———. 2000. *Bananas, Beaches, and Bases: Making Feminist Sense of International Politics*. Berkeley: University of California Press.

Eriksson Baaz, Maria. 2005. *The Paternalism of Partnership: A Postcolonial Reading of Identity in Development Aid*. London: Zed.

Escobar, Arturo. 1995. *Encountering Development: The Making and Unmaking of the Third World*. Princeton: Princeton University Press.

Étienne, Sauveur Pierre. 1997. *Haiti: L'invasion des ONG*. Port-au-Prince: Centre de Recherche Sociale et de Formation Economique pour le Développement.

Evans-Pritchard, E. E. (1940) 1969. *The Nuer: A Description of the Modes of Livelihood and Political Institutions of a Nilotic People*. New York: Oxford University Press.

Eyma, Émile Jr. 1992. "Organisations non-gouvernementales (ONG), groupes de base et action politique." In *Association québécoise des organismes de coopération internationale (AQOCI)*, edited by J. Raymond, 54–59. Port-au-Prince: Association québécoise des organismes de coopération internationale.

Faludi, Susan. 1991. *Backlash: The Undeclared War Against American Women*. New York: Doubleday.

Farmer, Paul. 1992. *AIDS and Accusation: Haiti and the Geography of Blame*. Berkeley: University of California Press.

———. 2003. *The Uses of Haiti*. Monroe, ME: Common Courage Press.

———. 2004. "An Anthropology of Structural Violence." *Current Anthropology* 45:305–325.

———. 2008. "Haiti's Unnatural Disaster." *The Nation*, October 6.

———. 2011a. *Haiti After the Earthquake*. New York: Polity Press.

———. 2011b. "Partners in Help: Assisting the Poor Over the Long Term." *Foreign Affairs*. July 29. Available at http://www.foreignaffairs.com/articles/68002/paul-farmer/partners-in-help.

Farmer, Paul, Margaret Connors, and Janie Simmons. 1996. *Women, Poverty, and AIDS: Sex, Drugs, and Structural Violence*. Monroe, ME: Common Courage Press.

Fass, Simon M. 1988. *Political Economy in Haiti: The Drama of Survival*. New Brunswick, NJ: Transaction Books.

Fatton, Robert. 2002. *Haiti's Predatory Republic: The Unending Transition to Democracy.* Boulder: Lynne Reiner.

———. 2004. "The Haitian Authoritarian *Habitus* and the Contradictory Legacy of 1804." *Journal of Haitian Studies* 10:22–43.

———. 2007. *The Roots of Haitian Despotism.* Boulder: Lynne Rienner.

Ferguson, James. 1990. *The Anti-politics Machine: "Development," Depoliticization, and Bureaucratic Power in Lesotho.* New York: Cambridge University Press.

———. 2005. "Anthropology and Its Evil Twin: 'Development' in the Constitution of a Discipline." In *The Anthropology of Development and Globalization: From Classical Political Economy to Contemporary Neoliberalism,* edited by M. Edelman and A. Haugerud, 140–153. Malden, MA: Blackwell.

Ferguson, James. 1987. *Papa Doc, Baby Doc: Haiti and the Duvaliers.* Oxford: Basil Blackwell.

Ferguson, James, and Akhil Gupta. 2002. "Spatializing States: Toward an Ethnography of Neoliberal Governmentality." *American Ethnologist* 29:981–1002.

Fisher, Robert. 1994. *Let the People Decide: Neighborhood Organizing in America.* New York: Twayne.

Fisher, William. 1997. "Doing Good? The Politics and Antipolitics of NGO Practices." *Annual Reviews in Anthropology* 26:439–464.

Fortun, Kim, and Mike Fortun. 2000. "The Work of Markets: Filming Within Indian Mediascapes, 1997." In *Para-sites: A Casebook Against Cynical Reason,* edited by G. Marcus, 287–347. Chicago: University of Chicago Press.

Foucault, Michel. 1978. *The History of Sexuality, Volume 1: An Introduction.* Translated by R. Hurley. New York: Vintage.

———. 1979. *Discipline and Punish.* Translated by Alan Sheridan. New York: Vintage.

———. 1991. "Governmentality." In *The Foucault Effect: Studies in Governmentality,* edited by C. G. Graham Purchell and Peter Miller, 87–104. Chicago: University of Chicago Press.

Freire, Paulo. 1985. *Pedagogy of the Oppressed.* Translated by M. B. Ramos. New York: Continuum.

Friedman, Thomas. 2005. *The World Is Flat.* New York: Farrar, Straus and Giroux.

Gabaud, Pierre Simpson. 2000. *Associationnisme paysan en haïti: Effets de permanence et de rupture.* Port-au-Prince: Editions des Antilles.

Gaillard-Pourchet, Gusti Klara. 1990. *L'expérience haïtienne de la dette extérieure.* Port-au-Prince: Maison Henri Deschamps.

———. 2002. *L'expérience haitienne de la dette extérieure ou une production caféière pillée (1875–1915).* Port-au-Prince: Maison Henri Deschamps.

Gayle, Helene. 2006. "HIV Prevention: How Effective Is the President's Emergency Plan for AIDS Relief." U.S. House Committee on Government Reform, Subcommittee on National Security, Emerging Threats, and International Relations, House of Representatives, Washington.

Geertz, Clifford. 1973. *The Interpretation of Cultures.* New York: Basic.

George, Susan. 1992. *The Debt Boomerang.* Washington: Institute for Policy Studies.

Gibbons, Elizabeth D. 1999. *Sanctions in Haiti: Human Rights and Democracy Under Assault.* Westport, CT: Praeger.

Gill, Lesley. 2000. *Teetering on the Rim: Global Restructuring, Daily Life, and the Armed Retreat of the Bolivian State.* New York: Columbia University Press.

Girard, Phillipe R. 2004. *Clinton in Haiti: The 1994 U.S. Invasion of Haiti.* New York: Palgrave Macmillan.

———. 2005. *Paradise Lost: Haiti's Tumultuous Journey from the Pearl of the Caribbean to Third World Hot Spot.* New York: Palgrave Macmillan.

Gladwin, Christina. 1991. *Structural Adjustment and African Women Farmers*. Gainesville: University Press of Florida.

Glick Schiller, Nina, and Georges Eugene Fouron. 2001. *Georges Woke Up Laughing: Long Distance Nationalism and the Search for Home*. Durham: Duke University Press.

Global Fund. 2004. "A Force for Change: The Global Fund at 30 Months." Global Fund to Fight AIDS, Tuberculosis, and Malaria, Geneva.

———. 2006. "Annual Report, 2005." Global Fund to Fight AIDS, Tuberculosis, and Malaria, Geneva.

Gold, Herbert. 1991. *Best Nightmare on Earth: A Life in Haiti*. New York: Touchstone.

González, Roberto. 2004. *Anthropologists in the Public Sphere: Speaking Out on War, Peace, and American Power*. Austin: University of Texas Press.

Gootnick, David, and GAO. 2006. "Spending Requirement Presents Challenges for Allocating Prevention Funding Under the President's Emergency Plan for AIDS Relief: Testimony Before the Subcommittee on National Security, Emerging Threats, and International Relations, Committee on Government Reform, House of Representatives." Government Accounting Office, Washington.

Gourevitch, Philip. 2010. "Alms Dealers: Can You Provide Humanitarian Aid without Facilitating Conflicts?" *The New Yorker*. October 11.

Gramsci, Antonio. 1971. *Selections from the Prison Notebooks of Antonio Gramsci*. Edited and translated by Quintin Hoare and Geoffrey Nowell Smith. New York: International Publishers.

Griffin, Clifford E. 1992. "United Nations Best Hope for a Solution in Haiti?" *Caribbean Affairs* 5:124–134.

Gunewardena, Nandini. 2008. "Disrupting Subordination and Negotiating Belonging: Women Workers in the Transnational Production Sites of Sri Lanka." In *The Gender of Globalization: Women Navigating Cultural and Economic Marginalities*, edited by N. Gunewardena and A. Kingsolver, 35–60. Santa Fe: School of American Research Press.

Gupta, Akhil, and Aradhana Sharma. 2006. "Globalization and Postcolonial States." *Current Anthropology* 47:277–307.

Habermas, Jürgen. 1989. *The Structural Transformation of the Public Sphere: An Inquiry into a Category of Bourgeois Society*. Translated by Thomas Burger. London: Polity Press.

———. 1992. "Further Reflections on the Public Sphere." In *Habermas and the Public Sphere*, edited by C. Calhoun, 421–461. Cambridge: MIT Press.

Hachette, Dominique, and the World Bank. 1981. "Haiti: Economic Memorandum: Recent Economic, Industrial and Sector Developments." World Bank, Washington.

Hallward, Peter. 2007. *Damming the Flood: Haiti, Aristide, and the Politics of Containment*. London: Verso.

Hancock, Mary Elizabeth. 1999. *Womanhood in the Making: Domestic Ritual and Public Culture in Urban South India*. Boulder: Westview Press.

———. 2006. "Washington's Landscape of Fear: Banal, Sublime, and Dangerous." *City and Society* 18:1–6.

Harding, Sandra. 1991. *Whose Science? Whose Knowledge?* Ithaca: Cornell University Press.

Hardt, Michael, and Antonio Negri. 2001. *Empire*. Cambridge: Harvard University Press.

Harrison, Faye Venetia. 1991. *Decolonizing Anthropology: Moving Further Toward an Anthropology for Liberation*. Washington, DC: Association of Black Anthropologists, American Anthropological Association.

———. 1997. "The Gendered Politics and Violence of Structural Adjustment: A View from Jamaica." In *Situated Lives: Gender and Culture in Everyday Life*, edited by L. Lamphere, H. Ragone, and P. Zavella, 451–468. New York: Routledge.

———. 2002. "Race and Globalization: Global Apartheid, Foreign Policy, and Human Rights." *Souls* 4:48–68.

———. 2008. *Outsider Within: Reworking Anthropology in the Global Age.* Urbana: University of Illinois Press.

Hart, Roger. 1997. *Children's Participation: The Theory and Practice of Involving Young Citizens in Community Development and Environmental Care.* London: Earthscan.

Harvey, David. 2003. *The New Imperialism.* Oxford: Oxford University Press.

———. 2005. *A Brief History of Neoliberalism.* New York: Oxford University Press.

Hefferan, Tara. 2007. *Twinning Faith and Development: Catholic Parish Partnering in the US and Haiti.* Bloomfield, CT: Kumarian Press.

Heinl, Robert Debs, Nancy Gordon Heinl. 1996. *Written in Blood: The Story of the Haitian People, 1492–1995.* Revised and expanded by Michael Heinl. Lanham, MD: University Press of America.

Hellman, Judith Adler. 1992. "The Study of New Social Movements in Latin America and the Question of Autonomy." In *The Making of Social Movements in Latin America: Identity, Strategy, and Democracy,* edited by A. Escobar and S. E. Alvarez, 52–61. Boulder: Westview Press.

Hewamanne, Sandya. 2006. "'Participation? My Blood and Flesh Is Being Sucked Dry': Market-Based Development and Sri Lanka's Free Trade Zone Women Workers." *Journal of Third World Studies* 23:51–74.

Hickey, Samuel, and Giles Mohan, eds. 2004a. *Participation: From Tyranny to Transformation? Exploring New Approaches to Participation in Development.* London: Zed Books.

———. 2004b. "Towards Participation as Transformation: Critical Themes and Challenges." In *Participation: From Tyranny to Transformation? Exploring New Approaches to Participation in Development,* edited by S. Hickey and G. Mohan, 3–24. London: Zed.

Hilhorst, Dorothea. 2003. *The Real World of NGOs: Discourses, Diversity and Development.* London: Zed.

Hochschild, Arlie Russell. 1989. *The Second Shift: Working Parents and the Revolution at Home.* New York: Viking.

Houtart, François. 1995. *Le défi de la mondialisation pour le sud.* Port-au-Prince: CRESFED.

Howell, Jude. 1997. "NGO-State Relations in Post-Mao China." In *NGOs, States and Donors: Too Close for Comfort?,* edited by D. Hulme and M. Edwards, 202–215. New York: St. Martin's Press.

Hrycak, Alexandra. 2002. "From Mothers' Rights to Equal Rights: Post-Soviet Grassroots Women's Associations." In *Women's Activism and Globalization: Linking Local Struggles and International Politics,* edited by N. A. Naples and M. Desai, 64–82. London: Routledge.

Hulme, David, and Michael Edwards. 1997. "Conclusion: Too Close to the Powerful, Too Far from the Powerless?" In *NGOs, States, and Donors: Too Close for Comfort?,* 275–284. New York: St. Martin's Press.

Human Rights Watch–Americas Watch Committee, and National Coalition for Haitian Refugees. 1993. *Silencing a People: The Destruction of Civil Society in Haiti.* New York: Human Rights Watch.

Humanitarian Accountability Project, and International Organization for Migration. 2010. "Camp Committee Assessment: A Tool for Deciding How to Work with Camp Committees." Humanitarian Accountability Project, Port-au-Prince.

Illich, Ivan. 1997. "Development as Planned Poverty" and "Twenty-Six Years Later." In *The Post-development Reader,* edited by M. Rahnema and V. Bawtree, 94–110. London: Zed.

Institut Haïten de l'Enfance (IHE). 2002. "Indicateurs de la Santé Publique, 2002." Institut Haïtien de l'Enfance, Port-au-Prince.

Institut Haïten de Statistique et d'Informatique (IHSI). 2003. "Enquête sur les conditions de vie en Haïti." Institut Haïten de Statistique et d'Informatique, Port-au-Prince.

———. 2008a. "Enquête sur la Santé Publique." Institut Haïten de Statistique et d'Informatique, Port-au-Prince.

———. 2008b. "'Le coin de l'IPC': Indice des Prix à la consommation de novembre 2008." Institut Haïtien des Statistique et d'Information, Port-au-Prince.

Interim Government of Haiti [unattributed]. 2004. "Interim Cooperation Framework, 2004–2006: Summary Report." In cooperation with the World Bank, United Nations, European Commission, and Inter-American Development Bank, Washington.

Interim Haiti Recovery Commission. 2011. "Haiti One Year Later: The Progress to Date and the Path Forward." Interim Haiti Recovery Commission, New York.

International Labor Organization. 2008. "World of Work Report, 2008: Income Inequalities in the Age of Financial Globalization." International Institute for Labour Studies, Geneva.

International Monetary Fund. 2001. "IMF Concludes Article IV Consultation with Haiti." International Monetary Fund, Washington.

———. 2002. "Haiti: Selected Issues." International Monetary Fund, Washington.

———. 2005a. "Haiti: Selected Issues." International Monetary Fund, Washington.

———. 2005b. "Haiti: Use of Fund Resources—Request for Emergency Post-Conflict Assistance—Staff Report; Staff Supplement; Press Release on the Executive Board Discussion; and Statement by the Executive Director for Haiti." International Monetary Fund, Washington.

———. 2006. "Haiti: Interim Poverty Reduction Strategy Paper." International Monetary Fund, Washington.

Jacklin, Jean Paul. 2007. "Chute d'Aristide: Les révélations de Guy Philippe à Signal FM." Le Matin (Port-au-Prince), May 27.

Jackson, Stephen. 2005. "'The State Didn't Even Exist': Non-governmentality in Kivu, Eastern DR Congo." In Between a Rock and a Hard Place: African NGOs, Donors, and the State, edited by J. I. T. Kelsall, 165–196. Durham: Carolina Academic Press.

Jadotte, Evans. 2006. "Income Distribution and Poverty in the Republic of Haiti." Poverty Monitoring, Measurement and Analysis, Quebec.

James, Erica Caple. 2010. Democratic Insecurities: Violence, Trauma, and Intervention in Haiti. Berkeley: University of California Press.

James, Ian. 2004. "Haiti Rebels Bring in Reinforcements from Dominican Republic, Fortify Northern Stronghold." Associated Press, February 14.

Jayawardena, Kumari. 1994. Feminism and Nationalism in the Third World. London: Zed.

Jean, J. A. Gracien. 2002. In Sociétés civiles en mutation, edited by P. Fils-Aimé, 1–55. Port-au-Prince: Centre International de Politologie Appliquée-Haïti.

Jolly, Margaret. 1996. "Woman ikat raet long human raet o no? Women's Rights, Human Rights, and Domestic Violence in Vanuatu." Feminist Review 52:169–190.

Kaag, Mayke. 2008. "Transnational Islamic NGOs in Chad: Islamic Solidarity in the Age of Neoliberalism." Africa Today 54:3–18.

Kamat, Sangeeta. 2002. Development Hegemony: NGOs and the State in India. Delhi: Oxford University Press.

———. 2003. "The NGO Phenomenon and Political Culture in the Third World." Development 46:88–93.

———. 2004. "The Privatization of the Public Interest: Theorizing NGO Discourse in the Neoliberal Era." Review of International Political Economy 11:155–176.

Karim, Lamia. 2001. "Politics of the Poor: NGOs and Grass-Roots Political Mobilization in Bangladesh." Political and Legal Anthropology Review 24:92–107.

Katz, Jonathan. 2010a. "Billions for Haiti, a Criticism for Every Dollar." Associated Press, March 6.

———. 2010b. "Haiti Still Waiting for Pledged U.S. Aid." Associated Press, September 28.

Kim, Seung-Kyung. 1997. *Class Struggle or Family Struggle? The Lives of Women Factory Workers in South Korea.* Cambridge: Cambridge University Press.

Klarreich, Kathie. 2005. *Madame Dread: A Tale of Love, Vodou and Civil Strife in Haiti.* New York: Nation.

Klein, Naomi. 2007. *The Shock Doctrine: The Rise of Disaster Capitalism.* New York: Metropolitan.

Köhler, Gernot. 1978. "Global Apartheid." In *Talking About People: Readings in Contemporary Cultural Anthropology,* edited by W. A. Haviland and R. J. Gordon, 262–268. Mountain View, CA: Mayfield.

Kolbe, Athena R., and Royce A Hutson. 2006. "Human Rights Abuse and Other Criminal Violations in Port-Au-Prince, Haiti: A Random Survey of Households." *The Lancet* 368:864–873.

Kothari, Uma. 2001. "Power, Knowledge, and Social Control in Participatory Development." In *Participation: The New Tyranny?,* edited by B. Cooke and U. Kothari, 139–152. London: Zed.

Laguerre, Michel. 1982. *Urban Life in the Caribbean: A Study of a Haitian Urban Community.* Cambridge, MA: Schenkman.

Lamphere, Louise. 1993. "The Domestic Sphere of Women and the Public World of Men: The Strengths and Limitations of an Anthropological Dichotomy." In *Gender in Cross Cultural Perspective,* edited by C. Brettel and C. Sargent, 67–77. Englewood Cliffs, NJ: Prentice Hall.

———. 2004. "The Convergence of Applied, Practicing, and Public Anthropology in the 21st Century." *Human Organization* 63:431–443.

Lang, Sabine. 2000. "The NGO-ization of Feminism." In *Global Feminisms Since 1945,* edited by B. G. Smith, 290–304. London: Routledge.

Lawless, Robert. 1992. *Haiti's Bad Press.* Rochester, VT: Schenkman.

Ledan, Djenane. 2009. *Chronique de mes dix jours en captivité.* Port-au-Prince: Maison Henri Deschamps.

Lenin, Vladimir Ilich. (1922) 1965. "Role and Function of Trade Unions Under the New Economic Policy." In *Collected Works,* edited and translated by David Skvirsky and Goerge Hanna, 188–196. Moscow: Progress Publishers.

Leve, Lauren. 2001. "Between Jesse Helms and Ram Bahadur: Women, 'Participation,' and 'Empowerment' in Nepal." *Political and Legal Anthropology Review* 24: 108–128.

Leve, Lauren, and Lamia Karim. 2001. "Privatizing the State: Ethnography of Development, Transnational Capital, and NGOs." *Political and Legal Anthropology Review* 24:53–58.

Lind, Amy Conger. 1992. "Power, Gender, and Development: Popular Women's Organizations and the Politics of Needs in Ecuador." In *The Making of Social Movements in Latin America: Identity, Strategy, and Democracy,* edited by A. Escobar and S. E. Alvarez, 134–149. Boulder: Westview Press.

———. 2000. "Negotiating Boundaries: Women's Organizations and the Politics of Restructuring in Ecuador." In *Gender and Global Restructuring: Sighting, Sites, and Resistances,* edited by M. H. Marchand and A. S. Runyan, 161–175. New York: Routledge

Lorde, Audre. 1984. "The Master's Tools Will Never Dismantle the Master's House." In *Sister Outsider: Essays and Speeches,* 110–113. Berkeley: Crossing Press.

Louis-Juste, Jean Anil. 2007. "Haïti, l'Invasion des ONG: La thèse n'est pas aussi radicale que son sujet." Faculté des Sciences Humaines, Université d'État d'Haïti, Port-au-Prince.

Low, Setha M. 2000. *On the Plaza: The Politics of Public Space and Culture.* Austin: University of Texas Press.

———. 2006. "The Erosion of Public Space and the Public Realm: Paranoia, Surveillance and Privatization in New York City." *City and Society* 18:43–49.

Low, Setha, and Sally Engle Merry. 2010. "Engaged Anthropology: Diversity and Dilemmas, An Introduction to Supplement 2." *Current Anthropology* 51:S203–S226.

Luetchford, Peter. 2006. "Brokering Fair Trade: Relations Between Coffee Cooperatives and Alternative Trade Organizations—A View from Costa Rica." In *Development Brokers and Translators: The Ethnography of Aid and Agencies*, edited by D. Lewis and D. Mosse, 127–158. Bloomfield, CT: Kumarian Press.

Lundahl, Mats. 1984. "Papa Doc: Innovator in the Predatory State." *Scandia* 50:39–78.

———. 1989. "History as an Obstacle to Change: The Case of Haiti." *Journal of Interamerican Studies and World Affairs* 31:1–21.

Lwijis, Janil. 1993. *Entè OPD: Kalfou Pwojè.* Port-au-Prince: Imprimateur II.

———. 2009. *ONG: Ki gouvènman ou ye?* Port-au-Prince: Asosyasyon Invèsite ak Invèsitèz Desalinyèn.

Macdonald, Laura. 1997. *Supporting Civil Society: The Political Role of Non-governmental Organizations in Central America.* New York: St. Martin's Press.

MacKinnon, Catharine A. 1989. *Toward a Feminist Theory of the State.* Cambridge: Harvard University Press.

Macrae, Joanna, and Nicholas Leader. 2001. "Apples, Pears, and Porridge: The Origins and Impact of the Search for 'Coherence' Between Humanitarian and Political Responses to Chronic Political Emergencies." *Disasters* 25:290–307.

Maguire, Robert E. 2003. "U.S. Policy Toward Haiti: Engagement or Estrangement?" Programs in International Affairs at Trinity College, Washington.

Mangonès, Kathy. 1991. "Reflexion sur l'elaboration d'une politique de développement." In *Definition, Rôle et Fonction des ONG: Cahier 2*, edited by HAVA, 5–9. Port-au-Prince: HAVA et le Comité inter ONG.

Mansbridge, Jane. 1999. "On the Idea That Participation Makes Better Citizens." In *Citizen Competence and Democratic Institutions*, edited by S. Elkin and K. Soltan, 291–325. University Park: Pennsylvania State University Press.

Marcelin, Frédéric. (1897) 2004. *Haïti et l'indemnité française.* Port-au-Prince: Editions Fardin.

Marx, Karl. (1852) 1978. "The Eighteenth Brumaire of Louis Bonaparte." In *The Marx-Engels Reader*, edited by M. Tucker, 594–617. New York: Norton.

———. (1857) 1978. "The Grundrisse." In *The Marx-Engels Reader*, edited by M. Tucker, 221–293. New York: Norton.

Maternowska, M. Catherine. 2006. *Reproducing Inequities: Poverty and the Politics of Population in Haiti.* New Brunswick: Rutgers University Press.

Mathurin, Alliette, Ernst Mathurin, and Bernard Zaugg. 1989. *Implantation et impact des organisations non gouvernementales: Contexte général et étude de cas.* Port-au-Prince: GRAMIR.

Mbakwem, B. C., and D. J. Smith. 2009. "'Returned to Sender': Corruption in International Health in Nigeria." In *The Practice of International Health: A Case-Based Orientation*, edited by D. Perlman and A. Roy, 217–231. Oxford: Oxford University Press.

McIlwaine, Cathy. 1998. "Contesting Civil Society: Reflections from El Salvador." *Third World Quarterly* 19:651–672.

McLanahan, Sara S., Annemette Sorensen, and Dorothy Watson. 1989. "Sex Differences in Poverty, 1950–1980." *Signs* 15:102–122.

McMichael, Philip. 1996. "The Development Project (Late 1940s to Early 1970s)." In *Development and Social Change*, 15–43. Thousand Oaks, CA: Pine Forge.

Médecins sans Frontières (MSF). 2006. "New Wave of Violence Hits Port-au-Prince, Haiti." Médecins sans Frontières, Paris.

Mendez, Jennifer Bickham. 2002. "Gender and Citizenship in a Global Context: The Struggle for Maquila Workers' Rights in Nicaragua." *Identities* 9:7–38.

Mertes, Tom. 2004. *A Movement of Movements: Is Another World Really Possible?* London: Verso.

Michels, Robert. 1949. *First Lectures in Political Sociology*. Minneapolis: University of Minnesota Press.

Miller, Daniel. 1997. *Capitalism: An Ethnographic Approach*. Oxford: Berg.

Mills, C. Wright. 1959. *The Sociological Imagination*. New York: Oxford University Press.

Mills, Mary Beth. 2003. "Gender and Inequality in the Global Labor Force." *Annual Review of Anthropology* 32:41–62.

Mindry, D. 2001. "Nongovernmental Organizations, 'Grassroots,' and the Polities of Virtue." *Signs* 26:1187–1211.

Ministèr Agrikilti ak Resous Natirèl. 2000. "Òganizasyon Peyizan nan Depatman Lwès." Ministè Agrikilti ak Resous Natirèl, Port-au-Prince.

Ministèr de la Condition Féminine et des Droits des Femmes (MCFDF). 2004. "Une régard sur la violence fait aux femmes." Colloque—VIH/SIDA et La Violence Sexuelle: Une Double Problématique. Port-au-Prince: Hôtel Montana.

Mintz, Sidney. 2010. *Three Ancient Colonies: Caribbean Themes and Variations*. Cambridge: Harvard University Press.

Moghadam, Valentine M. 2005. *Globalizing Women: Transnational Feminist Networks*. Baltimore: Johns Hopkins University Press.

Mohan, Giles. 2001. "Beyond Participation: Strategies for Deeper Empowerment." In *Participation: The New Tyranny?*, edited by B. Cooke and U. Kothari, 153–167. London: Zed.

Mohanty, Chandra Talpade. 1988. "Under Western Eyes: Feminist Scholarship and Colonial Discourses." *Feminist Review* 30:61–88.

———. 2003. *Feminism Without Borders: Decolonizing Theory, Practicing Solidarity*. Durham: Duke University Press.

Molyneux, Maxine. 1985. "Mobilization Without Emancipation? Women's Interest, the State, and Revolution in Nicaragua." In *New Social Movements and the State in Latin America*, edited by D. Slater, 233–260. Amsterdam: CEDLA.

Moraga, Cherríe L., and Gloria E. Anzaldúa. 1983. *This Bridge Called My Back: Writings by Radical Women of Color*. New York: Kitchen Table: Women of Color Press.

MOREPLA and PAPDA. 2004. "Kòmansman Mobilizasyon pou Defann Pwodiksyon Nasyonal la." MOREPLA and PAPDA, Port-au-Prince.

Morton, Alice. 1997. "Haiti: NGO Sector Study." World Bank, Washington.

Mosse, David. 2005. *Cultivating Development: An Ethnography of Aid Policy and Practice*. Ann Arbor: Pluto Press.

Mosse, David, and David Lewis. 2006. "Theoretical Approaches to Brokerage and Translation in Development." In *Development Brokers and Translators: The Ethnography of Aid and Agencies*, edited by D. Lewis and D. Mosse, 1–26. Bloomfield, CT: Kumarian Press.

Muggah, Robert, and Athena Kolbe. 2011. "Haiti: Why an Accurate Count of Civilian Deaths Matters." *Los Angeles Times*, July 12.

Mulet, Edmund. 2007. "Speech at the Center for International and Strategic Studies." Center for International and Strategic Studies, Washington.

Mumm, Jesse. 2008. "Redoing Chicago: Gentrification, Race, and Intimate Segregation." *North American Dialogue* 11:16–19.

Nagar, Richa, and Sangtin Writers. 2006. *Playing with Fire: Feminist Thought and Activism Through Seven Lives in India*. Minneapolis: University of Minnesota Press.

Nash, June C., and María Patricia Fernández-Kelly. 1983. *Women, Men, and the International Division of Labor*. Albany: SUNY Press.

Ndegwa, Stephen N. 1996. *The Two Faces of Civil Society: NGOs and Politics in Africa*. West Hartford, CT: Kumarian Press.

Nelson, Paul J. 1995. "'Accountable to Whom?,' and Other Issues for NGOs." In *The World Bank and Non-governmental Organizations: The Limits of Apolitical Development*, 36–66. New York: St. Martin's Press.

Nicholls, David. 1974. "A Work of Combat: Mulatto Historians and the Haitian Past, 1847–1867." *Journal of Interamerican Studies and World Affairs* 16:15–38.

———. 1996. *From Dessalines to Duvalier: Race, Colour, and National Independence in Haiti*. New York: Cambridge University Press.

Notes from Nowhere. 2003. *We Are Everywhere: The Irresistible Rise of Global Anticapitalism*. London: Verso.

NYU School of Law Center for Human Rights and Global Justice. 2011. "Sexual Violence in Haiti's IDP Camps: Results of a Household Survey." NYU School of Law, Center for Human Rights and Global Justice, New York.

NYU School of Law Center for Human Rights and Global Justice, Partners in Health, RFK Memorial Center for Human Rights, and Zanmi Lasante. 2008. "Wòch Nan Soley: The Denial of the Right to Water in Haiti." NYU School of Law, Center for Human Rights and Global Justice, New York.

N'Zengou-Tayo, Marie-José. 1998. "Fanm se poto mitan: Haitian Women, the Pillar of Society." *Feminist Review* 59:118–142.

Ong, Aihwa, and Stephen J. Collier. 2005. *Global Assemblages: Technology, Politics, and Ethics as Anthropological Problems*. Malden, MA: Blackwell.

Organisation for Economic Co-operation and Development (OECD). 2006. "2006 Survey on Monitoring the Paris Declaration: Overview of the Results." Organisation for Economic Co-operation and Development, Paris.

Oxfam America. 2008. "Smart Development: Why U.S. Foreign Aid Demands Major Reform." Oxfam America, Boston.

Oxfam International. 2011. "From Relief to Recovery: Supporting Good Governance in Post-earthquake Haiti." Oxfam International, Oxford.

Padmore, George. 1969. *Africa: Britain's Third Empire*. New York: Negro Universities Press.

Paley, Julia. 2001. "The Paradox of Participation: Civil Society and Democracy in Chile." *Political and Legal Anthropology Review* 24:1–12.

Pan American Health Organization. 2005. "Report from Ministry of Health Transmitted to Area of Health Analysis and Information Systems (AIS) by PAHO/WHO Country Representative." Pan American Health Organization, Port-au-Prince.

Parpart, Jane. 1999. "Rethinking Participation, Empowerment, and Development from a Gender Perspective." In *Transforming Development: Foreign Aid for a Changing World*, edited by J. Freedman, 250–267. Toronto: University of Toronto Press.

Paul, Samuel, and Arturo Israel. 1991. "Nongovernmental Organizations and the World Bank: Cooperation for Development." *World Bank Regional and Sectoral Studies* 163. Washington, DC: World Bank.

Pearce, Jenny. 1997. "Between Co-option and Irrelevance? Latin American NGOs in the 1990s." In *NGOs, States, and Donors: Too Close for Comfort?*, edited by D. Hulme and M. Edwards, 257–274. New York: St. Martin's Press.

Perkins, John. 2006. *Confessions of an Economic Hit Man.* New York: Plume.

Petras, James. 1997. "Imperialism and NGOs in Latin America." *Monthly Review* 49:10–17.

———. 2003. *The New Development Politics: The Age of Empire Building and New Social Movements.* Burlington, VT: Ashgate.

Pierre-Louis, François. 2011. "Earthquakes, Nongovernmental Organizations, and Governance in Haiti." *Journal of Black Studies* 42:186–202.

Pollock, John. 2003. "Performance-Based Contracting with NGOs in Haiti." Management Sciences for Health, Boston.

Polman, Linda. 2010. *The Crisis Caravan: What's Wrong with Humanitarian Aid?* New York: Macmillan.

Preston, Caroline, and Nicole Wallace. 2011. "American Donors Gave $1.4 Billion to Haiti Aid." *Chronicle on Philanthropy.*

Polyné, Millery. 2010. *From Douglass to Duvalier: U.S. African Americans, Haiti, and Pan Africanism, 1870–1964.* Gainesville: University Press of Florida.

Potter, Amy. 2009. "Voodoo, Zombies, and Mermaids: U.S. Newspaper Coverage of Haiti." *Geographical Review* 99:208–230.

Program on International Policy Attitudes. 2001. "Americans on Foreign Aid and World Hunger: A Study of U.S. Public Attitudes." Program on International Policy Attitudes, University of Maryland, College Park, MD.

———. 2005. "Americans on Addressing World Poverty." Program on International Policy Attitudes, College Park, MD.

Putnam, Robert D. 2001. *Bowling Alone: The Collapse and Revival of American Community.* New York: Touchstone.

Racine, Marie M. B. 1995. "The Long Journey Toward Freedom." *Roots* 1:7–12.

———. 1999. *Like the Dew That Waters the Grass: Words from Haitian Women.* Washington, DC: EPICA.

Ray, Raka. 1999. *Fields of Protest: Women's Movements in India.* Minneapolis: University of Minnesota Press.

Regan, Jane. 2003. "ONG 'altènatif'—zanmi oswa ennmi lit radikal?" Port-au-Prince.

Renda, Mary. 2001. *Taking Haiti: Military Occupation and the Culture of U.S. Imperialism, 1915–1940.* Chapel Hill: University of North Carolina Press.

Reseau National de Defense des Droits Humains (RNDDH). 2006. *Regard sur la Situation Générale des Droits Humains en Haiti sous le Gouvernement Intérimaire.* Port-au-Prince: Reseau National de Defense des Droits Humains

Rey, Terry. 1999. *Our Lady of Class Struggle: The Cult of the Virgin Mary in Haiti.* Trenton, NJ: Africa World Press.

Rice, Condoleezza. 2006. "Remarks by Condoleezza Rice, U.S. Secretary of State: New Direction for U.S. Foreign Assistance." U.S. Department of State, Washington.

Richard, Analiese. 2009. "Mediating Dilemmas: Local NGOs and Rural Development in Neoliberal Mexico." *Political and Legal Anthropology Review* 32:166–194.

Richardson, Laurie, and Grassroots International. 1997. "Kenbe Peyi a sou Kontwòl, Demokrasi nan Grangou: Men Politik USAID an Ayiti." Grassroots International, Boston.

Riddell, Roger. 2007. *Does Foreign Aid Really Work?* Oxford: Oxford University Press.

Riordan, Cornelius, and Jaya Sarkar. 1998. "Building Social Capital in Non-governmental Organizations: Buffalo Banks and Borewells." *International Journal of Sociology and Social Policy* 18:55–69.

Robert, Arnaud. 2010. "Haïti est la preuve de l'échec de l'aide internationale." *Le Temps* (Genève). December 20.

Robins, Steven. 2006. "From 'Rights' to 'Ritual': AIDS Activism in South Africa." *American Anthropologist* 108:312–323.

———. 2009. *Mobilising and Mediating Global Medicine and Health Citizenship: The Politics of AIDS Knowledge Production in Rural South Africa*. Brighton: University of Sussex, Institute of Development Studies.

Robinson, Randall. 2007. *An Unbroken Agony: Haiti, from Revolution to the Kidnapping of a President*. New York: Basic Civitas.

Robinson, William I. 2004. *A Theory of Global Capitalism: Production, Class, and State in a Transnational World*. Baltimore: Johns Hopkins University Press.

Rossi, Benedetta. 2006. "Aid Policies and Recipient Strategies in Niger: Why Donors and Recipients Should Not Be Compartmentalized into Separate 'Worlds of Knowledge.'" In *Development Brokers and Translators: The Ethnography of Aid and Agencies*, edited by D. Lewis and D. Mosse, 27–49. Bloomfield, CT: Kumarian Press.

Rostow, W. W. 1952. *The Process of Economic Growth*. New York: Norton.

———. 1960. *The Stages of Economic Growth: A Non-Communist Manifesto*. Cambridge: Cambridge University Press.

Rotberg, Robert. 1997. "Preface: Haiti's Last Best Chance." In *Haiti Renewed: Political and Economic Prospects*, edited by R. I. Rotberg, vii–xiii. Washington, DC: Brookings Institution Press.

———. 2003. "Haiti's Turmoil: Politics and Policy Under Aristide and Clinton." World Peace Foundation, Cambridge, MA.

———. 2004. "The Failure and Collapse of Nation-States: Breakdown, Prevention, and Repair." In *When States Fail: Causes and Consequences*, edited by R. Rotberg, 3–5. Princeton: Princeton University Press.

Ryan, William. 1971. *Blaming the Victim*. New York: Pantheon.

Sacks, Karen. 1975. "Engels Revisited: Women, the Organization of Production, and Private Property." In *Toward an Anthropology of Women*, edited by R. Reiter, 211–234. New York: Monthly Review Press.

Salemink, Oscar. 2006. "Translating, Interpreting, and Practicing Civil Society in Vietnam: A Tale of Calculated Misunderstandings." In *Development Brokers and Translators: The Ethnography of Aid and Agencies*, edited by D. Lewis and D. Mosse, 101–126. Bloomfield, CT: Kumarian Press.

Sampson, Steven. 1996. "The Social Life of Projects: Importing Civil Society to Albania." In *Civil Society: Challenging Western Models*, edited by C. Hann and E. Dunn, 121–142. London: Routledge.

Sampson, Steven, and Julie Hemment. 2001. "NGO-graphy: The Critical Anthropology of NGOs and Civil Society." Panel at the American Anthropological Association annual meeting, Washington, DC.

Sanday, Peggy Reeves. 2003. "Public Interest Anthropology: A Model for Engaged Social Science." School of American Research Workshop, Chicago.

Sandoval, Chela. 2000. *Methodology of the Oppressed*. Minneapolis: University of Minnesota Press.

San Martin, Nancy. 2002. "Joint Military Maneuvers Set for Dominican Republic." *Miami Herald*, December 3.

Sassen, Saskia. 1998. *Globalization and Its Discontents: Essays on the New Mobility of People and Money*. New York: New Press.

———. 2001. *The Global City: New York, London, Tokyo*. Princeton: Princeton University Press.

Schade, Jeanette. 2005. "Between Projectitis and the Formation of Countervailing Power: NGOs in Nation-Building Processes." In *Nation-Building: A Key Concept for Peaceful Conflict Transformation?*, edited by J. Hippler, 125–136. London: Pluto Press.

Scheper-Hughes, Nancy. 1995. "The Primacy of the Ethical: Towards a Militant Anthropology." *Current Anthropology* 36:409–420.

Scholte, Jan Aart, and Albrecht Schnabel. 2002. *Civil Society and Global Finance.* New York: Routledge.

Schuller, Mark. 2006a. "Break the Chains of Haiti's Debt." Jubilee USA, Washington.

———. 2006b. "Jamming the Meatgrinder World: Lessons Learned from Tenants Organizing in St. Paul." In *Homing Devices: The Poor as Targets of Public Housing Policy and Practice,* edited by M. Thomas-Houston and M. Schuller, 159–180. Lanham, MD: Lexington Press.

———. 2007a. "Haiti's 200-Year Ménage-à-Trois: Globalization, the State, and Civil Society." *Caribbean Studies* 35:141–179.

———. 2007b. "Killing with Kindness? Impacts of International Development Aid on Participation and Autonomy within Women's NGOs in Post-coup Haiti." PhD diss., University of California, Santa Barbara.

———. 2008. "'Haiti Is Finished!': Haiti's End of History Meets the Ends of Capitalism." In *Capitalizing on Catastrophe: Neoliberal Strategies in Disaster Reconstruction,* edited by N. Gunewardena and M. Schuller, 191–294. Lanham, MD: AltaMira Press.

———. 2009. "Gluing Globalization: NGOs as Intermediaries in Haiti." *Political and Legal Anthropology Review* 32:84–104.

———. 2010a. "Mister Blan: The Incredible Whiteness of Being (an Anthropologist)." In *Fieldwork Identities,* edited by E. Taylor, 125–150. Coconut Creek, FL: Caribbean Studies Press.

———. 2010b. "Unstable Foundations: The Impact of NGOs on Human Rights for Port-au-Prince's 1.5 Million Homeless." City University of New York and l'Université d'État d'Haïti, New York and Port-au-Prince.

———. 2011. "Mèt Ko Veye Ko: Foreign Responsibility in the Failure to Protect Against Cholera and Other Man-Made Disasters." City University of New York and l'Université d'État d'Haïti, New York and Port-au-Prince.

Schuller, Mark, and Pablo Morales, eds. 2012. *Tectonic Shifts: Impacts of Haiti's Earthquake.* Sterling, VA: Kumarian Press.

Schwartz, Timothy. 2008. *Travesty in Haiti: A True Account of Christian Missions, Orphanages, Fraud, Food Aid, and Drug Trafficking.* Charleston: Book Surge Publishing.

Schwartz, Timothy, with Yves-François Pierre and Eric Calpas. 2011. "BARR Survey Report: Building Assessments and Rubble Removal in Quake-Affected Neighborhoods in Haiti." USAID, Washington.

Scott, James C. 1990. *Domination and the Arts of Resistance: Hidden Transcripts.* New Haven: Yale University Press.

Sen, Amartya Kumar. 1999. *Development as Freedom.* New York: Anchor.

Sen, Gita, Caren Grown, and Development Alternatives with Women for a New Era. 1987. *Development, Crises, and Alternative Visions: Third World Women's Perspectives.* New York: Monthly Review Press.

Sharma, Aradhana. 2008. *Logics of Empowerment: Development, Gender, and Governance in Neoliberal India.* Minneapolis: University of Minnesota Press.

Sheller, Mimi. 2004. "'You Signed My Name, but Not My Feet': Paradoxes of Peasant Resistance and State Control in Post-revolutionary Haiti." *Journal of Haitian Studies* 10:72–86.

Simmons, David. 2010. "Structural Violence as Social Practice: Haitian Agricultural Workers, Anti-Haitianism, and Health in the Dominican Republic." *Human Organization* 69:10–18.

Sklair, Leslie. 2001. *The Transnational Capitalist Class.* Malden, MA: Blackwell.

Smith, Jennie Marcelle. 2001. *When the Hands Are Many: Community Organization and Social Change in Rural Haiti.* Ithaca: Cornell University Press.

——. 2004. "Singing Back: The *Chan Pwen* of Haiti." *Ethnomusicology* 48:105–126.

Smith, Matthew. 2009. *Red and Black in Haiti: Radicalism, Conflict, and Political Change, 1934–1957.* Chapel Hill: University of North Carolina Press.

Smith, Valerie. 1990. "Split Affinities: The Case of Interracial Rape." In *Conflicts in Feminism*, edited by M. Hirsch and E. F. Keller, 271–287. New York: Routledge.

SOFA, PAPDA, and SAKS. 2004. "Deuxieme déclaration des organisations de la société civile haïtienne sur le processus du CCI." SOFA, PAPDA, and SAKS, Port-au-Prince.

de Soto, Hernando. 2000. *The Mystery of Capital: Why Capitalism Triumphs in the West and Fails Everywhere Else.* New York: Basic.

Spivak, Giyatri. 1988. "Can the Subaltern Speak?" In *Marxism and the Interpretation of Culture*, edited by C. Nelson and L. Grossberg, 271–313. Urbana: University of Illinois Press.

Sprague, Jeb. 2007. "The Overthrow of Popular Democracy in Haiti, 2001–2004." Master's diss., California State University Long Beach.

Starr, Amory. 2005. *Global Revolt: A Guide to the Movements Against Globalization.* London: Zed.

Stiglitz, Joseph E. 2002. *Globalization and Its Discontents.* New York: Norton.

Strathern, Marilyn. 1985. "Kinship and Economy: Constitutive Orders of a Provisional Kind." *American Ethnologist* 12:191–209.

Susser, Ida. 2009. *AIDS, Sex, and Culture: Global Politics and Survival in Southern Africa.* Malden, MA: Wiley-Blackwell.

Tamayo, Juan. 2004. "U.S. Allegedly Blocked Extra Bodyguards." *Miami Herald*, March 1.

Terry, Fiona. 2002. *Condemned to Repeat?: The Paradox of Humanitarian Action.* Ithaca, NY: Cornell University Press.

Thayer, Millie. 2001. "Transnational Feminism: Reading Joan Scott in the Brazilian *Sertão*." *Ethnography* 2:243–271.

Thomas-Slayter, Barbara P. 1992. "Implementing Effective Local Management of Natural Resources: New Roles for NGOs in Africa." *Human Organization* 51:136–143.

Tiano, Susan. 1994. *Patriarchy on the Line: Labor, Gender, and Ideology in the Mexican Maquila Industry.* Philadelphia: Temple University Press.

Tocqueville, Alexis de. (1835) 2000. *Democracy in America.* Translated by Stephen D. Grant. Indianapolis: Hackett.

Trouillot, Michel-Rolph. 1977. *Ti dife boule sou Istoua Ayiti.* Brooklyn: Koleksyon Lakansyèl.

——. 1990. *Haiti, State Against Nation: The Origins and Legacy of Duvalierism.* New York: Monthly Review Press.

——. 1994a. "Culture, Color, and Politics in Haiti." In *Race*, edited by S. Gregory and R. Sanjek, 146–174. New Brunswick: Rutgers University Press.

——. 1994b. "Haiti's Nightmare and the Lessons of History." *NACLA Report on the Americas* 27:46–52.

——. 1995. *Silencing the Past: Power and the Production of History.* Boston: Beacon Press.

——. 2003. *Global Transformations: Anthropology and the Modern World.* New York: Palgrave Macmillan.

Tsing, Anna Lowenhaupt. 2005. *Friction: An Ethnography of Global Connection.* Princeton: Princeton University Press.

Turner, Victor. 1969. "Liminality and Communitas." In *The Ritual Process: Structure and Anti-structure*, edited by V. Turner, 94–130. Chicago: Aldine.

Udall, Morris K. 1961. "The Foreign Assistance Act of 1961: A Special Report." Retrieved December 29, 2011, from http://www.library.arizona.edu/exhibits/udall/special/foreign.html.

Ulysse, Gina Athena. 2002. "Conquering Duppies in Kingston: Miss Tiny and Me, Fieldwork Conflicts, and Being Loved and Rescued." *Anthropology and Humanism* 27:10–26.

———. 2008. *Downtown Ladies: Informal Commercial Importers, a Haitian Anthropologist, and Self-Making in Jamaica.* Chicago: University of Chicago Press.

United Nations. 1949. "Mission to Haiti: Report of the United Nations Mission of Technical Assistance to the Republic of Haiti." United Nations, Lake Success, NY.

———. 2011. "MINUSTAH: United Nations Stabilization Mission in Haiti." United Nations, New York.

United Nations Comité Inter-agences Femmes et Développment, and Mirielle Neptune Anglade. 1992. *La Situation des Femmes Haïtiennes.* Port-au-Prince: Comité Inter-agences Femmes et Développement.

UNNOH, SOFA, and PAPDA. 2004. "Troisième déclaration des Organisations de la société civile haïtienne relative au processus d'élaboration du CCI et à la conférence des bailleurs de fonds tenue à Washington les 19 et 20 juillet 2004." UNNOH, SOFA, and PAPDA, Port-au-Prince.

United Nations Programme on HIV/AIDS (UNAIDS). 2007. "Haiti: 2007 Country Progress Report." United Nations Programme on HIV/AIDS, Geneva.

Uphoff, Norman. 1993. "Grassroots Organizations and NGOs in Rural Development: Opportunities with Diminishing States and Expanding Markets." *World Development* 21:607–622.

USAID. 1997. "USAID Strategic Plan for Haiti, Fiscal Years 1999–2004." USAID–Haiti, Port-au-Prince.

———. 1999. "FY 2001 Results Review and Resources Request (R4)." USAID–Haiti, Port-au-Prince.

———. 2001. "USAID Development Efforts Benefit U.S. Economy." *Frontlines*, March/April.

———. 2003. "Fiscal Year 2004 Budget Justification-Haiti." USAID, Washington.

———. 2004a. "$100 Million in Abstinence-Focused Grants for HIV/AIDS Prevention Awarded Under President Bush's Emergency Plan for AIDS Relief." USAID, Washington.

———. 2004b. "U.S. Foreign Aid: Meeting the Challenges of the Twenty-First Century." USAID, Washington.

———. 2005a. "Fiscal Year 2006 Budget Justification." USAID, Washington.

———. 2005b. "Fiscal Year 2006 Budget Justification: Haiti." USAID, Washington.

———. 2005c. "Fragile States Strategy." USAID, Washington.

———. 2006a. "Policy Framework for U.S. Bilateral Aid." USAID, Washington.

———. 2006b. "USAID History." USAID, Washington.

Uvin, Peter. 1996. "Paths to Scaling Up: Alternative Strategies for Local Nongovernmental Organizations." *Human Organization* 55:344–354.

Vincent, Fernand. 2006. "NGOs, Social Movements, External Funding, and Dependency " *Development* 49:22–28.

Wallace, Tina. 2003. "NGO Dilemmas: Trojan Horses for Global Neoliberalism?" In *The Socialist Register 2004: The New Imperial Challenge*, edited by L. Panitch and C. Leys, 202–219. New York: Monthly Review Press.

Wallerstein, Immanuel Maurice. 1974. *The Modern World-System.* Vol. 1: *Capitalist Agriculture and the Origins of the European World-Economy in the Sixteenth Century.* New York: Academic Press.

———. 2003. *The Decline of American Power: The U.S. in a Chaotic World.* New York: New Press.

———. 2004. *World Systems Analysis: An Introduction.* Durham: Duke University Press.

Weber, Max. 1946a. "Class, Status, Party." In *From Max Weber: Essays in Sociology*, edited by H. H. Gerth and C. Wright Mills, 180–195. New York: Oxford University Press.

———. 1946b. "On Bureaucracy." In *From Max Weber: Essays in Sociology*, edited by H. H. Gerth and C. Wright Mills, 196–204. New York: Oxford University Press.

Weisbrot, Mark. 1997. "Structural Adjustment in Haiti." *Monthly Review* 48:25–39.

Weisbrot, Mark, and Luis Sandoval. 2007. "Debt Cancellation for Haiti: No Reason for Further Delays." Center for Economic and Policy Research, Washington.

Williams, Patricia J. 1995. "*Metro Broadcasting Inc. v. FCC*: Regrouping in Singular Times." In *Critical Race Theory*, edited by Kimberle Williams Crenshaw, Gary Peller, and Kendall Thomas, 191–200. New York: New Press.

Wils, Frits. 1996. "Scaling Up, Mainstreaming, and Accountability: The Challenge for NGOs." In *Beyond the Magic Bullet: NGO Performance and Accountability in the Post–Cold War World*, edited by M. Edwards and D. Hulme, 67–79. West Hartford, CT: Kumarian Press.

World Bank. 1998. "Post-conflict Reconstruction: The Role of the World Bank." World Bank, Washington.

———. 2002a. "Haiti: Country Assistance Evaluation." World Bank, Operations Evaluation Department, Washington.

———. 2002b. "Haiti: External Financing Report: October 1, 2000–September 30, 2001." World Bank, Washington.

World Bank, and International Monetary Fund. 2008. "Haiti: Poverty Reduction Strategy Paper." World Bank and International Monetary Fund, Washington.

World Health Organization. 2009. "World Health Statistics, 2009." World Health Organization, Geneva.

Yang, Mayfair Mei-hui. 1999. *Spaces of Their Own: Women's Public Sphere in Transnational China*. Minneapolis: University of Minnesota Press.

Young, Iris Marion. 1997. *Intersecting Voices: Dilemmas of Gender, Political Philosophy, and Policy*. Princeton: Princeton University Press.

Zinn, Howard. 1995. *A People's History of the United States: 1492–Present*. New York: Harper Perennial.

INDEX

1825 indemnity, 19–20
2004 coup, 6, 22, 30, 40, 45, 112, 157, 158

abstinence, 56, 70, 101–102, 119, 137–139, 150–152, 167
accountability, 133–134, 149, 156, 164, 176, 183
AIDS: faith-based response, 43, 151; and gender, 40–41, 46, 59, 61–62; local understandings of, 42–44, 56–58, 73, 112, 119, 129; prevention, 42–44, 46–52, 73, 81, 85–86, 100–102, 117–121, 124, 139, 149–152, 169, 185; social causes of, 40–41, 50, 67, 119, 150–151
Aristide, Jean-Bertrand, 2, 4, 6, 17, 22–5, 30, 39, 67, 77, 109, 111, 138, 144, 157–160, 168, 175; forced removal of, 1–4, 22–24, 111, 157–160; U.S. role in ouster, 2, 4, 6, 17, 22, 23, 159, 160
assemblages, 9, 178
autonomy, 9, 12, 76, 99–106, 125, 127–130, 133–135, 138, 153, 156, 167–170, 173, 177–179, 184; from donors, 127–130, 138, 153, 167; *granmoun tèt li*, 127–128, 135, 168, 177; local definitions of, 133–135, 167; of staff, 99–101, 103–106

Black feminism, 38–40
"blame the victim," 151
blan [foreigner], 10, 18, 113, 162
boomerang effect, 148, 151
bureaucracy, 88–90, 99–103, 141–143
Bush, George H. W., 22, 157, 158
Bush, George W., 4, 134, 139, 143, 149–151, 153, 155, 158, 193

Cadre de Coopèration Intèrimaire (CCI), 160–163
Carnival, *see* Kanaval
Caravan (Sove Lavi), 56–58, 114–117, 150, 168, 185
Central Intelligence Agency (CIA), 22, 23, 159
cholera, 172–176
civic infrastructure, 9, 45, 108, 135, 138, 170, 177–179
civil society, 12, 23, 24, 52, 148, 155, 161
class, 4, 10, 17, 18, 19, 21, 28, 38–40, 41, 49, 54, 58, 75, 88–91, 104, 166–167, 179–182; class distinctions, 54, 58
classification, of NGOs, 40, 59, 181
clientelism, 59–60, 63, 92

Clinton, Bill, 6, 19, 51, 134, 143–144, 148, 152, 154, 156, 157–158, 172, 173, 175, 183, 190
Cold War, 11, 12, 20, 135, 143–148, 175
communication, 51, 62–63, 73, 91, 101, 103–104, 106, 141, 164–165, 175–176, 183
Community Action Councils (CACs), 43–44, 49–51
consciousness-raising, 49
constituency, 38, 142, 143, 146–148, 149, 164, 180, 191–192
coordination, 67, 109, 123, 153, 155–156, 160, 173, 174, 176, 190, 192
Country Coordinating Mechanism (CCM), 123, 152
coup d'état, 1–4, 14–18, 20–34, 156–163

Danticat, Edwidge, 32
debt, 21, 162
dependency, 6, 23, 99–102, 119, 125, 135, 154, 173
development, 6–9, 12, 18–20, 21–23, 28, 60, 79, 80, 91, 94, 104, 109, 116, 121–122, 127, 132–170, 174, 176–181, 183, 187, 191–194; human, 45, 86; gender and, 40–41, 49–50, 141; and participation, 67–68, 71
disaster capitalism, 30, 138, 159–163
discipline, 56, 182, 184
divisions, between staff members, 74–106
Duvalier, François, 18, 20–22, 49
Duvalier, Jean-Claude, 20–21, 22, 40, 42, 49, 157

earthquake, 4–6, 65, 73, 110, 151, 161, 171–174
empowerment, 11, 79, 91, 116, 130, 139, 180, 182
Etienne, Sauveur Pierre, 9, 22, 109, 110
export-processing zone, 36–38, 45–49, 64, 76–78, 155, 157

family, ideology of, 75–6, 92
family planning, 45, 47, 85–6, 128–30, 142, 146–7
Farmer, Paul, xi-xiii, 6, 10, 11, 19, 21, 23, 27, 28, 40, 41, 119, 151, 155, 159, 191
feminism, 17, 34, 38–39, 49, 92, 111, 129; critiques of, 17, 38–39, 111, 166; local understandings of, 34, 38–40, 130; professionalization, 38, 40, 111. *See also* Black feminism; third world feminism

ABOUT THE AUTHOR

MARK SCHULLER is an assistant professor at York College, CUNY, and an affiliate of l'Université d'État d'Haïti. Besides publishing twenty scholarly articles and book chapters, Schuller writes for the *Huffington Post*. He codirected the documentary *Poto Mitan: Haitian Women, Pillars of the Global Economy* and coedited four books, including *Tectonic Shifts: Impacts of Haiti's Earthquake*.

CPSIA information can be obtained
at www.ICGtesting.com
Printed in the USA
LVOW11s0146211216
518128LV00003B/199/P